CW01025248

Laparoscopic Surgery for Benign Gynaecology

Advanced Skills Series

Edited by Alfred Cutner and Sanjay Vyas

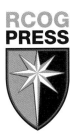

RCOG
PRESS

Contents

About the authors

Valentine Akande MRCOG
Consultant Obstetrician and Gynaecologist, Bristol Centre for Reproductive Medicine and Division of Women's Health, Southmead Hospital, Bristol, UK

Naaila Aslam MRCOG
Consultant Gynaecologist, Department of Obstetrics and Gynaecology, University College London Hospitals, London, UK

Karen Ballard PhD
Programme Director, MSc in Advanced Gynaecological Endoscopy, and Senior Lecturer in Women's Health, University of Surrey, Surrey, UK

Wei Jin Chua
Consultant Urologist and Clinical Director, Department of Urology, National University Hospital, Singapore

Kevin G Cooper MRCOG
Consultant Gynaecologist, Department of Obstetrics and Gynaecology, Aberdeen Royal Infirmary, Aberdeen, Scotland

Sarah M Creighton FRCOG
Consultant Gynaecologist, University College London Hospitals, Elizabeth Garrett Andersen Wing, London, UK

Alfred S Cutner FRCOG
Consultant Gynaecologist, University College London Hospitals, Elizabeth Garrett Andersen Wing, London, UK

Simon Edmonds MRCOG FRCSEd
Consultant Gynaecologist, Department of Gynaecology, Benenden Hospital Trust, Cranbrook, UK

Jim English MRCOG
Consultant Gynaecologist, Brighton & Sussex University Hospital, Brighton, UK

John Erian FRCOG
Consultant Gynaecologist, Princess Royal University Hospital, Farnborough, UK

Alan Farthing FRCOG
Consultant Gynaecological Surgeon, Queen Charlotte's Hospital, Imperial NHS Trust, London, UK

Jonathan Frappell FRCOG
Consultant Obstetrician and Gynaecologist, Derriford Hospital, Plymouth, UK

Mary Gooch
Theatre Manager, Benenden Hospital Trust, Cranbrook, UK

Mohamed Hefni FRCOG
Consultant Gynaecologist, Department of Gynaecology, Benenden Hospital Trust, Cranbrook, UK

Hayden Homer PhD MRCOG
Wellcome Trust Clinician Scientist, Cell and Developmental Biology, University College London, and Subspecialist in Reproductive Medicine, University College London Hospitals, Elizabeth Garrett Anderson Wing, London, UK

Wee-Liak Hoo MBBS
Clinical Research Fellow, University College Hospital London, London, UK

Davor Jurkovic FRCOG
Consultant Gynaecologist, Department of Obstetrics and Gynaecology, University College Hospital, London, UK

Francis Keeley FRCS (Urol)
Consultant Urologist, Bristol Urological Institute, Southmead Hospital, Bristol, UK

Andrew Kent FRCOG
Consultant Gynaecologist and Director of Gynaecological Surgery, Minimal Access Therapy Training Unit, Postgraduate Medical School, University of Surrey, Surrey, UK

Adrian M Lower FRCOG
Consultant Gynaecologist, The London Fibroid Clinic and Women's Health Partnership Ltd, Princess Grace Hospital, London, UK

Adam Magos FRCOG
Consultant Gynaecologist, Minimally Invasive Therapy Unit and Endoscopy Training Centre, University Department of Obstetrics and Gynaecology, The Royal Free Hospital, London, UK

Lina Michala MRCOG
Lecturer in Paediatric and Adolescent Gynaecology, University of Athens, Athens, Greece

Adam Moors FRCOG
Consultant Gynaecologist and Director, Laparoscopic Surgery Unit, Princess Anne Hospital, Southampton, UK

Anastasios Pachydakis MRCOG
Consultant Obstetrician and Gynaecologist, Iaso Hospital Minimal Access Unit, Athens, Greece

George Pandis MRCOG
Consultant Gynaecologist, University College London Hospitals, Elizabeth Garrett Anderson Wing, London, UK

Kevin Phillips FRCOG
Consultant Obstetrician and Gynaecologist, Castle Hill Hospital, Hull and East Yorkshire NHS Trust, Cottingham, UK

Nikita Rawal MRCOG
Research Fellow, Minimal Access Surgery, Women's Health Department, Castle Hill Hospital, Hull and East Yorkshire NHS Trust, Cottingham, UK

Karen I Rose MRCOG
Clinical Research Fellow in Urogynaecology, St Mary's Hospital, Manchester, UK

Ertan Saridogan FRCOG
Consultant Gynaecologist, University College London Hospitals, Elizabeth Garrett Anderson Wing, London, UK

Anthony RB Smith FRCOG
Consultant Urogynaecologist, St Mary's Hospital, Manchester, UK

Benjamin Thomas MRCOG
Senior Specialist Registrar, Minimally Invasive Therapy Unit and Endoscopy Training Centre, University Department of Obstetrics and Gynaecology, The Royal Free Hospital, London, UK

Geoffrey H Trew MRCOG
Consultant in Reproductive Medicine and Surgery, Hammersmith Hospital, London, UK and Honorary Senior Lecturer, Imperial College London, London, UK

Sameer Umranikar MRCOG
Consultant Obstetrician and Gynaecologist, Princess Anne Hospital, Southampton, UK

Sanjay Vyas FRCOG
Consultant Gynaecologist, Bristol Centre for Reproductive Medicine and Division of Women's Health, Southmead Hospital, Bristol, UK

Natasha Waters FRANCOG
Senior Clinical Research Fellow in Minimal Access Surgery, Minimal Access Therapy Training Unit, Postgraduate Medical School, University of Surrey, Surrey, UK

Sanjay Wijeyekoon FRCS
Consultant Colorectal Surgeon, Homerton University Hospital NHS Foundation Trust, London, UK

Alastair Windsor FRCS
Consultant Colorectal Surgeon, University College London Hospitals, London, UK

Jeremy Wright FRCOG
Clinical Director, MSc in Advanced Gynaecological Endoscopy, Department of Women's Health, University of Surrey, Surrey, UK

Acknowledgements

Chapter 4
The authors would like to thank Sarah Johnson, Surgical Care Practitioner, and all the theatre staff at Benenden Hospital for their help and support, in particular with the image acquisition.

Chapter 9
Hayden Homer is supported by a Wellcome Trust Clinical Fellowship (082587/z/07/z), The Wellcome Trust, Gibbs Building, 215 Euston Road, London NW1 2BE.

Chapter 15
The authors would like to thank Mr Eric Nyarko for editing the images and videos.

Abbreviations

APR	abdominal perineal resection
ATSM	Advanced Training Skills Module
BMI	body mass index
BSGE	British Society for Gynaecological Endoscopy
CAIS	complete androgen insensitivity syndrome
CASH	classic abdominal serrated-edge macromorcellator hysterectomy
CE	Conformité Européenne
CI	confidence interval
CLASICC trial	Conventional versus Laparoscopically assisted Surgery in Colorectal Cancer trial
CO_2	carbon dioxide
COLOR trial	Cancer Laparoscopic or Open Resection trial
COST study	Clinical Outcomes of Surgical Therapy study
CT	computed tomography
DMSA	dimercaptosuccinic acid
eVALuate study	evaluating the relative roles of Vaginal, Abdominal, and Laparoscopic hysterectomy study
FIGO	International Federation of Gynecology and Obstetrics
GnRH	gonadotrophin-releasing hormone
HeNe	helium–neon
ICIQ-VS	International Consultation on Incontinence Questionnaire – vaginal symptoms module
IP	infundibulopelvic
IVF	in vitro fertilisation
IVU	intravenous urogram
KTP	potassium–titanyl–phosphate
LAM	laparoscopically assisted myomectomy
LAR	low anterior resection
LASER	light amplification by the stimulated emission of radiation

LAVH	laparoscopically assisted vaginal hysterectomy
LLETZ	large loop excision of the transformation zone
LM	laparoscopic myomectomy
LUAL	laparoscopic uterine artery ligation
LUAO	laparoscopic uterine artery occlusion
LUNA	laparoscopic uterine nerve ablation
MAG3	mercaptoacetyltriglycine
MAS	minimal access surgery
MRI	magnetic resonance imaging
Nd:YAG	neodynium: yttrium–aluminium–garnet
NICE	National Institute for Health and Clinical Excellence
NPV	negative predictive value
OR	odds ratio
OSATS	objective structured assessment of technical skills
POI	point of impact
POP-Q	pelvic organ prolapse quantification
PPV	positive predictive value
rAFS	revised American Fertility Society criteria
RALM	robot-assisted laparoscopic myomectomy
RCOG	Royal College of Obstetricians and Gynaecologists
RCT	randomised controlled trial
RMI	risk of malignancy index
RR	relative risk
RVS	rectovaginal septum
TAH	total abdominal hysterectomy
TLH	total laparoscopic hysterectomy
TVT	tension-free vaginal tape
UAE	uterine artery embolisation
USL	uterosacral ligament
VALUE trial	Vaginal, Abdominal or Laparoscopic Uterine Excision trial

Preface

There is now no doubt that laparoscopic surgery benefits patients. It results in a shorter hospital stay, reduced need for analgesia and a quicker return to normal activity. In addition, the increased visualisation makes some operations less complicated than the open equivalent. The value of a diagnostic laparoscopy was quickly realised, and the potential for laparoscopic surgery followed. The number and complexity of laparoscopic operations have steadily increased following developments in imaging technology and surgical instruments. Gynaecologists have led this development. Despite all of this, we are aware that many operations which could be performed by the laparoscopic approach are still being performed by laparotomy. Sadly, this is to the detriment of women's health.

The disparity between what can be done and what is being done is, we believe, attributable to deficiencies in training. Thus, although UK trainees are exposed to some laparoscopic surgery, competence is required only in the most basic procedures. If laparoscopic surgery is to benefit more women, it is imperative that more gynaecologists are able to perform the surgery. This has been recognised by the British Society for Gynaecological Endoscopy and the Royal College of Obstetricians and Gynaecologists. As a result, an Advanced Training Skills Module in advanced laparoscopic surgery has been introduced. Trainees who complete this module will be in the vanguard of laparoscopic surgeons in the UK. However, there are many other trainees and established consultants whose practice needs to change. We believe it is no longer acceptable for a woman to have a laparotomy when there are laparoscopic alternatives which would be to her greater benefit. We are proud that this book, which encompasses all aspects of benign laparoscopic surgery in gynaecology, demonstrates the wealth of experience that is available.

We hope that what follows in print and video will help trainees and consultants develop their skills in laparoscopic surgery and lead to better care for women.

Alfred Cutner
Sajnay Vyas

1 Overview of laparoscopic surgery

Benjamin Thomas and Adam Magos

Introduction

Abdominopelvic surgery has seen a revolution in the last 30 years. The diagnosis and treatment of many conditions that in the past required a large incision may now be managed by laparoscopy – the introduction of a viewing device and surgical instruments through comparatively minute access points. Laparoscopy is perhaps the single most important change in gynaecological surgical practice to date as it offers less postoperative pain, shorter hospitalisation and a faster return to normal activities compared with laparotomy.

Gynaecologists may be said to have led this change of practice towards minimal access surgery (MAS). Whereas laparoscopic procedures such as ovarian cystectomy, salpingo-oophorectomy and myomectomy were described by Semm as early as 1979, the first comparable general surgical procedure, laparoscopic cholecystectomy, was only described several years later in 1985. Indeed, it was Semm, a gynaecologist, who performed the first laparoscopic appendicectomy in 1980.

Much more than in the case of conventional surgery, endoscopic surgery relies heavily on technology – optics, illumination, video technology and instrumentation. This technology is borne of decades of cooperation between pioneering surgeons and surgical equipment manufacturers. Laparoscopy requires distinct surgical expertise, given the limited tactile feedback and the fact that there is little direct access to tissue. However, its other major strength is that with appropriate laparoscopic training for a given procedure in a well selected woman who is adequately prepared, there is a decreased risk of complications compared with open surgery.

Laparoscopic surgery has affected diagnosis and management in virtually every area of gynaecology, from reproductive medicine to urogynaecology to oncology. As a result, 250 000 gynaecological laparoscopic procedures are performed in Britain annually.[1]

While the widespread adoption of endoscopic surgery has not always been based on proof of its efficacy and safety compared with traditional surgery, it is equally true to say that MAS has introduced a scientific rigour into surgical practice that was rarely seen in the past. Medical literature on MAS across all surgical specialties is extensive and growing by the day, and randomised controlled trials, cost–benefit analysis and quality-adjusted life years have become common currency among surgeons just as they have been for many years for physicians.[2]

History

The first known attempt at endoscopy was by Philip Bozzini (1773–1809) of Frankfurt, Germany, in 1805. He described the use of a double lumen urethral cannula to transmit candlelight into hollow organs.[3] However, the term 'endoscopy' did not appear in medical literature until 1867, when Segeles and Desormeaux described the concentration of light with a mirror through a genitourinary speculum.[4]

In 1901, Georg Kelling (1866–1945), a German gastroenterologist and surgeon from Dresden, visualised the peritoneal cavity of a dog through a Nitze cystoscope, having manually insufflated air through a Fiedler trocar using a sphygmomanometer.[5] His demonstration of what he called 'coelioscopy' at a meeting of the Society of German Natural Scientists and Physicians in Hamburg may be considered to be the birth of laparoscopy. Kelling ended his discussion of the method with a visionary remark:[6] 'I will now close, Gentlemen, by expressing the wish that the endoscopic method finds more usage than has been the case until now, considering the fact that it is truly more useful than the method of laparotomy used at present.'

Although disputed by Kelling, the Swedish internist Hans Christian Jacobæus (1879–1937) is widely held to have performed the first clinical laparoscopy and he indeed coined the term. The pioneer of therapeutic pneumothorax and thoracoscopic adhesiolysis with electrocautery, he published his experiences with the first laparoscopic operations in Stockholm in 1910, with the title 'On the possibility of performing cystoscopy for the examination of serous cavities'.[7] In 17 women with ascites, after cocainisation, he punctured the abdominal wall and inserted a Stille trocar into the abdomen with local anaesthesia. After partially draining the ascites and insufflating filtered air, he examined the cavity using a cystoscope inserted through the trocar.

In 1912, Jacobæus differentiated between laparoscopy in the presence and absence of ascites and recognised the significantly higher risk of intestinal injury in the latter group of women. He advocated operating with the utmost care to avoid visceral injury and ending the operation should this occur. Jacobæus also promoted the development of specialised instruments to optimise and simplify the procedure, and suggested the use of animals and corpses during initial endoscopic training. To decrease unnecessary complications, he recommended that the indications for laparoscopy should be ascertained cautiously. He favoured diagnostic laparoscopy over primary laparotomy, with conversion to an open procedure only when required, similar to today's philosophy. Jacobæus clearly appreciated the huge diagnostic and therapeutic potential of this approach despite its limitations.[8]

The procedure was subsequently developed in many other surgical centres. Rendle Short, working in Bristol, published the first English paper on laparoscopy in 1925.[9] He observed malignant nodules on the liver, tuberculosis, peritonitis, pelvic tumours and ectopic pregnancy. Difficulties and dangers discouraged most gynaecologists until 1944, when Decker and Cherry placed a woman in the knee–chest position and induced a spontaneous pneumoperitoneum through an incision in the posterior vaginal fornix.[10] Called 'culdoscopy', this technique became the standard in the USA for over two decades and was performed with only local anaesthesia through a natural orifice. However, many found the position rather clumsy and, compared with laparoscopy, it offered only a limited view of the pelvis and comparatively little opportunity for intervention.

The Parisian surgeon Raoul Palmer (1904–1985) made improvements to this transvaginal surgical approach in 1949. However, his main contribution to endoscopy took place 3 years earlier when in 1946 he reintroduced laparoscopy, inducing an artificial pneumoperitoneum in the Trendelenburg position under general anaesthesia. In 1952, Fourestier, Gladu and Vulmiere revolutionised endoscopy by introducing the transmission of light through a quartz rod from a light source outside the body.[11] Improvements such as this led to the acceptance of diagnostic laparoscopy and laparoscopic sterilisation in gynaecology. More extensive therapeutic procedures were regarded as simply too dangerous, given that laparoscopy afforded a lesser view than laparotomy and no direct manual contact with tissue.

Here begins the inspiring story of pioneer Kurt Karl Stephan Semm (1927–2003), who had trained as a toolmaker before qualifying as a physician in 1951. His early experience in gynaecological endocrinology was followed by work in the treatment of infertility. While assistant physician to Richard Fikentscher, chief at the Second Gynaecological Clinic at the University of Munich, he made his first innovative contribution; as a trained toolmaker with a father and brother in the medical instrument manufacturing business,[12] Semm's design and construction of an apparatus for carbon dioxide (CO_2) insufflation of the fallopian tubes was presented at the Second World Congress on Sterility and Fertility in Naples in 1956. There, Semm met Palmer, who introduced him to laparoscopy, the technique to which Semm would dedicate the rest of his professional life.

Semm refined his CO_2 insufflator for use in laparoscopy by automating it with the 'CO$_2$-Pneu-Automatik', which maintained a steady-state intra-abdominal pressure. The measurement of pressure gave an early warning to the surgeon should the insufflation needle be incorrectly placed, outside the peritoneal cavity. Further safety features were added, and Semm also developed a vacuum intrauterine sound especially for gynaecological peritoneoscopy, allowing manipulation of the uterus and chromopertubation.[13] Semm was also involved with improving the performance of the laparoscope. From 1970, as the director of the Department of Obstetrics and Gynaecology at Kiel University Hospital, Semm introduced therapeutic laparoscopy in earnest. He developed thermocoagulation, adapted the Roeder loop originally used for tonsillectomy and, most importantly, was the first to describe extra- and intra-corporeal endoscopic knotting to achieve endoscopic haemostasis.[14]

However, his colleagues at Kiel received these innovations with not simply scepticism, but scorn and ridicule. Semm was thought to exaggerate the morbidity associated with postoperative adhesions minimised by his surgical approach. He was famously induced to have a brain scan, perhaps to provide some explanation for his bold deviation from accepted practice. Furthermore, when presenting the enucleation of an ovarian cyst, his slide projector was abruptly unplugged amid calls that the surgery was unethical. The first fully laparoscopic appendicectomy was performed by Semm in 1980 at Kiel University Hospital, and was later presented at a surgical meeting. As a result of this, the then president of the German Surgical Society called for Semm's suspension from medical practice. In addition, the paper describing this operation was rejected by the *American Journal of Obstetrics and Gynecology*, again on the grounds that the operation was unethical.[15,16]

Semm sailed against this tide of disapproval and small-mindedness, treating ectopic pregnancy and performing uterine myomectomy and, finally, hysterectomy. He was later praised for the development of an approach that is now the gold standard for certain operations, and the University of Kiel became a leading centre of laparoscopy. Semm's tireless teaching and design of such training aids as the 'pelvi-trainer' hugely contributed to the spread of endoscopic skill on both sides of the Atlantic. Owing to his lecturing extensively abroad to both gynaecologists and general surgeons, publishing in several languages and film making, laparoscopy gained acceptance in the USA through the 1980s and later in Europe.[14,17]

With the development in the mid-1980s of video cameras that could be coupled to a laparoscope, the surgeon was finally released from direct visualisation through the instrument. This decreased fatigue and allowed all present in theatre a view of the operation. Subsequently, microelectronic advances enabled cameras to become smaller, lighter and of higher resolution.[18] There were many other pioneers of laparoscopy such as, in alphabetical order: Maurice Bruhat (France), James Daniell (USA), Hans Frangenheim (Germany), Victor Gomel (Canada), Richard Kleppinger (USA), Harry Reich (USA), Patrick Steptoe (England) and Chris Sutton (England). Their work culminated in general surgeons taking note and, in 1985, Erich Mühe in Böblingen, Germany, carried out the first laparoscopic cholecystectomy using some of Semm's techniques.[19] The large majority (85%) of cholecystectomies are now performed this way.[20]

Subsequently, laser technology and the concept of keyhole surgery captured the attention of the media and the imagination of the public, making operative laparoscopy one of the first truly consumer-driven technological medical advances. As a result, the 1990s saw rapid advances in laparoscopic procedures for urinary incontinence, pelvic organ prolapse and gynaecological cancer.

The case for laparoscopy

Patrick Steptoe (1913–1988), the English gynaecologist well known for the development of in vitro fertilisation, said: 'Laparoscopy … can allow a detailed and accurate examination of the female pelvic organs. In properly selected cases, and particularly in the field of infertility investigations, laparoscopy can be the most important and indeed the only method of assessing certain factors. The proof of the absence of organic lesions … can often avoid laparotomy, saving patients pain and distress, and the hospital services time, bed occupancy and money.'[11]

General advantages of laparoscopy over laparotomy

Many situations exist in which laparoscopy may be indicated (Table 1.1). The next section deals with some aspects of these indications and the advantages of laparoscopy to their specific circumstances. However, there are some benefits that are applicable to most procedures.

Laparoscopy undoubtedly affords a more detailed and magnified view of the peritoneal cavity, which facilitates more precise surgery, akin to microsurgery; for example, coagulation of bleeding points and ablation of diseased tissue may cause less collateral damage to surrounding structures. Areas less

TABLE 1.1 **Indications and contraindications for diagnostic laparoscopy**

Indications	Relative and absolute contraindications
Acute or chronic pelvic pain	Mechanical or paralytic bowel obstruction
Ectopic pregnancy	Generalised peritonitis
Pelvic inflammatory disease (including tuberculosis)	Diaphragmatic hernia
Endometriosis	Major intraperitoneal haemorrhage (for example shock)
Adnexal torsion	Severe cardiorespiratory disease
Subfertility	Massive obesity
Congenital pelvic abnormality	Inflammatory bowel disease
Abnormal pelvic scan	Large abdominal mass
Unexplained pelvic mass	Advanced pregnancy
Staging for ovarian malignancy	Multiple abdominal incisions
	Irreducible external hernia

accessible by laparotomy such as the pouch of Douglas, the posterior aspect of the broad ligaments and the upper abdomen may be more thoroughly evaluated. Indeed, the approach offers the opportunity to identify coincident disease. The presence of a pneumoperitoneum decreases bleeding and hence provides a cleaner operating field, and the use of thermal energy can render the operation bloodless. As a result of these factors, procedures that are technically difficult by conventional surgery may become easier.

As video monitoring is an integral part of the operating equipment, a complete and permanent record of the operation is possible at laparoscopy without hindering or slowing surgery; this record can be invaluable for teaching, for explanation to the woman and for medico-legal purposes.

There is a wealth of evidence that laparoscopy generally gives rise to less postoperative pain and permits an earlier discharge from hospital compared with laparotomy. Less pain allows faster mobilisation and discharge of the woman after a laparoscopic sterilisation[21] and also after the treatment of an ectopic pregnancy.[22–24] In addition, an earlier return to work is usually possible.

A large meta-analysis has concluded that there is overwhelmingly decreased wound haematoma, febrile morbidity and infection after laparoscopy compared with laparotomy.[25] It may be predicted that swifter mobilisation decreases the likelihood of venous thromboembolism and that a shorter hospital stay presents less opportunity for hospital-acquired infections.

The advantages of avoiding a laparotomy remain even with more complex operative laparoscopic procedures as it is the route of surgery that seems to confer the benefit rather than the procedure itself. For example, after benign ovarian cystectomy, there was less pain and febrile morbidity compared with laparotomy (odds ratio 0.34).[26] The pooled incidence of intraoperative and postoperative complications was also decreased (odds ratio 0.26), as was hospital stay (by almost 3 days). Hysterectomy remains the most common major gynaecological operation and performing it laparoscopically rather than by laparotomy leads to less pain, shorter hospital stay (by 1 day), faster convalescence and better short-term quality of life measured at 6 weeks (this advantage is not seen if laparoscopic hysterectomy is compared with vaginal hysterectomy).[27] An earlier return to work is possible (by 1 week in the case of hysterectomy).[28] This is of particular personal benefit to the self-employed. Remarkably, the degree of postoperative pain and the length of convalescence are not significantly related to the type of any resective surgery performed.[29]

Bowel is handled less at laparoscopy and so the degree of postoperative ileus is decreased, with most women being able to tolerate a light diet from recovery of consciousness. Given that endoscopic procedures are associated with less intraoperative tissue trauma, it has long been held that fewer de novo adhesions will arise,[30,31] which will decrease the incidence of postoperative bowel obstruction and lessen the risk of visceral injury during any subsequent abdominal operation. There is evidence that the incidence of postoperative adhesion formation after laparoscopic sterilisation and tubal surgery for ectopic pregnancy is lower than that after laparotomy,[32] although more recently this has been disputed for other procedures.[33]

Obviously, less significant wound dehiscence occurs when incisions are 5mm and the risk of 'burst abdomen' is eliminated. Postoperative hernias are also rare with laparoscopic port incisions less than 10mm in size and uncommon even with larger incisions if repaired correctly.[34] There is clearly also a cosmetic advantage with smaller incisions. The impact of laparoscopy compared with open surgery on sexual behaviour and function has yet to be fully evaluated.

Laparoscopic surgery is usually cost-effective except when using predominantly expensive disposable instruments. Taking into account operative costs, hospital stay and management of surgical complications, laparoscopic surgery both for ectopic pregnancy[35] and for benign ovarian cysts[26] has been shown to be highly cost-effective compared with laparotomy. We elaborate on these considerations later in this chapter.

Indications

The panoply of procedures possible using a laparoscopic approach is the subject of this book. We have tried to outline only a few here in discussing principles pertinent to MAS, as well as mentioning groups of women who may particularly benefit from laparoscopic surgery.

Diagnosis

The favourable complication profile of laparoscopy has lowered the threshold for direct visualisation of the abdominopelvic organs for diagnostic purposes. However, the Royal College of Obstetricians and Gynaecologists (RCOG) recommends that gynaecologists who perform laparoscopy for suspected pathology are competent at intermediate-level (Level 2; see Table 1.2) laparoscopic surgery, which may then be performed concurrently with diagnosis – the so-called 'see and treat' principle.[36] Women may be classified preoperatively as follows:

- Unlikely to have pelvic pathology, or likely to have pathology that may be treated adequately without surgery, so avoiding a woman's exposure to any unnecessary risk in the first instance.

- Unlikely to have severe endometriosis; may be treated adequately by an intermediate-level laparoscopist should pathology be found.

- Likely to have severe endometriosis; may benefit most from referral to a specialist centre for complex primary surgery, which possibly halves the risk of at least entry-related laparoscopic complications through one rather than two operations. In practice, however, this may be an inefficient use of a tertiary referral given that many women referred will have a mild appearance to their disease (as is the unpredictable nature of endometriosis) without a prior laparoscopy by a general gynaecologist. The decision to refer should clearly be made on an individual basis.

Emergency diagnosis / treatment

Much has been published on treatment of the most common life-threatening gynaecological emergency, ectopic pregnancy – a topic that will be addressed in a chapter of its own, but save it to mention that 30% of ectopic pregnancies are still treated by laparotomy even in developed countries.[20] For any further

TABLE 1.2 **Royal College of Obstetricians and Gynaecologists classification of laparoscopic procedures**

Level 1	Level 2	Level 3
Diagnostic laparoscopy	Division of filmy adhesions	Division of thick adhesions
Sterilisation	Linear salpingotomy or salpingectomy for ectopic pregnancy	LAVH with significant associated pathology
Aspiration of ovarian cyst	Salpingostomy for infertility	Total laparoscopic hysterectomy
Ovarian biopsy	Ovarian cystectomy	Myomectomy for intramural fibroids
	Treatment of endometrioma	Treatment of rAFS stage III and IV endometriosis
	Salpingo-oophorectomy	Pelvic and aortic lymphadenectomy
	Ovarian drilling with laser or diathermy for polycystic ovaries	Pelvic sidewall and ureteric dissection
	Treatment of rAFS stage I and II endometriosis	Presacral neurectomy
	Myomectomy for pedunculated subserous fibroid	Incontinence procedures
	Uterosacral nerve ablation	Prolapse procedures
	LAVH without significant associated pathology	

Abbreviations: LAVH = laparoscopically assisted vaginal hysterectomy | rAFS = revised American Fertility Society criteria.

significant decrease in operative morbidity, earlier diagnosis and, in particular, more widely available MAS skills are required.

The clinical presentation of fertility-threatening ovarian torsion is non-specific and so its diagnosis is missed preoperatively in about 50% of affected women. A promptly performed ultrasound scan showing ovaries that are less than 5 cm in diameter may help exclude the diagnosis, although no investigation is perfect. Early laparoscopy with detorsion and cystectomy with ovarian conservation, if at all possible, offers an obvious fertility advantage over the traditional approach of laparotomy and ovarian extirpation,[37] but relies on gynaecologists on call having adequate training in MAS.

Even routine early laparoscopy has been shown to promptly and accurately diagnose – and efficiently manage – the acute abdomen.[38] Changing the clinical diagnosis in 30% of cases, early laparoscopy reduces the rate of unnecessary laparotomy and provides a less traumatic approach if an operation is required for treatment. Laparoscopy is likely to have a less deleterious effect on fertility compared with laparotomy, and this is why 69% of consultant general surgeons reserve laparoscopy use to women of reproductive age.[39]

Emergency surgery in intrauterine pregnancy

Approximately 0.2% of women with intrauterine pregnancies require intra-abdominal surgery for nongynaecological or gynaecological conditions, most commonly appendicitis, cholecystitis, adnexal torsion, ovarian cyst and, very rarely, heterotopic pregnancy. The incidence of fetal loss increases from 1.5% to 35% if an uncomplicated appendicitis is allowed to rupture, to say nothing of maternal morbidity. In general, laparoscopy in pregnancy is associated with a good maternal and fetal outcome. Miscarriage, preterm labour and fetal death are related more to the pathology treated than to the operative intervention. Beyond the first trimester, an open laparoscopic entry[40] is prudent to decrease the risk of uterine injury. Thought should be given to insertion of all trocars in a more cephalad position with prior insertion of a nasogastric tube, the administration of steroids depending on gestation, and tocolysis. A left lateral tilt and maintenance of intra-abdominal pressure at less than 12 mmHg for the shortest required time will decrease the theoretical risk of hypercarbia and fetal acidosis.[41] The complication rate of laparoscopy in pregnancy seems to be similar to that while not pregnant.[42] Laparoscopic splenectomy[43,44] and retroperitoneal adrenalectomy[45] have been reported in pregnant women without complication.

Sterilisation

After diagnostic endoscopy, where laparoscopy began, sterilisation was the first laparoscopic intervention. Tubal sterilisation is the most requested method of contraception worldwide. While in developing countries 'mini-laparotomy' is the most common approach, in developed countries it is interval laparoscopic sterilisation. The laparoscopic approach should be chosen where available. Indeed, after a normal pregnancy and delivery, there is little justification for delaying laparoscopic sterilisation beyond 5 days after delivery because, surprisingly, complication rates including uterine injury are similar regardless of whether the procedure is performed at 5 days or after the traditional interval of 6 weeks.[46]

Laparoscopic hysterectomy and its variants

In the presence of adhesions, endometriosis or adnexal pathology, or if salpingo-oophorectomy would be otherwise technically challenging, laparoscopic assistance may permit completion of hysterectomy vaginally. For instance, an Italian multicentre prospective randomised study has shown that there is reduced blood loss, pain and hospital stay after laparoscopically assisted vaginal hysterectomy than after total abdominal hysterectomy, with fewer complications.[47]

Other technical variants include total and subtotal laparoscopic hysterectomy, each with its own champions. Whatever the precise technique, there is no evidence that the use of a laparoscope for hysterectomy offers any advantages over vaginal hysterectomy in the absence of extrauterine pathology, and many gynaecologists feel that vaginal hysterectomy should be the default route for removing the uterus.[27]

Adolescence

Whereas imaging has improved to largely obviate the need for diagnostic laparoscopy in rare congenital anatomical anomalies, treatment for these and advanced endometriosis laparoscopically may be of particular benefit to the young. In addition to a favourable complication profile relative to laparotomy, a minimally invasive approach is likely to have positive effects on education through an earlier return to school, fertility through decreased adhesion formation, and cosmetic result.[48] Meticulous handling of tissue and surface reconstruction of ovaries after cystectomy is of particular importance. The success of such operations should perhaps be determined by the woman's future fertility rather than solely by the length of hospitalisation.[19]

Endometriosis

The gold standard for the diagnosis of endometriosis, laparoscopy is also the modality of choice for the treatment of infertility associated with mild or moderate endometriosis. Good evidence exists for improving pain and fertility with laparoscopic laser ablation of endometriotic deposits and excision of endometriomas. Excision of deeply invasive endometriosis eradicates diseased tissue, which tends to respond poorly to medical treatment, while preserving reproductive function (unlike hysterectomy, which in any event would not treat endometriosis in the rectovaginal pouch).[49] A further use of laparoscopy is in chronic pelvic pain, where conscious pain mapping may permit more focused treatment where symptoms are most severe.[50]

Treatment of subfertility

Although diagnostic laparoscopy is no longer recommended as a standard investigation for all infertile couples,[51] the detection rate for unexpected conditions such as endometriosis and pelvic adhesions is about 20%.[52] There is ample evidence to support the use of ovarian drilling in polycystic ovary syndrome refractory to clomifene citrate[53] on grounds of effectiveness, treatment of coexisting adhesions and endometriosis (and hence other symptoms) and diagnosis of tubal patency. Ovarian drilling considerably decreases the multiple pregnancy rate and has no risk of ovarian hyperstimulation, while simultaneously reducing direct and indirect costs compared with gonadotrophin therapy.[54] Women may welcome an approach to causes of infertility such as endometriosis that obviates the need for in vitro fertilisation and its association with poorer pregnancy outcome once pregnancy is achieved. Furthermore, laparoscopy also has a role in optimising fertility with assisted reproduction; for example, salpingectomy may be used to treat hydrosalpinges before in vitro fertilisation.[55] A passing mention of outpatient culdoscopy is of interest here, in that it has recently been shown to be a cost-effective alternative to laparoscopy in certain circumstances and may be employed in a one-stop fertility clinic.[56]

Urogynaecological and prolapse surgery

As in all surgical disciplines, evolution of techniques and procedures occurs as a result of a growing body of research and experience. Some procedures inevitably become obsolete, such as laparoscopic ventrosuspension of the uterus to the round ligaments for treatment of uterine prolapse,[57] and perhaps the same can be said for laparoscopic colposuspension, which has been largely superseded by procedures such as tension-free vaginal tape. In fact, the management of urinary incontinence and uterovaginal prolapse is undergoing major changes and it is unclear at present whether laparoscopic procedures or vaginal surgery with mesh will prove to be superior.

Cancer

While not the remit of this text, no overview of laparoscopy could omit mentioning that women diagnosed with gynaecological cancer stand to gain dramatically in quality of life from the use of less invasive surgery. From retroperitoneal lymph node sampling to radical laparoscopic hysterectomy with pelvic and para-aortic lymphadenectomy, first described in 1992,[58] great strides are being made in the avoidance of traumatic conventional surgery. Now, many endometrial, cervical and early ovarian cancers may be amenable to laparoscopic treatment[59] without increasing postoperative morbidity or recurrence risk.[60]

It is apparent from all of the above that the question is not so much 'What can be accomplished laparoscopically?' but 'What cannot?'. The answer is that most procedures performed by laparotomy can be performed laparoscopically, provided there is no large pelvic mass or extensive malignancy. This does not mean that laparoscopy is necessarily the best option in given circumstances. However, since the early days of this approach, attention has shifted from what technically may be achieved in terms of treating disease in its various forms to what will most benefit women. There is much debate about the more complex procedures. In many cases, the decision depends more on the particular skills of the gynaecologist, the presence of contraindications and the relative risks of complications.[61]

Expectations and complications, especially compared with laparotomy

Before any laparoscopy, discussion of realistic expectations and serious and frequent complications is most important, supported by concise written patient information. The RCOG has published consent guidelines for diagnostic laparoscopy,[62] although clearly counselling should be more extensive where complex therapeutic laparoscopy is planned. There is a common misconception among the lay public that keyhole surgery is minor surgery, whereas in reality the only difference is the incision size. Therefore, it is not surprising in the event of a complication that people often assume there has been negligence. As a result, endoscopic surgery has become one of the major areas of medical litigation in gynaecology.[63] All women should be made aware of the relative risks of MAS compared with conventional surgery. In particular, they should understand that any endoscopic operation may have to be converted to laparotomy and that bowel, bladder, ureter and major vessel injury are recognised risks with laparoscopy.

A meta-analysis of randomised controlled trials[25] showed that the risk of minor complications after benign gynaecological surgery is consistently 40% lower with laparoscopy than with laparotomy, regardless of surgical complexity. Minor complications in this analysis included fever, wound haematoma and infection. The combined risk of major complications (those that were life-threatening, resulted in long-term disability or required additional major surgery) was similar between the two routes.

Over 50% (25 764) of all laparoscopic procedures performed in The Netherlands in 1994 were studied prospectively,[64] further elucidating the risks. The most frequent complication of laparoscopy in general is haemorrhage from an

TABLE 1.3 **Complication rate according to surgical complexity**[64]

Category of laparoscopy	Complication rate (%)
Diagnostic laparoscopy	0.27
Laparoscopic sterilisation	0.45
Operative laparoscopy in general	1.79
Laparoscopically assisted hysterectomy	9.02

epigastric vein, followed by a gastrointestinal injury occurring during the set-up phase while creating a pneumoperitoneum and inserting the primary trocar. It was found that training reduces the incidence of these entry complications. Both the meta-analysis[25] and the Dutch study[64] clearly demonstrate that the complication rate increases with surgical complexity (Table 1.3), as might be expected in any form of surgery. This further supports the notion that specialised MAS training is required for all but the most straightforward procedures.

Major complications such as visceral or vascular injury are relatively uncommon during laparoscopic procedures, with a reported frequency of 0.1–0.5%, but trauma to the retroperitoneal vessels is almost unique to laparoscopy.[65] One in three complications is associated with the establishment of a pneumoperitoneum, and one in four complications is not diagnosed during the procedure.[66] Injury to retroperitoneal vessels usually requires immediate laparotomy, whereas complications such as bowel injury are increasingly managed laparoscopically provided any perforation is small and faecal soiling minimal.[67] Gynaecological laparoscopy in general has a mortality rate of 4.4–8/100 000, compared with a mortality rate of 150/100 000 after abdominal hysterectomy for benign indications.[65,68,69]

Certain procedures are of course associated with a relatively high risk of complication. By way of an example, laparoscopic hysterectomy procedures are charged as having an increased major complication rate (11.1%) compared with abdominal hysterectomy (6.2%) in the eVALuate study,[27] a prospective randomised trial of 1346 women. Crucially, however, conversion from laparoscopy to laparotomy (3.9%) was included as a major complication in this study, even though no other complication occurred in a large proportion of cases. We feel that this provides an unfair comparison, as the outcome is materially no worse for those converted to laparotomy than for those undergoing a primary laparotomy if performed for technical reasons when the woman has received adequate preoperative counselling. This said, it is generally believed that the risk of ureteric injury is greater during total hysterectomy when some or all of the operation has been performed laparoscopically.

Anecdotally, many women made aware of a greater complication profile still prefer laparoscopy to an open procedure because their recovery is probably faster. Nonetheless, safety is improved by careful patient selection and adequate patient preparation (for example bowel preparation), a level of surgical training appropriate for the intended procedure, recognition of any complication intraoperatively (although this can sometimes be difficult) and a high suspicion of complications in women whose recovery is longer than expected. Most importantly, surgeons must not consider conversion to laparotomy as failure, and must always consult colleagues from other specialties in the management of potentially serious complications.

Patient selection

Patient selection criteria largely depend on the specific laparoscopic procedure.[59] The principle mentioned previously is reiterated here: unless a woman is likely to benefit in some way from laparoscopy, its risks cannot be justified. As most operations performed are diagnostic and the most common complications occur during laparoscopic entry, it follows that reducing the number of operations that are less likely to benefit women will lead to greater benefit for less risk on a population basis.

Considerable additional risk is introduced by a previous laparotomy or peritonitis secondary to the presence of adhesions.[64] Therefore, extreme surgical care is required if laparoscopy is contemplated, including entry well clear of the scar through, for example, Palmer's point.

Morbid obesity is another relative contraindication to laparoscopy, as with other surgery: positioning may be difficult; the initial entry may be complicated; longer ports and instruments are required; access may be hindered by enlarged bowel and a fatty omentum; the operation is usually more technically challenging; to say nothing of the anaesthetic risk. However, these women may benefit most from a decrease in their significant risk of wound infection with an open procedure. Introduction of the Veress needle through the uterine fundus has allowed successful peritoneal insufflation in obese women, but this method is currently not routine.[70,71] Conversely, women who are underweight are at an increased risk of vascular injury even as the skin incision is made, as the aorta may bifurcate caudal to the umbilicus and underlie the skin by only 2 cm.[72,73]

Although sometimes influenced by the media and aggressive marketing, by no means the least of the considerations is the woman's preference. As with other treatment options, this will usually influence the operative decision.

Implementation/requirements for laparoscopy

The skeletal requirements for a laparoscopy service are skilled staff, training, equipment and time, which come at a certain cost.

Staff

A thorough knowledge of pelvic and abdominal anatomy, excellent hand–eye coordination and an appreciation of one's own limitations are essential to any laparoscopist. In addition, a full understanding of instrumentation is required to be a safe and effective operator, from basic physical principles to how equipment is assembled and connected, from when and how to use a particular instrument to what to do when it seems to be malfunctioning. Crucially, expertise must be developed through sufficient training and continuous exposure of the surgeon to laparoscopic procedures of a complexity appropriate to his or her practice. This said, such complex surgery is a team effort and assistants, anaesthetists, theatre staff, all other trainees and students present should be engaged mentally and involved in the operation by becoming familiar with patient positioning, equipment and the surgery itself, all of which are discussed later in this book.

Training

Endoscopic surgery is very different from conventional surgery and it probably takes longer to acquire the necessary skills to operate without the benefits of direct vision and tissue handling. As an acknowledgement of the importance of hysteroscopic and laparoscopic surgery to modern gynaecological care, coupled with a wish to improve and structure training in this area, the RCOG has made basic endoscopic surgery (Level 1 hysteroscopy and laparoscopy) a core curriculum subject for trainees, and there are Advanced Training Skills Modules for advanced hysteroscopic and laparoscopic surgery as a means of accreditation for those wishing to extend their skills. However, advanced (Level 3) procedures require a much higher degree of skill to be completed successfully and have a higher conversion rate even in experienced hands.[74] Hysterectomy is still the most common major gynaecological procedure and women's demand for the minimally invasive approach is increasing.[20] Although hysterectomy is defined as a Level 2 procedure by the RCOG, it may seem challenging for the general gynaecologist of the future to provide this operation without skills that go beyond what may be learned in an Advanced Training Skills Module. Although the RCOG recommends that any laparoscopist should effectively possess Level 2 skills to treat incidental disease concurrently with diagnosis, some argue that there should be distinct subspecialty training in MAS.

Equipment

Nowhere is technology having such a dramatic impact in surgery as in the development of newer and better instruments for endoscopy. Almost every week sees the introduction of yet another device, which is often more expensive than the last. However enticing, and quite apart from the cost implications, it is difficult to justify continuously changing one's surgical technique, and we believe that getting to know a few instruments well and using them to their potential is preferable to using many less efficiently.

Operating time

The more complex procedures tend to take longer and the operating time is less predictable.[75] For example, hysterectomy with a laparoscopic approach generally takes 30–35 minutes longer than either abdominal or vaginal hysterectomy.[27] Time is of course money, so there is a need for appropriate allocation of resources as a result.

Cost

Cost comparisons produce variable results, a longer operating time and the use of disposable instruments often outweighing any advantages of shorter hospitalisation and faster recovery. Whereas there is undoubtedly significant cost associated with implementing and sustaining an MAS service, there are financial gains at hospital level and advantage to the economy as a whole. The advantages to a given hospital are through decreased postoperative stay and perhaps decreased subsequent admissions for adhesion complications. The financial gain also goes far beyond an earlier return to work for a woman admitted for, say, ovarian cystectomy, but extends to the unpaid carer, social services and employer. If a specialist centre changes the life of just one average-earning 30-year-old woman with endometriosis annually, to the extent that she is able to work until retirement when previously she was not, this must have a dramatically beneficial effect at the macroeconomic level.

References

1 Sutton C J G, Philips K. *Preventing Entry-related Gynaecological Laparoscopic Injuries*. Green-top Guideline No. 49. London: Royal College of Obstetricians and Gynaecologists; 2008 [www.rcog.org.uk/womens-health/clinical-guidance/preventing-entry-related-gynaecological-laparoscopic-injuries-green-].

2 Magos A. Hysteroscopy and laparoscopy. In: *Dewhurst's Textbook of Obstetrics and Gynaecology*. 7th Edition. Oxford: Blackwell Publishing; 2007.

3 Bozzini P. [Light conductor, an invention for the viewing of internal parts and diseases with illustration]. *J Pract Arzneykunde Wundarzneykunst* 1805;24:107–4. Article in German.

4 Desormeaux A J. The endoscope and its application to the diagnosis and treatment of affections of the genitourinary passages. *Chicago Med J* 1867;24:177–94.

5 Kelling G. [On viewing the esophagus and stomach by means of flexible instruments]. *Verh Ges Dtsch Naturf Ärzte* 1902;73:117. Article in German.

6 Hatzinger M, Badawi K, Langbein S, Häcker A. The seminal contribution of Georg Kelling to laparoscopy. *J Endourol* 2005;19:1154–6.

7 Jacobæus H C. [On the possibility of performing cystoscopy for the examination of serous cavities]. *Münch Med Wochenschr* 1910;57:2090–2. Article in German.

8 Hatzinger M, Kwon S T, Langbein S, Kamp S, Häcker A, Alken P. Hans Christian Jacobaeus: Inventor of human laparoscopy and thoracoscopy. *J Endourol* 2006;20:848–50.

9 Short A R. The uses of coelioscopy. *Br Med J* 1925;2:254–5.

10 Decker A, Cherry T. Culdoscopy: a new method in diagnosis of pelvic disease. *Am J Surg* 1944;64:40–4.

11 Steptoe P C. Gynaecological endoscopy – laparoscopy and culdoscopy. *J Obstet Gynaecol Br Commonw* 1965;72:535–43.

12 Hackford S, personal communication.

13 Semm K. [Laparoscopy in gynecology]. *Geburtshilfe Frauenheilkd* 1967;27:1029–42. Article in German.

14 Litynski G S. Kurt Semm and the fight against skepticism: endoscopic hemostasis, laparoscopic appendectomy, and Semm's impact on the "laparoscopic revolution". *JSLS* 1998;2:309–13.

15 Moll F H, Marx F J. A pioneer in laparoscopy and pelviscopy: Kurt Semm (1927–2003). *J Endourol* 2005;19:269–71.

16 Morgenstern L. Against the tide: Kurt Karl Stephan Semm (1927–2003). *Surg Innov* 2005;12:5–6.

17 Smith J. Kurt Semm. A pioneer in minimally invasive surgery. *Br Med J* 2003;327:397.

18 Nezhat C, Nezhat F, Nezhat C. Operative laparoscopy. videolaparoscopy and videolaseroscopy. *Ann N Y Acad Sci* 1994;734:433–44.

19 Tadir Y, Fisch B. Operative laparoscopy: A challenge for general gynecology? *Am J Obstet Gynecol* 1993;169:7–12.

20 Jansen F W, Kolkman W. Implementation difficulties of advanced techniques in gynecological laparoscopy. *Gynecol Surg* 2008;5:261–4.

21 Filshie M. Laparoscopic sterilization. *Semin Laparosc Surg* 1999;6:112–7.

22 Brumsted J, Kessler C, Gibson C C, Nakajima S, Riddick D H, Gibson M. A comparison of laparoscopy and laparotomy for the treatment of ectopic pregnancy. *Obstet Gynecol* 1988;71:889–92.

23 Vermesh M, Silva P D, Rosen G F, Stein A L, Fossum G T, Sauer M V. Management of unruptured ectopic gestation by linear salpingostomy: a prospective, randomised clinical trial of laparoscopy versus laparotomy. *Obstet Gynecol* 1989;73:400–4.

24 Baumann R, Magos A L, Turnbull A. Prospective comparison of videopelviscopy with laparotomy for ectopic pregnancy. *Br J Obstet Gynecol* 1991;98:765–71.

25 Chapron C, Fauconnier A, Goffinet F, Bréart G, Dubuisson J B. Laparoscopic surgery is not inherently dangerous for patients presenting with benign gynaecologic pathology. Results of a meta-analysis. *Hum Reprod* 2002;17:1334–42.

26 Medeiros L R, Fachel J M G, Garry R, Stein A T, Furness S. Laparoscopy versus laparotomy for benign ovarian tumours. *Cochrane Database Syst Rev* 2005;(3): CD004751.

27 Garry R, Fountain J, Mason S, Napp V, Brown J, Hawe J, et al. The eVALuate study: two parallel randomised trials, one comparing laparoscopic with abdominal hysterectomy, the other comparing laparoscopic with vaginal hysterectomy. *Br Med J* 2004;328:129.

28 Persson P, Wijma K, Hammar M, Kjølhede P. Psychological wellbeing after laparoscopic and abdominal hysterectomy–a randomised controlled multicentre study. *BJOG* 2006;113:1023–30.

29 Mais V, Ajossa S, Guerriero S, Peiretti R F, Serri F, Melis G B. Postoperative pain and postoperative recovery following resective laparoscopy: no relation to the intra-abdominal surgical procedure. *Gynaecol Endosc* 2003;5:197–210.

30 Operative laparoscopy study group. Postoperative adhesion development after operative laparoscopy: evaluation at early second-look procedures. *Fertil Steril* 1991;55:700–4.

31 Nezhat C, Nezhat F, Metzger D A, Luciano A A. Adhesion reformation after reproductive surgery by videolaseroscopy. *Fertil Steril* 1990;53:1008–11.

32 Lundorff P, Hahlin M, Källfelt B, Thorburn J, Lindblom B. Adhesion formation after laparoscopic surgery in tubal pregnancy: a randomised trial versus laparotomy. *Fertil Steril* 1991;55:911–5.

33 Lower A M, Hawthorn R J, Clark D, Boyd J H, Finlayson A R, Knight A D, et al. Adhesion-related readmissions following gynaecological laparoscopy or laparotomy in Scotland: an epidemiological study of 24 046 patients. *Hum Reprod* 2004;19;1877–85.

34 Garry R. Towards evidence-based laparoscopic entry techniques: clinical problems and dilemmas. *Gynaecol Endosc* 1999;8:315–26.

35 Gray D T, Thorburn J, Lundorff P, Strandell A, Lindblom B. A cost-effectiveness study of a randomised trial of laparoscopy versus laparotomy for ectopic pregnancy. *Lancet* 1995;345:1139–43.

36 Ball E, Koh C, Janik G, Davis C. Gynaecological laparoscopy: 'see and treat' should be the gold standard. *Curr Opin Obstet Gynecol* 2008;20:325–30.

37 Lo L M, Chang S D, Horng S G, Yang T Y, Lee C L, Liang C C. Laparoscopy versus laparotomy for surgical intervention of ovarian torsion. *J Obstet Gynaecol Res* 2008;34:1020–5.

38 Golash V, Willson P D. Early laparoscopy as a routine procedure in the management of acute abdominal pain. A review of 1,320 patients. *Surg Endosc* 2005;19:882–5.

39 Stechman M J, Roy D, Mainprize K S. Current practice in the United Kingdom for the use of diagnostic laparoscopy in suspected acute appendicitis. *Colorectal Dis* 2009;11:817–20.

40 Hasson H M. Open laparoscopy as a method of access in laparoscopic surgery. *Gynaecol Endosc* 1999;8;353–62.

41 Al-Fozan H, Tulandi T. Safety and risks of laparoscopy in pregnancy. *Curr Opin Obstet Gynecol* 2002;14:375–9.

42 Fatum M, Rojansky N. Laparoscopic surgery during pregnancy. *Obstet Gynecol Surv* 2001;56:50–9.

43 Anglin B V, Rutherford C, Ramus R, Lieser M, Jones D B. Immune thrombocytopenic purpura during pregnancy: laparoscopic treatment. *JSLS* 2001;5:63–7.

44 Iwase K, Higaki J, Yoon H F, Mikata S, Tanaka Y, Takahashi T, et al. Hand-assisted laparoscopic splenectomy for idiopathic thrombocytopenic purpura during pregnancy. *Surg Laparosc Endosc Percutan Tech* 2001;11:53–6.

45 Aishima M, Tanaka M, Haraoka M, Naito S. Retroperitoneal laparoscopic adrenalectomy in a pregnant woman with Cushing's syndrome. *J Urol* 2000;164:770–1.

46 Huber A W, Mueller M D, Ghezzi F, Cromi A, Dreher E, Raio L. Tubal sterilization: Complications of laparoscopy and minilaparotomy. *Eur J Obstet Gynecol Reprod Biol* 2007;134:105–9.

47 Marana R, Busacca M, Zupi E, Garcia N, Paparella P, Catalano G F. Laparoscopically assisted vaginal hysterectomy versus total abdominal hysterectomy: a prospective, randomized multicenter study. *Am J Obstet Gynecol* 1999;180:270–5.

48 Pandis G K, Michala L, Creighton S M, Cutner A S. Minimal access surgery in adolescent gynaecology. *BJOG* 2009;116:214–9.

49 Garry R. Laparoscopic excision of endometriosis: the treatment of choice? *Br J Obstet Gynaecol* 1997;104:513–5.

50 Howard F M, El-Minawi A M, Sanchez R A. Conscious pain mapping by laparoscopy in women with chronic pelvic pain. *Obstet Gynecol* 2000;96:934–9.

51 National Institute for Health and Clinical Excellence. Assessment and treatment for people with fertility problems. London: NICE; 2004 [www.nice.org.uk/CG011].

52 Henig I, Prough S G, Cheatwood M, DeLong E. Hysterosalpingography, laparoscopy and hysteroscopy in infertility. A comparative study. *J Reprod Med* 1991;36:573–5.

53 Gant N F. Infertility and endometriosis: comparison of pregnancy outcomes with laparotomy versus laparoscopic techniques. *Am J Obstet Gynecol* 1992;166:1072–81.

54 Farquhar C M. An economic evaluation of laparoscopic ovarian diathermy versus gonadotrotrophin therapy for women with clomiphene citrate-resistant polycystic ovarian syndrome. *Curr Opin Obstet Gynecol* 2005;17:347–53.

55 Burney R O, Nezhat C. Infertility treatment: the viability of the laparoscopic view. *Fertil Steril* 2008;89:461–4.

56 Khouri A, Magos A. The cost of out-patient culdoscopy compared with in-patient laparoscopy in women with infertility. *J Obstet Gynaecol* 2005;21:160–5.

57 Lin L L, Ho M H, Haessler A L, Betson L H, Alinsod R H, Liu C Y, et al. A review of laparoscopic uterine suspension procedures for uterine preservation. *Curr Opin Obstet Gynecol* 2005;17:541–6.

58 Nezhat C R, Burrell M O, Nezhat F R, Benigno B B, Welander C E. Laparoscopic radical hysterectomy with paraaortic and pelvic node dissection. *Am J Obstet Gynecol* 1992;166:864–5.

59 DeSimone C P, Ueland F R. Gynecologic laparoscopy. *Surg Clin N Am* 2008;88:319–41.

60 Querleu D, Leblanc E, Ferron G, Narducci F. Laparoscopic surgery in gynaecological oncology. *Eur J Surg Oncol* 2006;32:853–8.

61 Jacobson T Z, Davis C J. Safe laparoscopy: is it possible? *Curr Opin Obstet Gynecol* 2004;16:283–8.

62 Ismail K M K. *Diagnostic Laparoscopy*. Consent Advice No. 2. London: Royal College of Obstetricians and Gynaecologists; 2008 [http://www.rcog.org.uk/diagnostic-laparoscopy].

63 Argent V P. Medico-legal problems in gynaecology. *Curr Obstet Gynaecol* 2003;13:294–9.

64 Jansen F W, Kapiteyn K, Trimbos-Kemper T, Hermans J, Trimbos J B. Complications of laparoscopy: a prospective multicentre observational study. *Br J Obstet Gynaecol* 1997;104:595–600.

65 Magrina J F. Complications of laparoscopic surgery. *Clin Obstet Gynecol* 2002;45:469–80.

66 Querleu D, Chapron C, Chevallier L, Bruhat M A. Complications of gynaecological laparoscopy. A French collaborative study. *N Engl J Med* 1993;328:1355.

67 Chapron C, Pierre F, Harchaoui Y, Lacroix S, Beguin S, Querleu D, et al. Gastrointestinal injuries during gynaecological laparoscopy. *Hum Reprod* 1999;14:333–7.

68 Gynaecological laparoscopy. The report of the working party of the confidential enquiry into gynaecological laparoscopy. *Br J Obstet Gynaecol* 1978;85:401–3.

69 Varol N, Healey M, Tang P, Sheehan P, Maher P, Hill D. Ten-year review of hysterectomy morbidity and mortality: can we change direction? *Aust N Z J Obstet Gynaecol* 2001;41:295–302.

70 Sanders R R, Filshie G M. Transfundal induction of pneumoperitoneum prior to laparoscopy. *J Obstet Gynaecol Br Commonw* 1974;81:829–30.

71 Santala M, Järvelä I, Kauppila A. Transfundal insertion of a Veress needle in laparoscopy of obese subjects: a practical alternative. *Hum Reprod* 1999;14:2277–8.

72 Hurd W W, Bude R O, DeLancey J O L, Pearl M L. The relationship of the umbilicus to the aortic bifurcation: implications for laparoscopic technique. *Obstet Gynecol* 1992;80:48–51.

73 Hanney R M, Carmalt H L, Merrett N, Tait N. Use of the Hasson cannula producing major vascular injury at laparoscopy. *Surg Endosc* 1999;13:1238–40.

74 Rosser J C Jr, Murayama M, Gabriel N H. Minimally invasive surgical training solutions for the twenty-first century. *Surg Clin North Am* 2000;80:1607–24.

75 Shushan A, Mohamed H, Magos A L. A case–control study to compare the variability of operating time in laparoscopic and open surgery. *Hum Reprod* 1999;14:1467–9.

2

Laparoscopic entry techniques

Kevin Phillips and Nikita Rawal

Introduction

Laparoscopy is a very common procedure in gynaecology and is increasingly used in other specialties. Approximately 250 000 women undergo laparoscopy in the UK every year.[1,2] Initially, the technique was used only to inspect the pelvis to make a diagnosis. It is now increasingly used to enable minimal access surgery. There is evidence that laparoscopic surgery provides significant benefits compared with laparotomy both for women requiring treatment and for healthcare providers.[3,4] The benefits for women include less visible scarring, less postoperative pain and quicker recovery. The benefits for healthcare providers include shorter hospital stays and thus reduced inpatient costs. The benefits for surgeons include a no-touch operative technique.

As with any surgical technique, the laparoscopic approach is associated with complications, which must be offset against the expected clinical benefits. Most complications are related to the method of entry of the laparoscope.[5–7] The most serious complications can be life-threatening and include bowel, major abdominal vessel injury and anterior abdominal wall vessel injury. Fortunately, these most serious complications are rare, with the incidence of bowel perforation reported as being 1.13–1.8/1000 procedures, and the incidence of major abdominal vessel perforation and anterior abdominal wall vessel perforation reported as being 0.9–1.05/1000 procedures.[1,6] While these low rates are heartening, it still implies that over 250 individuals in the UK will have a serious complication each year.[8] The relative infrequency of these accidents prevents an individual gynaecologist from gaining a true appreciation of their importance or frequency in the global situation. Each of these complications may lead to considerable physical and emotional suffering for the woman, relatives and doctors as well as financial costs. In the present climate, where the expectations from patients and the public are so high, many of these laparoscopic accidents will result in litigation.

The Middlesbrough consensus

With these risks in mind, various recommendations have been published regarding safe laparoscopic entry techniques.[4,5,8–11] One of the first was a consensus document[8] on laparoscopic entry techniques prepared by an international group of gynaecological and general surgeons who specialised in laparoscopic surgery. This group met in Middlesbrough, UK, in 1999 and critically evaluated the published evidence at the time. The resulting consensus document had the support of the International Society for Gynecologic Endoscopy, the European Society for Gynaecological Endoscopy, the Australian Gynaecological Endoscopy Society, the British Society for Gynaecological Endoscopy and the Minimal Access Surgical Training Group of the Royal College of Obstetricians and Gynaecologists (RCOG).

The Middlesbrough consensus emphasises the need for an intraumbilical incision and a sharp Veress needle. There is also a recommendation that all entry phases of laparoscopy be performed with the person under surgery lying level, with no Trendelenburg tilt, because this position rotates the sacral promontory and brings the aortic bifurcation close to the umbilicus, thus increasing the chances of vascular injury.[12] It also states that the intra-abdominal pressure, rather than the volume of infused carbon dioxide, should be used as a guide to determine when to site the primary trocar.

Following the Middlesbrough recommendations, two national surveys[13,14] were conducted to identify laparoscopic entry techniques employed by gynaecologists in the UK, to determine if the consensus technique was used and to observe whether the entry technique affected complications. Both surveys demonstrated variation in the laparoscopic entry techniques used by the gynaecologists and did not reveal any safety advantages of one technique over another. The authors of a Cochrane meta-analysis[15] on laparoscopic entry techniques have also concluded that there is no evidence of benefit of one technique over another in terms of safety. The most important adverse outcomes are damage to the gastrointestinal tract and the major blood vessels. These complications can occur during diagnostic or major surgical procedures.

It is therefore vital that the incidence, nature and causes of these complications are fully understood. It is also essential to identify the optimal methodology and equipment to ensure that the rate of these major complications is reduced to the unavoidable minimum.

The most effective way to reduce complications of laparoscopic entry is to optimise insertion of the primary trocar and cannula.

Closed entry

The classical or closed entry requires cutting of the abdominal skin with a scalpel and insertion of a Veress needle into the peritoneal cavity (Figure 2.1), followed by gas insufflation and then insertion of a trocar. Finally, the laparoscope is passed through the trocar once the obturator is removed.[16] The potential benefits of the closed technique are shorter operating times, immediate recognition of bowel or vascular injuries and near exclusion of entry failure.[17]

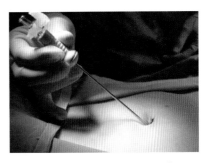

FIGURE 2.1 **Veress needle insertion in base of umbilicus**

Most practising gynaecologists worldwide use the Veress-needle pneumoperitoneum technique to access the abdominal cavity.[4,18] Creation of a pneumoperitoneum is the vital first step in any laparoscopic procedure and it is the one still associated with most complications.[5] As there are inherent problems with the blind insertion of the Veress needle and trocar into the peritoneal cavity, it is crucial that extreme caution be taken when the technique is used. The RCOG has produced a Green-top Guideline[2] explaining each step of laparoscopy. It is important to adhere to that instruction to minimise the risk of any complications.

According to the RCOG Green-top Guideline,[2] the following points should be observed when performing closed laparoscopy:

- The primary incision for laparoscopy should be vertical from the base of the umbilicus (not in the skin below the umbilicus). Care should be taken not to incise so deeply as to enter the peritoneal cavity.

- The Veress needle should be sharp, with a good and tested spring action. A disposable needle is recommended as it will fulfil these criteria.

- The operating table should be horizontal (not in the Trendelenburg tilt) at the start of the procedure.

- The abdomen should be palpated to check for any masses and for the position of the aorta before insertion of the Veress needle.

- The lower abdominal wall should be stabilised in such a way that the Veress needle can be inserted at right angles to the skin and should be inserted along the umbilical tube just sufficiently to penetrate the fascia and the peritoneum. Two audible clicks are usually heard as these layers are penetrated.

- An intra-abdominal pressure of 20–25 mmHg should be used for gas insufflation before inserting the primary port. The distension pressure is then reduced to 12–15 mmHg and the intra-abdominal contents are inspected.

Complications of the closed technique

Insertion of the Veress needle may seem simple to an observer but is full of challenges. Failure to gain entry into the peritoneal cavity at the first attempt is not uncommon. Studies have shown that the complications increase with each attempt. In their audit of entry techniques, Richardson and Sutton[19] reported a complication rate of 0.8–16.3% with one attempt, 16.3–37.5% with two attempts, 44.4–64.0% with three attempts and 84.6–100.0% with more than three attempts. Complications were extraperitoneal insufflations, bladder and bowel injuries and failed laparoscopy. It is recommended that after two failed attempts either the open Hasson technique or Palmer's point entry should be used to insert the Veress needle. Extraperitoneal insufflation is one of the most common complications of laparoscopy and frequently leads to abandonment of the procedure. Kabukoba and Skillern[20] described a technique to deal with extraperitoneal insufflation that requires the laparoscope to be left in the extraperitoneal space and the gas not evacuated. The Veress needle is then reintroduced into the extraperitoneal space in front of the telescope and visually guided into the peritoneal cavity.

Tests of safe entry

A single randomised trial[21] has investigated elevation versus no elevation of the abdominal wall before insertion of the Veress needle. The latter was associated with a reduced rate of failed entry.[15,21] Several tests have been advocated to determine the correct placement of the Veress needle. These include the double-click sound of the Veress needle, the aspiration test, the hanging drop test, the 'hiss' sound test and the syringe test.[22–25] The most reliable test uses initial pressure; if this is less than 8 mmHg, it is very unlikely that the Veress needle is in the wrong space. The fact that visceral and vascular injuries occur even when these tests are used shows that they are not 100% accurate. Failure to perform these tests should no longer be considered substandard care or negligence.[26] Excessive lateral movement of the needle should be avoided as this may convert a small needle-point injury in the wall of the bowel or vessel into a more complex tear. Moving the needle after insertion can enlarge a 1.6 mm puncture injury to an injury of up to 1 cm in viscera or blood vessels.[27]

Insufflation pressures

The high-pressure entry technique has been increasingly adopted worldwide and it is recommended that an insufflation pressure of 20–25 mmHg is achieved before inserting the trocar. The rationale is that it produces greater splinting of the anterior abdominal wall and a deeper intra-abdominal carbon dioxide bubble than the traditional volume-limited pneumoperitoneum. In a study by Phillips et al.,[28] if a constant force of 3 kg was applied to the abdominal wall at the umbilicus, with the abdominal cavity insufflated to a pressure of 10 mmHg, the depth between the 'indented' umbilicus and the intra-abdominal contents was only 0.6 cm. If the same force was applied to an abdomen insufflated to 25 mmHg, the depth was 5.6 cm (range 4–8 cm; Figures 2.2 and 2.3). The mean volume of carbon dioxide required to achieve this pressure was 5.58 l.[28] It has been determined that port insertion requires about 4 kg of force, but the newer disposable ports require only half the force of a reusable port, mainly because the trocar is sharper with the disposable ports.[29,30] No adverse effect on the circulation or respiratory function has been observed using these insufflation pressures, as long as the person undergoing the procedure is lying flat.[31]

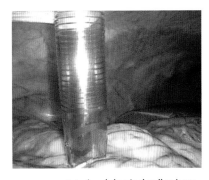

FIGURE 2.2 **Anterior abdominal wall to intra-abdominal contents with 15 mmHg pressure**

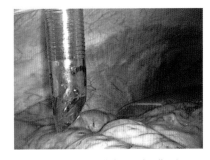

FIGURE 2.3 **Anterior abdominal wall to intra-abdominal contents with 20 mmHg pressure**

The combined results of three series involving 8997 laparoscopies using entry pressures of 25–30 mmHg included reports of four (0.04%) bowel and one (0.01%) major vessel injury.[5] In all instances of bowel injury, the bowel had been adherent to the entry site of the anterior abdominal wall (type 2 injury). The vascular injury occurred because of an inadvertent loss of the pneumoperitoneum during trocar insertion.

Insertion of the trocar

The primary trocar should be inserted in a controlled manner at 90° to the skin, through the incision at the thinnest part of the abdominal wall, in the base of the umbilicus. The insertion should be stopped immediately when the trocar is inside the abdominal cavity.[2] Once the laparoscope has been introduced through the primary cannula, it should be rotated through 360° to check visually for any adherent bowel. If this is present, it should be closely inspected for any evidence of haemorrhage, damage or retroperitoneal haematoma. If there is concern that the bowel may be adherent under the umbilicus, the primary trocar site should be visualised from a secondary port site, preferably with a 5 mm laparoscope. On completion of the procedure, the laparoscope should be used to check that there has not been a through-and-through injury of bowel adherent under the umbilicus by visual control during removal.

Open entry

Hasson first described the open-entry technique in 1971.[32] The suggested benefits are prevention of gas embolism, of preperitoneal insufflation and, possibly, of visceral and major vascular injury. The technique involves the use of a cannula fitted with a cone-shaped sleeve, a blunt obturator and, possibly, a second sleeve to which stay sutures can be attached.[33]

A small incision is made transversely or longitudinally at the umbilicus. This incision should be long enough to be able to dissect down to the fascia, incise it and enter the peritoneal cavity under direct vision. To minimise the risks of damage using this procedure, it is important to ensure that, following the placement of a skin incision at the lower border of the umbilicus, the deep fascia is elevated with suitable graspers, such as Littlewood forceps, to separate the abdominal wall from its contents. A small incision is made in the fascia and expanded with blunt-ended forceps. This usually effects entry. If it does not, the abdomen is raised and the peritoneum incised with care to ensure that the risk of bowel injury is minimised. Entry is confirmed by visualising the bowel or omentum. A blunt-tipped cannula is then inserted into the abdomen.

The trocar insertion should be guided between thin retractors to prevent displacement of the cannula. The fascial sutures can be used to ensure that the trocar remains in place during the surgery. These sutures can then be tied at the end of the procedure to close the fascial defect. Gas is insufflated through the cannula to produce the pneumoperitoneum. Newer disposable blunt trocars have been specifically designed to make this technique quicker and easier, but there is no clear evidence of a safety advantage.

General surgeons have embraced the open method of entry and suggest that it is safer than closed laparoscopy. However, there is little evidence to back this assertion,[34–37] the main problem being the lack of power of randomised clinical trials. Ahmad et al.[15] in their Cochrane meta-analysis failed to identify any safety advantage of using an open technique as opposed to a closed method of entry in terms of both visceral and major vascular injury.

At this time, there is no convincing evidence that the open-entry technique is superior or inferior to the other entry techniques currently available.

The open-entry technique does have a lower incidence of vascular injuries, but this is balanced by a potentially higher incidence of bowel injury,[4] although this can be mitigated if alternative entry sites are chosen in high-risk women. Instead of dissecting down at the umbilicus in people with suspected bowel adhesions, an alternative site of entry may be more appropriate, such as the left upper quadrant or the ninth/tenth intercostal spaces. This could possibly decrease the rate of bowel injury because these sites are rarely affected by adhesions and, if the stomach is empty and there is no hepatosplenomegaly, using these sites of entry seems to be safe.

Direct trocar entry

The direct trocar entry technique was developed to overcome the difficulty associated with grasping the abdominal wall already distended by the pneumoperitoneum.[38] The suggested advantage of this method of entry is the avoidance of complications related to the use of a Veress needle, a failed pneumoperitoneum, extraperitoneal insufflation, intestinal insufflation or the more serious carbon dioxide embolism.[39] Laparoscopic entry is initiated with only one blind step instead of three (Veress needle, insufflation and trocar). Sharp disposable trocars are commended for a direct insertion technique because reusable trocars are rarely sharpened. If the equipment is not optimal, more strength may be required to adequately elevate the abdominal wall and to make a controlled forward thrust with the trocar, thus increasing the risk of complications.

This is the quickest method of laparoscopic entry and it may be safe in experienced hands. However, it is not widely used in gynaecological practice. A meta-analysis[15] of six randomised controlled trials[40–45] that have compared Veress-needle with direct trocar entry demonstrated an advantage for the direct trocar entry technique in terms of reducing extraperitoneal insufflation and failed entry into the abdomen, but there was no advantage in terms of avoiding solid organ injury.

Alternative entry devices

EndoTip® visual cannula

The endoscopic threaded imaging port EndoTip® (Karl Storz, Tuttlingen, Germany) is a reusable visual cannula system that allows direct visualisation of insertion of the primary port.[46] This laparoscopic access system was devel-

TABLE 2.1 **Classification of laparoscopic injuries**

Type of injury	Description
Type 1	Injury with the Veress needle or trocar to normally sited bowel and blood vessels
Type 2a	Injury with the Veress needle or trocar to bowel loosely adherent to the anterior abdominal wall
Type 2b	Injury with the Veress needle or trocar to bowel firmly adherent to the anterior abdominal wall

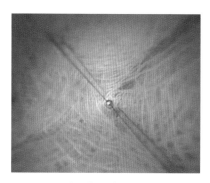

FIGURE 2.4 **View down the laparoscope in a direct visualisation port; a swab has been held against the tip of the trocar**

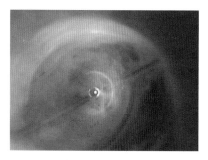

FIGURE 2.5 **The direct visualisation port being inserted through the anterior abdominal wall; fat, sheath and rectus muscle layers can be seen; the peritoneum is also visible at the tip of the trocar**

oped for primary port insertion. The cannula requires no trocar and no axial penetration force during insertion. It provides magnified visualisation through the scope on the monitor during access and exit. The device has a proximal valve section and a distal cannula section with a single thread winding around its outer surface, ending in a blunt tip. After umbilical incision and insufflation, a 0° laparoscope is mounted in the cannula. The tip of the cannula is inserted into a tiny fascial incision and rotated clockwise. The fascia and then the muscle fibres spread radially and are transposed onto the cannula's outer thread. The thin peritoneum transilluminates; bowel, vessels and/or adhesions are visualised before entry into the peritoneum.

In theory, the routine use of this device will reduce the incidence of type 2a injuries by displacing rather than penetrating bowel and avoid all type 1 injuries (Table 2.1). This is entirely speculative and as yet not backed by significant data, but this technology certainly warrants further investigation as a potentially promising approach.

Other disposable optical trocar systems have been produced that allow the primary trocar to be inserted under direct visualisation, with the laparoscope inserted into a channel in the trocar. These systems allow the individual layers of the abdominal wall to be identified and should make it immediately obvious when the abdominal cavity has been entered. They should also make it obvious if the bowel has inadvertently been entered. They may reduce the rate of both type 1 and type 2 lesions but will probably not avoid either type of lesion entirely (Figures 2.4 and 2.5).

The Step™ radially expanding device

The radially expanding access system Step™ (Covidien, Mansfield, MA, USA) was developed to minimise tissue trauma.[47] This system uses a pneumo-peritoneum needle with a polymeric sleeve. Following routine insufflation, the needle is removed, leaving the outer sleeve in situ. Direct dilatation of the sleeve results in a port 5–12 mm in size. The suggested benefits are that only one sharp instrument enters the abdominal cavity, less tissue trauma occurs and, possibly, fewer bowel and vascular injuries occur.[48,49] The Cochrane meta-analysis by Ahmad et al.[15] failed to demonstrate any advantage of using Step with reference to major complications. However, it did demonstrate a decreased incidence of trocar site bleeding when the Step trocar was used for port entry. These trocars do have blunt tips that may provide some protection from injuries.

Shielded trocar

This trocar is designed with a shield that partially retracts and exposes the sharp tip as it encounters resistance through the abdominal wall.[50] As the shield enters the abdominal cavity, it springs forward and covers the sharp tip of the trocar. Although called a safety trocar, many injuries have occurred using such instruments.[51] It has been observed that even when this trocar is used as per specification, there is a brief moment when the sharp trocar tip is exposed and unprotected as it enters the abdominal cavity.[52,53]

Alternative sites of insertion

Palmer's point

When periumbilical adhesions are suspected, the most rational alternative site is in the left upper quadrant at Palmer's point, which is situated 3 cm below the left costal margin in the midclavicular line.[54] Left upper quadrant insufflation requires emptying of the stomach by nasogastric suction and introduction of a Veress needle perpendicular to the skin. Correct placement is confirmed by use of the pressure/flow test. Carbon dioxide is then introduced to achieve a pressure of 25 mmHg and the internal surface of the anterior abdominal wall is inspected in the area beneath the umbilicus, with a laparoscope. If there are no adhesions, the trocar and cannula can be inserted under visual guidance of the laparoscope. If adhesions are present, they can be dissected free via secondary ports in the lower left abdomen or via a visually selected alternative entry site. This technique could be considered in obese and very thin women, but should be considered in all women with a previous midline laparotomy. Women with previous splenic or gastric surgery, significant hepatosplenomegaly, portal hypertension or gastropancreatic masses should be excluded.[55]

Other entry sites have been tried but, in general, are to be avoided. According to the RCOG,[2] 'suprapubic insertion of the Veress needle puts the bladder at risk of damage and is associated with the highest rate of failure due to preperitoneal insufflation of gas. ... Entry through the posterior fornix could cause serious problems if the woman was found to have deep infiltrating endometriosis with obliteration of the cul-de-sac and the rectum adherent to the back of the cervix.[56] A low rectal perforation at this site could be particularly dangerous and it should only be used when imaging techniques have clearly shown that the posterior cul-de-sac is free from deep infiltrating endometriosis and adherent bowel.' Another entry technique is transuterine entry using a long Veress needle through the fundus of the uterus transvaginally.[57,58] This technique has been especially helpful in obese women. A single randomised controlled trial compared the transuterine route of entry with the infraumbilical route and did not reveal any advantage of one route over another.[58] No major complications were reported in either group. The transuterine approach was not associated with an increased risk of trauma or infection of pelvic organs.

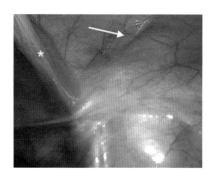

FIGURE 2.6 **Lateral umbilical ligament (*) and inferior epigastric vessels (arrow)**

Secondary ports

Secondary ports should always be introduced under direct laparoscopic guidance to precisely control the depth and direction of the trocar insertion.[2] Secondary ports are inserted perpendicular to the skin while maintaining the pneumoperitoneum at 20–25 mmHg. Once the tip of the trocar has pierced the peritoneum, it should be angled towards the anterior pelvis under careful visual control until the sharp tip has been removed. The superficial vessels should be located by transillumination and the inferior epigastric vessels by direct laparoscopic inspection. Lateral trocars should be inserted with both transillumination and direct laparoscopic guidance. The inferior epigastric arteries and the venae comitantes running beside them can be visualised just lateral to the lateral umbilical ligaments (the obliterated hypogastric arteries) in all but the most obese women (Figure 2.6). In a woman who is obese, the incision should be made well lateral to the edge of the rectus sheath, taking care to avoid injury to vessels on the pelvic sidewall. It is recommended that removal of the ports is also performed under direct vision so that any haemorrhage can be observed and treated if present. Any nonmidline port over 7 mm and any midline port greater than 10 mm requires formal deep sheath closure to avoid the occurrence of port-site hernia.[59,60]

Counselling

Complications in surgery can be reduced by selection of the right surgical technique for the right patient, use of good-quality, well-maintained instruments and careful attention to the minutiae of the technique. Nevertheless, not all complications can be avoided and women should be made aware of this.

Women must be informed of the risks and potential complications associated with laparoscopy. This should include discussion of the risks of the entry technique used (specifically, injury to the bowel, urinary tract and major blood vessels). On present evidence, the risk of all three may be in the region of 1–4/1000 procedures.[1,3,7] Women should also be informed that with any laparoscopic procedure there is a possibility of laparotomy and that on very rare occasions a temporary colostomy may be required. The discussion should also include later complications associated with the entry ports, specifically hernia formation. Women and their doctors should expect a progressive and maintained improvement after laparoscopic surgery. Increasing pain or vomiting is not usual after this type of procedure and either occurrence should alert the woman and doctor to the real risk of complications. Increasing pain should be assumed to be a consequence of bowel damage until proven otherwise. It is essential that all concerned maintain a very high index of suspicion about these rare but potentially very serious complications. The woman and her family should leave hospital with written information about the recognition of complications and the action to be taken in the event of these developing.

Challenges

Women with previous abdominal surgery

Detailed surgical history and proper assessment are required before planning any laparoscopic procedure in women with previous abdominal surgery. Adhesions are a problem and the frequency is related to the type of previous surgery (Figure 2.7); it is 0–15% with previous laparoscopic surgery, 20–28% with previous laparotomy with horizontal suprapubic incision and 50–60% in

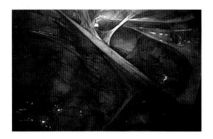

FIGURE 2.7 **Adhesions to the anterior abdominal wall following previous surgery**

those who have had previous laparotomy with a vertical incision.[61-64] The rate of severe adhesions containing bowel near the umbilicus is 5%. Of these, 92% occurred after previous laparotomy and more than two-thirds of the latter followed midline incision. These figures are important when counselling women with previous abdominal surgery.

Most of the adhesions can be predicted from the surgical history. The distribution of anterior wall adhesions can be accurately and safely mapped using a minilaparoscope inserted at another site, usually Palmer's point.[65]

Obese women

Laparoscopic surgery is of particular benefit to obese women compared with laparotomy because the latter has significant risks of complications. The RCOG[2] recommends performance of an open (Hasson) technique for primary entry in morbidly obese women. However, this can still be difficult. Palmer's point entry is another favoured entry technique in obese women because there is significantly less subcutaneous fat in the left upper quadrant compared with the umbilical area. The guidance provided by the RCOG[2] further states: 'If a Veress needle approach is used in the woman who is morbidly obese, it is important to make the vertical incision as deep as possible in the base of the umbilicus, since this is the area where skin, deep fascia and parietal peritoneum of the anterior abdominal wall will meet. In this area, there is little opportunity for the parietal peritoneum to tent away from the Veress needle and allow extraperitoneal insufflation and surgical emphysema. If the needle is inserted vertically, the mean distance from the lower margin of the umbilicus to the peritoneum is 6 cm (±3 cm). This allows placement of a standard length needle even in extremely obese women.[66] Insertion at 45°, even from within the umbilicus, means that the needle has to traverse distances of 11–16 cm, which is too long for a standard Veress needle.'[67]

Very thin women

The RCOG advice is as follows:[2] 'Women at highest risk of vascular injury are the young, thin, nulliparous women with well-developed abdominal musculature; women with severe anorexia are at particular risk. The aorta may lie less than 2.5 cm below the skin in these women. Great care, therefore, must be taken when performing first entry and a Hasson approach or insertion at Palmer's point is preferable in this situation.'

The gravity of this high-risk situation is further emphasised by Levy,[68] who also discusses its management. It is prudent to have a plan in theatre of what to do if there is a major vascular injury during laparoscopy; all theatre staff should be aware of this plan. It should include rapid conversion to laparotomy, at least compression over the injury and a call to vascular surgeons for advice and assistance.

Conclusion

Laparoscopic access is normally without incident whatever technique is used. However, serious injury can occur. The circumstances under which there is a greater risk of complications are known and the risk can be reduced with simple measures. Women should also be informed of the risks of laparoscopic entry, quite apart from the risks and benefits of any surgical procedure undertaken once laparoscopic entry has been obtained.

References

1 Chamberlain G, Brown C. *Gynaecological Laparoscopy. The Report of the Working Party of the Confidential Enquiry into Gynaecological Laparoscopy.* London: Royal College of Obstetricians and Gynaecologists; 1978.

2 Royal College of Obstetricians and Gynaecologists. *Preventing Entry-related Gynaecological Laparoscopic Injuries.* Green-top Guideline No. 49. London: RCOG; 2008 [www.rcog.org.uk/womens-health/clinical-guidance/preventing-entry-related-gynaecological-laparoscopic-injuries-green-].

3 Chapron C, Fauconnier A, Goffinet F, Breart G, Dubuisson J B. Laparoscopic surgery is not inherently dangerous for patients presenting with benign gynecologic pathology: results of a meta-analysis. *Hum Reprod* 2002;17:1334–42.

4 Garry R. Towards evidence-based laparoscopic entry techniques: clinical problems and dilemmas. *Gynaecol Endosc* 1999;8:315–26.

5 Jansen F W, Kapiteyn K, Trimbos-Kemper T, Hermans J, Trimbos J B. Complications of laparoscopy: a prospective multicentre observational study. *Br J Obstet Gynaecol* 1997;104:595–600.

6 Harkki-Siren P, Kurki T. A nationwide analysis of laparoscopic complications. *Obstet Gynecol* 1997;89:108–12.

7 Jansen F W, Kolkman W, Bakkum E A, de Kroon C D, Trimbos-Kemper T C M, Trimbos J B. Complications of laparoscopy: an inquiry about closed versus open-entry technique. *Am J Obstet Gynecol* 2004;190;634–8.

8 A consensus document concerning laparoscopic entry techniques: Middlesbrough, March 19–20 1999. *Gynaecol Endosc* 1999;8:403–6.

9 Ewen S. Avoiding complications of the laparoscopic approach. *Obstet Gynecol* 1999;1:34–6.

10 Kalu G, Wright J. Laparoscopic surgery and the law. *Obstet Gynecol* 2001;3:141–6.

11 Vilos G A, Vilos A G. Safe laparoscopic entry guided by Veress needle CO_2 insufflation pressure. *J Am Assoc Gynecol Laparosc* 2003;10:415–20.

12 Pasic R, Mullins F, Gable D R, Levine R L. Major vascular injuries in laparoscopy. *J Gynecol Surg* 1998;14:123–8.

13 Ahmad G, Duffy J M N, Watson A J S. Laparoscopic entry techniques and complications. *Int J Gynecol Obstet* 2007;99:52–5.

14 Lalchandani S, Phillips K. A survey of practices of consultant gynaecologists. *Gynecol Surg* 2005;22:245–9.

15 Ahmad G, Duffy J M N, Phillips K, Watson A. Laparoscopic entry techniques. *Cochrane Database Syst Rev* 2008;(2): CD006583.

16 Palmer R. Safety in laparoscopy. *J Reprod Med* 1974; 13:1–5.

17 Copeland C, Wing R, Hulka J F. Direct trocar insertion at laparoscopy: an evaluation. *Obstet Gynecol* 1983;62:655–9.

18 Lingam K, Cole R. Laparoscopy entry port visited: a survey of practices of consultant gynaecologists in Scotland. *Gynaecol Endosc* 2001;10:335–42.

19 Richardson R F, Sutton C J G. Complications of first entry: a prospective laparoscopic audit. *Gynaecol Endosc* 1999;8:327–34.

20 Kabukoba J J, Skillern L H. Coping with extraperitoneal insufflation during laparoscopy: a new technique. *Obstet Gynecol* 1992;80:144–5.

21 Briel J W, Plaisier P W, Meijer W S, Lange J F. Is it necessary to lift the abdominal wall when preparing a pneumoperitoneum? A randomised study. *Surg Endosc* 2000;14:862–4.

22 Munro M G. Laparoscopic access: complications, technologies and techniques. *Curr Opin Obstet Gynecol* 2002;14:365–74.

23 Brill A J, Cohen B M. Fundamentals of peritoneal access. *J Am Assoc Gynecol Laparosc* 2003;10:287–97.

24 Fear R E. Laparoscopy: a valuable aid in gynecologic diagnosis. *Obstet Gynecol* 1968;31:297–309.

25 Marret H, Harchaoui Y, Chapron C, Lansac J, Pierre F. Trocar injuries during laparoscopic gynaecological surgery. Report from the French Society of Gynecological Laparoscopy. *Gynaecol Endosc* 1998;7:235–41.

26 Teoh B, Sen R, Abbott J. An evaluation of four tests used to ascertain Veress needle placement at closed laparoscopy. *J Minim Invasive Gynecol* 2005;12:153–8.

27 Brosens I, Gordon A. Bowel injuries during gynaecological laparoscopy: a multinational survey. *Gynaecol Endosc* 2001;10:141–5.

28 Phillips G, Garry R, Kumar C, Reich H. How much gas is required for initial insufflation at laparoscopy? *Gynaecol Endosc* 1999;8:369–74.

29 Corson S L, Batzer F R, Gocial B, Maislin G. Measurements of the force necessary for laparoscopic trocar entry. *J Reprod Med* 1989;34:282–4.

30 Tarney C M, Glass K, Munro M G. Entry force and intra-abdominal pressure associated with six laparoscopic trocar cannula systems: a randomized comparison. *Obstet Gynecol* 1999;94:83–8.

31 Tsaltas J, Pearce S, Lawrence A, Meads A, Mezzatesta J, Nicolson S. Safer laparoscopic trocar entry: it is all about pressure. *Aust N Z J Obstet Gynaecol* 2004;44:349–50.

32 Hasson H M. A modified instrument and method for laparoscopy. *Am J Obstet Gynecol* 1971; 110:886–7.

33 Hasson H M. Open laparoscopy as a method of access in laparoscopic surgery. *Gynaecol Endosc* 1999;8:353–62.

34 Wolfe B M, Gardiner B N, Leary B F, Frey C F. Endoscopic cholecystectomy. An analysis of complications. *Arch Surg* 1991;126:1192–8.

35 Crist D W, Gadacz T R. Complications of laparoscopic surgery. *Surg Clin North Am* 1993;73:265–89.

36 Merlin T, Maddern G J, Jamieson G G, Hiller J E, Brown A R, Kolbe A. *A systematic review of the methods used to establish laparoscopic pneumoperitoneum.* ASERNIP-S Report No. 13. Adelaide, South Australia: Australian Safety and Efficacy Register of New Interventional Procedures – Surgical; 2001 [www.surgeons.org/racs/ research-and-audit/asernip-s/asernip-s-publications/ systematic-reviews/methods-used-to-establish-laparoscopic-pneumoperitoneum].

37 Molloy D, Kalloo P D, Cooper M, Nguyen T V. Laparoscopic entry: a literature review and analysis of techniques and complications of primary port entry. *Aust N Z J Obstet Gynaecol* 2002;42:246–54.

38 Dingfelder J R. Direct laparoscopic trocar insertion without prior pneumoperitoneum. *J Reprod Med* 1978;21:45–7.

39 Catarci M, Carlini M, Gentileschi P, Santoro E, for the Lap Group Roma. Major and minor injuries during the creation of pneumoperitoneum: a multicenter study on 12,919 cases. *Surg Endosc* 2001;15:566–9.

40 Agresta F, De Simone P, Ciardo L F, Bedin N. Direct trocar insertion versus Veress needle in nonobese patients undergoing laparoscopic procedures: a randomised prospective single centre study. *Surg Endosc* 2004;18:1778–81.

41 Borgatta L, Gruss L, Barad D, Kaali S G. Direct trocar insertion vs. Veress needle use for laparoscopic sterilisation. *J Reprod Med* 1990;35:891–4.

42 Byron J W, Markenson G, Miyazawa K. Randomized comparison of Verres needle and direct trocar insertion for laparoscopy. *Surg Gynecol Obstet* 1993;177:259–62.

43 Gunenc M Z, Yesilgedlar N, Bingöl B, Onalan G, Tabak S, Gökmen B. The safety and efficacy of direct trocar insertion with elevation of the rectus sheath instead of the skin for pneumoperitoneum. *Surg Laparosc Endosc Percutan Tech* 2005;15:80–1.

44 Tansatit T, Wisawasukmonchol W, Bunyavejchevin S. A randomized, prospective study comparing the use of the missile trocar and the pyramidal trocar for laparoscopy. *J Med Assoc Thai* 2006;89:941–7.

45 Bemelman W A, Dunker M S, Busch O R, Den Boer K T, de Wit L T, Gouma DJ. Efficacy of establishment of pneumoperitoneum with Veress needle, Hasson Trocar, and modified blunt trocar (TrocDoc): a randomized study. *J Laparoendosc Adv Surg Tech A* 2000;10:325–30.

46 Ternamian A M. A second-generation laparoscopic port system: Endotip™. *Gynecol Endosc* 1999;8:397–401.

47 Turner D J. Making the case for the radially expanding access system. *Gynecol Endosc* 1999;8:391–5.

48 Ternamian A M. Laparoscopy without trocars. *Surg Endosc* 1997;11:815–8.

49 Ternamian A M. A trocarless, reusable, visual-access cannula for safer laparoscopy; an update. *J Am Assoc Gynecol Laparosc* 1997;5:197–201.

50 Fuller J, Scott W, Ashar B, Corrado J. Laparoscopic trocar injuries: a report from a U.S. Food and Drug Administration (FDA) Center for Devices and Radiological Health (CDRH) Systematic Technology Assessment of Medical Products (STAMP) Committee. Washington, DC: FDA; 2003 [www.fda.gov/medicaldevices/safety/alertsandnotices/ucm197339.htm].

51 Soderstrom R M. Bowel injury litigation after laparoscopy. *J Am Assoc Gynecol Laparosc* 1993;1:74–7.

52 Trocars: safety and selection. Emergency Care Research Institute. *Health Devices* 1998;27:376–99.

53 Trocars: new data on safety and selection. *Health Devices* 2000;29:67–71.

54 Palmer R. Safety in laparoscopy. *J Reprod Med* 1974;13:1–5.

55 Tulikangas R K, Nicklas A, Falcone T, Price L L. Anatomy of the left upper quadrant for cannula insertion. *J Am Assoc Gynecol Laparosc* 2000;7:211–4.

56 Neely M R, McWilliams R, Makhlouf H A. Laparoscopy: routine pneumoperitoneum via the posterior fornix. *Obstet Gynecol* 1975;45:459–60.

57 Trivedi A N, MacLean NE. Transuterine insertion of Veress needle for gynecological laparoscopy at Southland Hospital. *NZ Med J* 1994;107:316–7.

58 Santala M, Jarvela I, Kauppila A. Transfundal insertion of a Veress needle in laparoscopy of obese subjects: a practical alternative. *Hum Reprod* 1999;14:2277–8.

59 Rabinerson D, Avrech O, Neri A, Schoenfield A. Incisional hernia after laparoscopy. *Obstet Gynecol Surv* 1997;52:701–3.

60 Kadar N, Reich H, Lui C Y. Incisional hernias after major laparoscopic procedures. *American J Obstet Gynecol* 1993;168:1493–7.

61 Audebert A J, Gomel V. Role of microlaparoscopy in the diagnosis of peritoneal and visceral adhesions and in the prevention of bowel injury associated with blind trocar insertion. *Fertil Steril* 2000;73:631–5.

62 Agarwala N, Liu C Y. Safe entry technique during laparoscopy: left upper quadrant entry using the ninth intercostal space: a review of 918 procedures. *J Minim Invasive Gynecol* 2005;12:55–61.

63 Levrant S G, Bieher E J, Barnes R B. Anterior abdominal wall adhesions after laparotomy or laparoscopy. *J Am Assoc Gynecol Laparosc* 1997;4:353–6.

64 Brill A, Nezhat F, Nezhat C H, Nezhat C. The incidence of adhesions after prior laparotomy: A laparoscopic appraisal. *Obstet Gynecol* 1995;85:269–72.

65 Garry R. Complications of laparoscopic entry. *Gynaecol Endosc* 1997;6:319–29.

66 Holtz G. Insufflation of the obese patient. In: Diamond M P, Corfman R S, DeCherney A H, editors. *Complications of Laparoscopy and Hysteroscopy*. 2nd ed. Oxford: Blackwell Science; 1997. p. 22–5.

67 Hurd W H, Bude R O, DeLancey J O, Gauvin J M, Aisen A M. Abdominal wall characteristics with magnetic resonance imaging and computed tomography. The effect of obesity on the laparoscopic approach. *J Reprod Med* 1991;36:473–6.

68 Levy B S. Perforation of large vascular structures. In: Diamond M P, Corfman R S, DeCherney A H, editors. *Complications of Laparoscopy and Hysteroscopy*. 2nd ed. Oxford; Blackwell Science; 1997. p. 26–9.

3 Preoperative imaging

Wee-Liak Hoo, Naaila Aslam and Davor Jurkovic

Introduction

A detailed preoperative gynaecological ultrasound examination, when performed by a skilled operator, is helpful in selecting women for surgical treatment, planning the operation and deciding on the level of surgical expertise which is required to complete the operation safely and successfully.

Ultrasound is a diagnostic method that enables the noninvasive diagnosis of a wide range of gynaecological conditions. Transvaginal ultrasound in particular has greatly increased our ability to examine the pelvic anatomy. This method of examination allows the assessment of mobility and tenderness of pelvic organs in addition to their detailed morphological analysis. The improved resolution of high-frequency probes, together with closer proximity of the ovaries to the ultrasound probe, has resulted in better image quality compared with transabdominal ultrasound. Transabdominal ultrasound with a full bladder is usually reserved for women who have not been sexually active in the past and those who decline transvaginal examination. Transabdominal ultrasound with an empty bladder is an important adjunct to transvaginal scanning in women with large pelvic tumours extending above the symphysis pubis and in those with the ovaries displaced outside the lesser pelvis.

In the last decade, the use of laparoscopy in gynaecological surgery has gained popularity as a result of rapid technical progress and increased surgical skills. Laparoscopic surgery has become accepted as the best method for surgical excision of benign adnexal masses.[1] Many laparoscopic operations are now performed as day surgery procedures where women are discharged home a few hours after their procedure. To optimise the use of day surgery facilities and reduce the risk of conversion to a laparotomy, careful patient selection is crucial.

It is widely recognised that suspected malignancies are best treated by gynaecological oncologists working in cancer centres.[2] Correctly characterising adnexal masses is therefore vital in determining optimal patient management. Ultrasound is also an effective triage tool in the management of

TABLE 3.1 **Diagnostic accuracy of pattern recognition achieved with various scoring systems**

Diagnostic test	Sensitivity (%)	Specificity (%)
Pattern recognition technique[8]	85	90
Tailor model[8] (*n*=133)	69	88
Timmerman model[8] (*n*=82)	62	79
Lerner et al.[10] (*n*=312)	97	77
Sassone et al.[9] (*n*=143)	100	83

endometriosis. General gynaecologists may operate on women with mild or moderate endometriosis, but severe endometriosis should be referred to tertiary endometriosis centres.

The ability to correctly classify pelvic pathology on the basis of ultrasound scanning is dependent upon the skill and expertise of the operator.[3] Expert ultrasound operators using clinical information and their subjective assessment of the greyscale morphology (also known as the pattern recognition technique) can differentiate malignant from benign masses with a high degree of accuracy.[4] Timmerman et al.[3] have shown that expert ultrasound operators are often able to distinguish between benign and malignant adnexal masses with an accuracy of up to 92%. This makes it possible to optimise and individualise patient management, which includes the option of expectant management in asymptomatic women with benign pathology. Conversely, an ultrasound performed by an examiner with limited skills and knowledge or with inappropriate equipment will inevitably be of poor quality. Poor-quality gynaecological ultrasound may cause harm by resulting in an incorrect diagnosis and thus inappropriate treatment.[5] It is therefore fundamental that any person performing gynaecological ultrasound examinations is adequately supervised and trained in using the appropriate equipment.

Assessment of adnexal tumours

Ultrasound is the investigation of choice in the initial assessment of women with suspected pelvic pathology. It is widely available and relatively inexpensive compared with other imaging modalities. Although the role of ultrasound in the assessment of adnexal pathology is well established, accurate preoperative discrimination between benign and malignant adnexal tumours remains difficult. This is largely because of the considerable overlap between the sonographic features of benign and malignant tumours. The differentiation between benign and malignant tumours is critical for planning a woman's care because malignant tumours warrant urgent management by a gynaecological oncologist. Benign ovarian cysts, however, may be managed conservatively and are usually suitable for minimal access surgery.

Determining the risk of malignancy

The more complex the appearance of a cyst on an ultrasound scan, the greater the likelihood of malignancy. Studies assessing ovarian morphology using B-mode greyscale ultrasound showed that small unilocular simple cysts (Figure 3.1) have a low probability of being malignant.[6] However, the presence of papillary projections and solid areas within the cyst (Figure 3.2) increases the probability of ovarian malignancy.[7] Furthermore, the risk of malignancy increases with increasing locularity and size of the cyst. These features are not exclusive to malignancy, however, and can also be found in benign tumours.

To improve the accuracy of ultrasound diagnosis, several morphological scoring systems have been designed. These systems assign scores to each tumour depending on the presence or absence of certain morphological features on greyscale ultrasound. However, the diagnostic accuracy of these scoring systems (Table 3.1) has not been high enough to allow their implementation into routine clinical practice.[8–10]

With the advent of transvaginal colour Doppler imaging, it was hoped that it would become possible to assess vascular changes within the ovary and that this would subsequently lead to better detection of malignant changes (Figure 3.3). However, significant variation exists in the reported results of colour and pulsed Doppler studies for the assessment of adnexal masses.[11–13] This variation may result from the angiogenic properties of the ovaries, the complex vasculature of ovarian neoplasms and the potential sources of error involved in Doppler assessment. Overall, the addition of colour Doppler imaging has not been shown to improve the accuracy of the assessment significantly compared with greyscale morphology alone.

The availability of serum tumour markers has stimulated further work on improving the diagnostic accuracy of ultra-

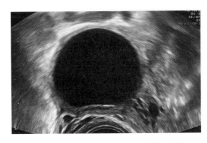

FIGURE 3.1 **Simple ovarian cyst with a thin and smooth inner wall and anechoic fluid**

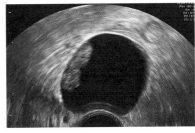

FIGURE 3.2A **Large papillary projection arising from the inner wall of an ovarian cyst**

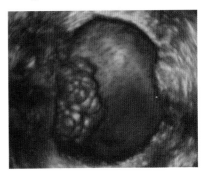

FIGURE 3.2B **Three-dimensional scan of the surface of the papillary projection in the same cyst**

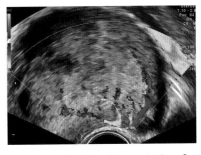

FIGURE 3.3 **Colour Doppler examination of an ovarian tumour, which demonstrates high blood supply to the lesion**

sound. By far the most commonly used tumour marker is the serum CA125 level, which is raised in nearly 80% of women with advanced (stage III) ovarian cancers but in only 40–44% of women with stage I disease.[14–17] Serum CA125 levels used in isolation are relatively nonspecific and therefore require interpretation in conjunction with clinical and ultrasound findings.[18–20] Jacobs et al.[21,22] were one of the first groups to describe a multiparameter scoring system. Their risk of malignancy index (RMI) has been widely adopted in the UK to facilitate the triage of women with ovarian tumours for referral to tertiary gynaecological oncology units. The risk of malignancy is calculated using the following formula:

$$RMI = U \times M \times CA125$$

In this formula, U is the ultrasound score, M is the menopausal status and CA125 is the serum CA125 level in kU/l. Each of the following greyscale morphological features is given 1 point if present: bilateral lesions, multilocular lesions, solid areas, intra-abdominal metastases and ascites. If the sum of the points is 0 or 1, the ultrasound score is 1, whereas a sum of 2 or more is represented by an ultrasound score of 3. Premenopausal women have a menopausal score of 1 and postmenopausal women a menopausal score of 3. At an RMI cut-off level of 200, a sensitivity of 85% and a specificity of 97% were reported for distinguishing benign from malignant tumours.[21]

Although the RMI is a relatively simple test to use in clinical practice, it has significant false-negative and false-positive rates when tested prospectively.[23–25] We prospectively evaluated the original RMI (RMI1) and the revised RMI (RMI2) in 61 women.[26] Both models missed 26% of all invasive ovarian cancers and had false-positive rates of 15% and 20%, respectively. The fact that these results differ from those of the original studies [21,23] could be explained by differences in the study populations, inconsistencies in the definitions used for various morphological features and the variety of morphological appearances within tumours of different histological types.

A novel approach to the examination of ovarian tumours involves complex diagnostic models such as multivariable logistic regression and artificial neural networks that incorporate demographic, sonographic and biochemical data to improve the ultrasound diagnosis of ovarian cancer.[27–31] Again, when tested prospectively, the diagnostic accuracy of these models remains inferior to the assessment of tumour morphology (pattern recognition) by an experienced ultrasound operator.[8]

TABLE 3.2 **Sensitivity and specificity of a diagnosis based on greyscale ultrasound imaging (pattern recognition) achieved by an expert ultrasound operator**[4]

Diagnosis	Sensitivity (%)	Specificity (%)
Malignancy	88 (21/24)	96 (143/149)
Endometriosis	92 (24/26)	97 (143/147)
Dermoid cyst	90 (18/20)	98 (150/153)
Ovarian fibroma or fibrothecoma	56 (5/9)	100 (164/164)
Hydro-, pyo- or haematosalpinx	100 (8/8)	100 (165/165)
Myoma	86 (6/7)	99 (165/166)
Paraovarian or paratubal cyst	83 (5/6)	99 (166/167)
Peritoneal cyst	100 (3/3)	99 (169/170)
Abscess	33 (1/3)	99 (169/170)

Pattern recognition

Pattern recognition is the use of greyscale ultrasound morphology to characterise adnexal tumours and is superior to all other ultrasound methods, for example simple classification systems, scoring systems and mathematical models, in discriminating between benign and malignant adnexal tumours (Video 3.1).

Greyscale ultrasound images provide us with the same information that is obtained by the surgeon or pathologist when he or she cuts a surgical specimen to examine the contents. Many pelvic masses have a typical macroscopic appearance that allows for a fairly confident diagnosis to be made based on their greyscale ultrasound appearance alone. This is true of most dermoid cysts, endometriomas, corpora lutea, hydrosalpinges, peritoneal pseudocysts, paraovarian cysts and benign solid ovarian tumours (Table 3.2). An expert ultrasound operator can confidently and correctly distinguish between benign and malignant adnexal masses by this method with or without the use of colour Doppler ultrasound examination, with a sensitivity ranging from 88% to 98% and a specificity ranging from 89% to 96%.[8,32]

A mass that has a completely smooth internal wall is almost certainly benign, whereas a mass with irregularities should always evoke suspicion of malignancy.[4,8,32] Papillary projections are considered to be strong indicators of malignancy, although these are more common in borderline tumours than in invasive cancers (Video 3.2).[32] However, they may also be present in benign tumours such as cystadenofibromas. Papillary projections are responsible for many false-positive ultrasound diagnoses of malignancy.

Features of ovarian tumours that are considered suspicious include the presence of ascites and peritoneal tumour deposits within the pelvis, the presence of extensive papillarities (defined as the presence of multiple papillary projections of more than 3 mm in diameter, covering large sections of the inner cyst wall) that arise from the inner cyst wall, the presence of an irregular solid component within the cyst with evidence of necrosis (ill-defined anechoic areas within a predominantly solid lesion) and the absence of any healthy ovarian tissue adjacent to the cyst (negative 'ovarian crescent' sign).[32–34] There is a consensus in the UK that optimal care for these women involves a laparotomy by a gynaecological oncologist in a regional cancer centre.[2]

Role of ultrasound in benign adnexal tumours

Determination of the nature and extent of benign disease with ultrasound enables us to optimise and individualise treatment. An accurate assessment enables us to plan the most appropriate management, including the option of conservative management in benign adnexal tumours. If surgery is deemed necessary, ultrasound enables us to plan the best surgical approach (laparoscopic versus open surgery) and the level of surgical expertise required.

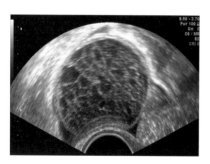

FIGURE 3.4 **Typical ultrasound image of a fresh haemorrhagic cyst filled with a blood clot**

In women with benign pathology, the option of expectant management should be considered if appropriate. The ovary undergoes constant morphological changes as part of its normal physiology. The possibility of a benign functional cyst, such as a corpus luteum or follicular cyst, must always be considered during ultrasound assessment. The typical vascular 'ring of fire' sign as seen in a corpus luteum or the typical morphological appearance of a haemorrhagic cyst (thin cobweb-like appearance; Figure 3.4) are features that would suggest a functional lesion.[32,35] It is therefore imperative to complement the scan findings with the clinical history and presenting complaint of the woman.

The incidental finding of a benign adnexal tumour during routine ultrasound examination presents a novel clinical dilemma. In these women, there is no compelling reason for surgical intervention and expectant management is often seen as the preferred option. However, in the absence of clinical symptoms, some women choose to have surgical intervention for fear of risk of malignancy or anxiety about possible complications such as torsion or cyst rupture.

Pelvic endometriosis

The diagnosis of endometriosis is traditionally established by visual inspection of the pelvis during laparoscopic surgery or laparotomy. The dependence on such invasive diagnostic tools has led to considerable interest in the use of non-invasive techniques such as ultrasound and magnetic resonance imaging (MRI) to detect the presence and extent of endometriosis. MRI is a complex and expensive method that is usually reserved for a select group of women with proven pelvic pathology. By contrast, ultrasound is widely available and is routinely used in the assessment of women presenting with gynaecological complaints.

When assessing women with endometriosis, ultrasound allows us to assess not only the morphology of the pelvic organs but also their mobility and tenderness (Video 3.3). It is widely acknowledged that the success of surgery for pelvic endometriosis is highly dependent on the expertise and training of the operating surgeon.[36,37] Factors increasing the risk of conversion to laparotomy include severe pelvic adhesions and severe pelvic endometriosis. Whereas mild to moderately severe endometriosis can be treated by medium-level laparoscopic surgeons, severe pelvic disease should be operated on by surgeons with considerable laparoscopic expertise, particularly if the disease involves the rectovaginal septum.[36–38] In an attempt to optimise the treatment of severe pelvic endometriosis, tertiary referral endometriosis centres have been established in the UK.[36] However, the capacity of these tertiary centres is limited, so the ability to triage women with severe disease for expert care is crucial. Ultrasound has the ability to diagnose severe disease with a high level of accuracy and therefore allows better triaging of women with pelvic endometriosis for referral to regional endometriosis centres.

Peritoneal endometriosis, ovarian endometriosis and deep infiltrating endometriosis have been distinguished as three clinicopathological entities with different origins.[39,40] There is now a general consensus that peritoneal endometriotic lesions can be attributed to the survival, adhesion, proliferation, invasion and vascularisation of endometrial tissue regurgitated through the fallopian tubes during menstruation, an idea referred to as implantation theory.[41] However, the pathogenesis of ovarian endometriosis and deep infiltrating endometriosis remains controversial.[42] Certainly, one of the main debates remains whether the different forms of disease have a common aetiology or whether they represent separate entities with different pathogeneses.

Superficial peritoneal endometriosis is not detectable by transvaginal ultrasound. However, transvaginal ultrasonography has become an important tool for the diagnosis of ovarian endometriosis or endometriomas. Asymptomatic endometriomas are increasingly diagnosed in young women. The pref-

TABLE 3.3 **Accuracy of ultrasound in the diagnosis of endometriosis**[44]

Study	Number of cysts	Sensitivity (%)	Specificity (%)	LR+ (95% CI)	LR− (95% CI)
STUDIES USING GREYSCALE ULTRASOUND					
Jain et al.[70]	37	64	100	−	0.4 (0.2–0.8)
Melis et al.[71]	93	83	89	7.6 (3.7–15.6)	0.2 (0.09–0.4)
Kurjak and Kupesic[72]	656	84	97	29.8 (18.2–49)	0.2 (0.1–0.3)
Guerriero et al.[73,74]	219	84	95	18 (8.7–37.4)	0.2 (0.1–0.3)
Alcazar et al.[75]	82	89	91	9.8 (4.2–22.8)	0.1 (0.04–0.4)
Guerriero et al.[76]	170	81	96	22.6 (8.6–59.6)	0.2 (0.1–0.3)
STUDIES USING DOPPLER ULTRASOUND					
Alcazar et al.[75]	57	90	22	1.2 (0.8–1.4)	0.4 (0.09–1.7)
Guerriero et al.[76]	170	90	97	33.5 (10.9–103)	0.1 (0.05–0.2)

Abbreviations: LR+ = positive likelihood ratio | LR− = negative likelihood ratio.

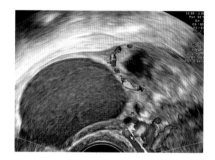

FIGURE 3.5 **Typical ultrasound image of an endometrioma showing hyperechoic fluid and well defined inner walls**

erential site for an endometrioma is the left ovary.[43] Moore et al.[44] conducted a systematic review of literature investigating the accuracy of transvaginal ultrasonography to diagnose ovarian endometriomas (Table 3.3). They concluded that transvaginal greyscale ultrasound is an effective test both to rule in and to rule out the diagnosis of an ovarian endometrioma in a woman with an adnexal mass.

The characteristic features of endometriomas include well-circumscribed thick-walled cysts that contain homogeneous low-level internal echoes described as 'ground glass' in appearance (Figure 3.5).[45,46] The fluid is often hypoechoic, so in some instances it may be necessary to increase the gain setting to detect the low-level echogenicity. 'Solid masses' can be seen protruding from the cyst wall into the cyst lumen like solid papillary projections, but these probably represent blood clots or fibrin.[32,47] False positives include corpus luteum and lutein cysts, teratomas, ovarian fibromas, tubo-ovarian abscesses and carcinomas.

Physical examination to evaluate the extent of posterior pelvis infiltration is frequently inadequate.[48] Imaging techniques are therefore increasingly being applied to diagnose posterior pelvis, bowel and bladder endometriosis. Although transvaginal ultrasound is very accurate in diagnosing endo-

TABLE 3.4 **Accuracy of clinical examination, transvaginal ultrasound and magnetic resonance imaging in the diagnosis of deep endometriosis** [52]

Diagnostic modality	Sensitivity (%)	Specificity (%)	PPV	NPV
RECTOSIGMOID ENDOMETRIOSIS				
Transvaginal ultrasound	98	100	100	98
MRI	83	98	98	84
Vaginal digital examination	72	54	63	64
RETROCERVICAL ENDOMETRIOSIS				
Transvaginal ultrasound	95	98	98	97
MRI	76	68	61	81
Vaginal digital examination	68	46	45	69

Abbreviations: MRI = magnetic resonance imaging | NPV = negative predictive value | PPV = positive predictive value.

metriomas, its accuracy in the assessment of deep infiltrating endometriosis is variable. Deep infiltrating endometriosis is defined by the presence of endometrial implants, fibrosis and muscular hyperplasia under the peritoneum and can involve the uterosacral ligaments, the rectosigmoid colon (Figure 3.6), the vagina and the bladder. On ultrasound, the endometriotic nodules appear as hypoechoic linear thickening and solid areas with or without regular contours.[49,50]

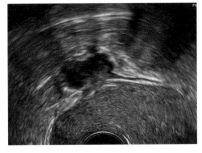

FIGURE 3.6 **Deep infiltrating endometriosis (endometriotic nodule) of the rectosigmoid colon seen as a solid hypoechoic lesion**

In the diagnosis of deep endometriosis, the sensitivity of transvaginal ultrasonography has been reported to range from 30% to 97% and the specificity from 81% to 100%.[49–51] The most encouraging results were obtained by Abrao et al.,[52] who compared the accuracy of transvaginal ultrasonography, clinical examination and MRI in diagnosing rectosigmoid and retrocervical endometriosis (Table 3.4). They reported a sensitivity and specificity of 98% and 100%, respectively, for ultrasound in the diagnosis of rectosigmoid endometriosis and of 95% and 98%, respectively, in retrocervical disease. The greater accuracy reported by Abrao et al.[52] could partly be explained by their use of bowel preparation before ultrasound scanning, which reduces the number of artefacts on ultrasound. Bazot et al.[50] found that transvaginal ultrasound offered an adequate view of the rectal wall and particularly the rectosigmoid junction

TABLE 3.5 **Accuracy of transvaginal sonography and rectal endoscopic sonography in the diagnosis of deep infiltrating endometriosis** [51]

Site of endometriosis	Transvaginal sonography		Transrectal sonography	
	Sensitivity (%)	Specificity (%)	Sensitivity (%)	Specificity (%)
USL	80.8 (59/73)	75.0 (6/8)	46.6 (34/73)	50.0 (4/8)
Vagina	50.0 (13/26)	96.4 (53/55)	7.7 (2/26)	98.2 (54/55)
RVS	11.1 (1/9)	100 (72/72)	22.2 (2/9)	93.1 (67/72)
Intestine	92.6 (50/54)	100 (27/27)	88.9 (48/54)	92.6 (25/27)
Ovary	94.3 (33/35)	84.8 (39/46)	68.6 (24/35)	91.3 (42/46)

Abbreviations: RVS = rectovaginal septum | USL = uterosacral ligament.

located near the retrocervical area, which was a common site of colorectal involvement (in up to 75% of instances).

The main limitation reported for transvaginal ultrasonography is its inability to measure the distance between the lower limit of the lesion and the anal margin. Moreover, it can fail to identify deep pelvic endometriosis in the sigmoid colon, which is typically located higher in the pelvis.[49,50]

Some authors have advocated the use of transrectal scans to improve the ultrasound diagnosis of deeply infiltrating endometriosis, particularly the diagnosis of uterosacral and intestinal endometriosis.[53–56] Bazot et al.,[51] however, achieved a better diagnosis of uterosacral and rectosigmoid endometriosis with transvaginal ultrasonography than with the transrectal approach (Table 3.5). This group also showed that transvaginal ultrasonography is very accurate in the diagnosis of intestinal and bladder endometriosis, but less so in detecting uterosacral, vaginal and rectovaginal septum involvement.[50] The limitation of transrectal scans lies in their poor sensitivity for the diagnosis of endometriomas and obliteration of the pouch of Douglas.[49]

Studies have showed that the accuracy of high-quality transvaginal ultrasound is comparable and possibly even superior to that of MRI in the diagnosis of deep pelvic endometriosis.[52,57] Abrao et al.[52] found sensitivity and specificity rates of 83% and 98% for the detection of rectosigmoid endometriosis with MRI and rates of 76% and 68% for the detection of retrocervical disease (Table 3.4). These values were inferior to those achieved with transvaginal ultrasound.

Furthermore, transvaginal ultrasound allows examination for the presence of adhesions by use of dynamic manipulation of the pelvic organs. This is an advantage over MRI. Ultrasound can also be used to assess the uterus for the presence of adenomyosis in this group of women. Adenomyosis is an indicator of severe disease. The presence of 'kissing ovaries' on an ultrasound scan is another sign of severe disease.[58] The presence of tubal pathology, which is particularly important in women seeking fertility advice, may also be assessed using ultrasound (Figure 3.7). Finally, the pouch of Douglas may be examined for the presence of adhesions.

Dermoid cysts

Mature cystic teratomas or dermoid cysts (Figure 3.8) are commonly detected during ultrasound examination of the pelvis. Improvements in the quality of the ultrasound equipment and increases in experience among ultrasound operators have improved the accuracy of dermoid cyst diagnosis by ultrasound. The resulting increase in confidence in an ultrasound-based diagnosis has largely eliminated the possibility of cancer as an indication for surgery in this context. In the majority of women, these cysts are diagnosed incidentally and are not the cause of the woman's presenting complaint and yet their presence is often considered to be an indication for surgery. In asymptomatic women with a diagnosis of a dermoid cyst, the possible benefits of surgical intervention are not clear and the risks and costs of surgery are hard to justify. Expectant management is a feasible option in this group of women.

Hoo et al.[59] looked at 93 asymptomatic women who underwent expectant management of their ultrasound-diagnosed ovarian dermoid cysts. After a mean follow-up period of 20.5 months, expectant management was successful in 69/93 (74.2%) women. The remaining 24 (25.8%) women underwent surgery after the period of expectant management. Half of the surgical interventions were performed on request of the women. Only nine (9.7%) women developed symptoms attributable to their cyst during the follow-up period and underwent surgery. Three (3.2%) women had an opportunistic ovarian cystectomy during an unrelated operation. Logistic regression analysis showed that the risk of surgical intervention was increased in younger women, in those with a parity of two or more and in those with no previous history of ovarian cysts, larger cyst diameters or bilateral dermoid cysts. Multiparous women had at least 12 times the risk of surgical intervention compared with nulliparous women and women with bilateral dermoid cysts had an 18-fold higher risk of having an operation than women with unilateral ovarian cysts.

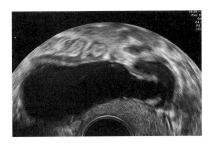

FIGURE 3.7 **Typical ultrasound image of a hydrosalpinx**

The hydrosalpinx is characterised by the sausage-shaped cyst with incomplete septations.

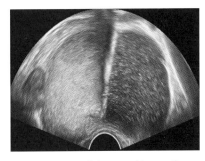

FIGURE 3.8 **Typical ultrasound image of a dermoid cyst**

Dermoid cyst characterised by a fluid level and hyperechoic materials within the cyst.

Dermoid cysts have been shown to grow slowly over a period of time, with various studies reporting a similar mean cyst growth rate of up to 1.8 mm/year.[60] The tendency of dermoid cysts to grow continuously may justify surgery in younger women. Our recommendation is that expectant management is a feasible option in older, nulliparous women, especially in those with small unilateral cysts. However, intermittent monitoring of dermoid cysts should be performed to ensure that laparoscopic surgical intervention can be offered before the cyst becomes too large. It is widely recognised that spillage of cyst contents can occasionally cause severe peritonitis, so it should be avoided.[61–63] Some authors advocate open surgery for large dermoid cysts with a mean diameter of more than 10 cm because these cysts are difficult to remove from the abdominal cavity without rupture.[64]

Pelvic adhesions

Ultrasound is a dynamic investigation that can be used to assess the mobility of pelvic organs and the presence of adhesions. Guerriero et al.[65] found that the mobility of the ovary could be evaluated using transvaginal imaging. The positive predictive value (PPV) of transvaginal ultrasound in diagnosing adhesions was reported as 81%. The inability to separate the ovary from the uterus during targeted palpation using a transvaginal ultrasound probe was more accurate in predicting adhesions than other indicators such as blurring of the margins of the ovary (PPV 65%). Okaro et al.[66] assessed ovarian mobility by applying pressure with the ultrasound probe. They reported a good correlation (kappa 0.81) between ovarian mobility on transvaginal ultrasound and at laparoscopy. However, most of the women in their series had normal ovaries, which are much easier to assess for mobility than large pelvic tumours are.

Yazbek et al.[67] conducted a study involving the preoperative transvaginal ultrasound assessment of 137 women. The diagnosis of severe pelvic adhesions was made with a sensitivity of 44% (95% CI 17–69%), a specificity of 98% (95% CI 94–99%) and a PPV of 67% (95% CI 30–90%). The sensitivity and PPV of ultrasound examination for the diagnosis of pelvic adhesions was not as high as expected. Five occurrences of severe adhesions were missed and there were two false-positive diagnoses of adhesions. Only 3/113 (2.7%) women who had laparoscopy had severe adhesions at surgery that had not been detected on the scan. However, in this study, undiagnosed severe pelvic adhesions accounted for 5/13 (38.5%) of failed laparoscopies that were converted to laparotomy. The presence of adhesions was particularly difficult to predict in obese women and in those with large tumours.

Role of ultrasound in surgical triage

There is no doubt that ultrasound has a role in the preoperative triage of women. Its potential role includes not only the correct differentiation between benign and malignant tumours, but also assessment of the severity of disease such as endometriosis and the extent of pelvic adhesions. Ultrasound can be used to identify women in whom surgery is likely to be difficult. This allows discussion with the relevant surgical teams when planning surgery.

In the study of 137 women by Yazbek et al.,[67] an attempt was made to establish a likely histological diagnosis by use of the pattern recognition method. All tumours suspected to be malignant were operated on by a gynaecological oncologist. The selection criteria for laparoscopic surgery were: no ultrasound features suggestive of ovarian cancer, evidence of a predominantly cystic lesion with no solid foci of more than 5 cm in mean diameter, evidence of a dermoid cyst of less than 10 cm in mean diameter and no evidence of severe pelvic endometriosis or severe pelvic adhesions. Severe endometriosis was suspected in women with ultrasound-diagnosed ovarian endometriomas in whom the ovaries were firmly adherent to the posterolateral aspect of the uterus or in whom the pouch of Douglas was completely obliterated with adhesions.[58,68] Pouch of Douglas obliteration was diagnosed when there was an absence of free movement between the posterior uterine surface and the large bowel. Pelvic adhesions were suspected when the adnexal tumours could not be mobilised by gentle palpation using the transvaginal or transabdominal probe or in women with evidence of peritoneal pseudocysts (Figure 3.9).

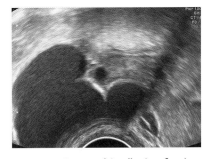

FIGURE 3.9 **Severe pelvic adhesions forming a peritoneal pseudocyst**

This peritoneal pseudocyst contains moderately echogenic fluid and incomplete septations. A normal ovary with an antral follicle is seen adjacent to the pseudocyst.

Of the 137 women with adnexal tumours included in the study, 113 (82.5%) were selected for laparoscopy and 24 (17.5%) for laparotomy. Laparoscopy was successfully completed in 107/113 (94.7%) women. Preoperative ultrasound assessment with the previously mentioned selection criteria was shown to predict successful outcomes of laparoscopic surgery with a sensitivity of 98% (95% CI 94–99%) and a specificity of 79% (95% CI 60–90%). The PPV was 95% (95% CI 89–98%), the positive likelihood ratio 4.58 (95% CI 2.25–9.32) and the negative likelihood ratio 0.02 (95% CI 0.01–0.09).[67]

These selection criteria for performing laparoscopic surgery may be used to identify women in whom the risk of conversion to laparotomy is low and who are suitable for day surgery.

Does a better ultrasound diagnosis lead to better patient management?

A common problem in the management of women with adnexal masses is that the ultrasound operator is unable to reach a confident preoperative diagnosis. Instead, operators tend to provide a summary of the morphological tumour characteristics as seen on the ultrasound scan. Infrequently, they do attempt to differentiate between benign and malignant ovarian tumours or try to predict a histological diagnosis. The interpretation of the ultrasound findings is often left to clinicians who have little or no experience in using ultrasonography for the diagnosis and who feel compelled to undertake surgery to ensure that women with ovarian cancer are not managed incorrectly. As a result, many women with benign cysts are treated as having potentially malignant disease and are routinely referred to regional cancer centres for further management.

Yazbek et al.[69] assessed the outcome of 150 women with suspected adnexal tumours who were referred to a tertiary gynaecological cancer centre. The women were randomised to having a routine ultrasound assessment by a nonexpert ultrasonographer ($n=73$) or to having an ultrasound assessment performed by an expert ultrasonographer ($n=77$). In the expert group, 99% of the women received a likely histological diagnosis, compared with 52% in the nonexpert group. The sensitivity achieved by the expert operator was much higher than that achieved by the nonexpert operator (88% versus 40%), whereas the specificity values were similar (96% versus 100%). The improved sensitivity in the expert group led to a significant reduction in the number of major surgical staging procedures performed for presumed ovarian cancer. As a result, more women underwent minimally invasive procedures, which contributed to a significantly reduced length of hospital stay in the expert operator group. Thus, the ability of an expert ultrasound operator to diagnose benign adnexal pathology leads to a greater reduction in the number of women treated as potentially having ovarian cancer and promotes the use of more conservative management options.

Conclusion

Detailed preoperative transvaginal ultrasound examination is helpful for assessing the feasibility of laparoscopic surgery in women with benign adnexal lesions. The assessment of tumour morphology and mobility helps to identify women in whom the risk of conversion to laparotomy is minimal and surgery may be performed as day surgery. Ultrasound assessment of women with suspected endometriosis has greatly improved in the last 10 years. The introduction of high-resolution transvaginal scanning combined with targeted palpation enables accurate diagnosis and staging of pelvic endometriosis. This has facilitated the referral of women to minimal access surgeons who are highly skilled in the management of severe pelvic endometriosis. The quality of an ultrasound examination in gynaecology, however, remains highly dependent on the experience of the operator. The skill level of the operator not only affects the accuracy of the ultrasound diagnosis, but also has a measurable impact on the management of women with evidence of adnexal abnormalities on the scan.

References

1 Yuen P M, Yu K M, Yip S K, Lau W C, Rogers M S, Chang A. A randomized prospective study of laparoscopy and laparotomy in the management of benign ovarian masses. *Am J Obstet Gynecol* 1997;177:109–14.

2 Junor E J, Hole D J, McNulty L, Mason M, Young J. Specialist gynaecologists and survival outcome in ovarian cancer: a Scottish national study of 1866 patients. *Br J Obstet Gynaecol* 1999;106:1130–6.

3 Timmerman D, Schwärzler P, Collins WP, Claerhout F, Coenen M, Amant F, et al. Subjective assessment of adnexal masses with the use of ultrasonography: an analysis of interobserver variability and experience. *Ultrasound Obstet Gynecol* 1999;13:11–6.

4 Valentin L. Pattern recognition of pelvic masses by gray-scale ultrasound imaging: the contribution of Doppler ultrasound. *Ultrasound Obstet Gynecol* 1999;14:338–47.

5 Valentin L. Transvaginal sonography in gynaecology. *Rev Gynaecol Pract* 2004;4:50–7.

6 Granberg S, Wikland M, Jansson I. Macroscopic characterization of ovarian tumors and the relation to histological diagnosis: criteria to be used for ultrasound evaluation. *Gynecol Oncol* 1989;35:139–44.

7 Granberg S, Norstrom A, Wikland M. Tumors in the lower pelvis as imaged by vaginal sonography. *Gynecol Oncol* 1990;37:224–9.

8 Valentin L, Hagen B, Tingulstad S, Eik-Nes S. Comparison of 'pattern recognition' and logistic regression models for discrimination between benign and malignant pelvic masses: a prospective cross validation. *Ultrasound Obstet Gynecol* 2001;18:357–65.

9 Sassone A M, Timor-Tritsch I E, Artner A, Carolyn W, Warren WB. Transvaginal sonographic characterization of ovarian disease: evaluation of a new scoring system to predict ovarian malignancy. *Obstet Gynecol* 1991; 78:70–6.

10 Lerner J P, Timor-Tritsch I E, Federman A, Abramovich G. Transvaginal ultrasonographic characterization of ovarian masses with an improved, weighted scoring system. *Am J Obstet Gynecol* 1994;170:81–5.

11 Rehn M; Lohmann K, Rempen A. Transvaginal ultrasonography of pelvic masses: Evaluation of B-mode technique and Doppler ultrasonography. *Am J Obstet Gynecol* 1996;175:97–104.

12 Buy J N, Ghossain M A, Hugol D, Hassen K, Sciot C, Truc J B, et al. Characterization of adnexal masses: combination of color Doppler and conventional sonography compared with spectral Doppler analysis alone and conventional sonography alone. *Am J Roentgenol* 1996;166:385–93.

13 Valentin L, Sladkevicius P, Marsal K. Limited contribution of Doppler velocimetry to the differential diagnosis of extrauterine pelvic tumors. *Obstet Gynecol* 1994;83:425–33.

14 Vergote I B, Børmer O, Abeler V M. Evaluation of C A 125 in the monitoring of ovarian cancer. *Am J Obstet Gynecol* 1987;157:88–92.

15 Cuckle H S, Wald N J. Screening for ovarian cancer. In: Miller A B, Chamberlain U, Day N E, Hakama M, Prorok P C, editors. *Cancer Screening*. Cambridge: Cambridge University Press; 1991. p. 228–39.

16 Bourne T H, Campbell S, Reynolds K, Hampson J, Bhatt L, Crayford T J, et al. The potential role of serum C A 125 in an ultrasound-based screening program for familial ovarian cancer. *Gynecol Oncol* 1994;52:379–85.

17 Maggino T, Gadducci A, D'Addario V, Pecorelli S, Lissoni A, Stella M, et al. Prospective multicenter study on C A 125 in postmenopausal pelvic masses. *Gynecol Oncol* 1994;54:117–23.

18 Di-Xia C, Schwartz P E, Xinguo L, Zhan Y. Evaluation of C A 125 levels in differentiating malignant from benign tumours in patients with pelvic masses. *Obstet Gynecol* 1988;72:23–7.

19 Niloff J M, Knapp R C, Schoetzl E M. C A 125 antigen levels in obstetric and gynecologic patients. *Obstet Gynecol* 1984;64:703–7.

20 Vasilev S A, Schaerth J B, Campeau J, Morrow C P. Serum C A 125 levels in preoperative evaluation of pelvic masses. *Obstet Gynecol* 1988;71:751–6.

21 Jacobs I, Oram D, Fairbanks J, Turner J, Frost C, Grudzinskas J G. A risk of malignancy index incorporating C A 125, ultrasound and menopausal status for the accurate preoperative diagnosis of ovarian cancer. *Br J Obstet Gynaecol* 1990;97:922–9.

22 Davies A P, Jacobs I, Woolas R, Fish A, Oram D. The adnexal mass: benign or malignant? Evaluation of a risk of malignancy index. *Br J Obstet Gynaecol* 1993;100:927–31.

23 Tingulstad S, Hagen B, Skjeldestad F E, Onsrud M, Kiserud T, Halvorsen T, et al. Evaluation of a risk of malignancy index based on serum C A 125, ultrasound findings and menopausal status in the pre-operative diagnosis of pelvic masses. *Br J Obstet Gynaecol* 1996;103:826–31.

24 Morgante G, la Marca A, Ditto A, De Leo V. Comparison of two malignancy risk indices based on serum C A 125, ultrasound score and menopausal status in the diagnosis of ovarian masses. *Br J Obstet Gynaecol* 1999;106:524–7.

25 Andersen E S, Knudsen A, Rix P, Johansen B. Risk of malignancy index in the preoperative evaluation of patients with adnexal masses. *Gynecol Oncol* 2003;90:109–12.

26 Aslam N, Tailor A, Lawton F, Carr Y J, Savvas S M, Jurkovic D. Prospective evaluation of three different models for the pre-operative diagnosis of ovarian cancer. *BJOG* 2000;107:1347–53.

27 Tailor A, Jurkovic D, Bourne T H, Collins W P, Campbell S. Sonographic prediction of malignancy in adnexal masses using multivariate logistic regression analysis. *Ultrasound Obstet Gynecol* 1997;10:41–7.

28 Timmerman D, Bourne T H, Tailor A, Collins W P, Verrelst H, Vandenberghe K, et al. A comparison of methods for preoperative discrimination between malignant and benign adnexal masses: the development of a new logistic regression model. *Am J Obstet Gynecol* 1999;181:57–65.

29 Tailor A, Jurkovic D, Bourne TH, Collins WP, Campbell S. Sonographic prediction of malignancy in adnexal masses using an artificial neural network. *Br J Obstet Gynaecol* 1999;106:21–30.

30 Timmerman D, Verrelst H, Bourne T H, De Moor B, Collins W P, Vergote I, et al. Artificial neural network models for the pre-operative discrimination between malignant and benign adnexal masses. *Ultrasound Obstet Gynecol* 1999;13:17–25.

31 Clayton R D, Snowden S, Weston M J, Mogensen O, Eastaugh J, Lane G. Neural networks in the diagnosis of malignant ovarian tumours. *Br J Obstet Gynaecol* 1999;106:1078–82.

32 Valentin L. Use of morphology to characterize and manage common adnexal masses. *Best Pract Res Clin Obstet Gynaecol* 2004;18:71–89.

33 Jokubkiene L, Sladkevicius P, Valentin L. Does three-dimensional power Doppler ultrasound help in discrimination between benign and malignant ovarian masses? *Ultrasound Obstet Gynecol* 2007;29:215–25.

34 Timmerman D, Valentin L, Bourne T H, Collins W P, Verrelst H, Vergote I. Terms, definitions and measurements to describe the sonographic features of adnexal tumors: a consensus opinion from the International Ovarian Tumor Analysis (IOTA) Group. *Ultrasound Obstet Gynecol* 2000;16:500–5.

35 Aleem F, Pennisi J, Zeitoun K, Predanic M. The role of color Doppler in diagnosis of endometriosis. *Ultrasound Obstet Gynecol* 1995;5:51–4.

36 Kennedy S, Bergqvist A, Chapron C, D'Hooghe T, Dunselman G, Greb R, et al. ESHRE guideline for the diagnosis and treatment of endometriosis. *Hum Reprod* 2005;20:2698–704.

37 Jacobson TZ, Duffy JM, Barlow D, Koninckx PR, Garry R. Laparoscopic surgery for pelvic pain associated with endometriosis. *Cochrane Database Syst Rev* 2009;(4): CD001300.

38 Royal College of Obstetricians and Gynaecologists. *The Investigation and Management of Endometriosis*. Green-top Guideline No. 24. London: RCOG; 2006 [www.rcog.org. uk/womens-health/clinical-guidance/investigation-and-management-endometriosis-green-top-24].

39 Nisolle M, Donnez J. Peritoneal endometriosis, ovarian endometriosis, and adenomyotic nodules of the rectovaginal septum are three different entities. *Fertil Steril* 1997;68:585–96.

40 Matarese G, De Placido G, Nikas Y, Alviggi C. Pathogenesis of endometriosis: natural immunity dysfunction or autoimmune disease? *Trends Mol Med* 2003;9:223–8.

41 Sampson JA. Peritoneal endometriosis due to the menstrual dissemination of endometrial tissue into the peritoneal cavity. *Am J Obstet Gynecol* 1927;14:422–69.

42 Vignali M, Infantino M, Matrone R, Chiodo I, Somigliana E, Busacca M, et al. Endometriosis: novel aetiopathogenetic concepts and clinical perspectives. *Fertil Steril* 2002;78:665–78.

43 Vercellini P, Aimi G, De Giorgi O, Maddalena S, Carinelli S, Crosignani PG. Is cystic ovarian endometriosis an asymmetric disease? *Br J Obstet Gynaecol* 1998;105:1018–21.

44 Moore J, Copley S, Morris J, Lindsell D, Golding S, Kennedy S. A systematic review of the accuracy of ultrasound in the diagnosis of endometriosis. *Ultrasound Obstet Gynecol* 2002;20:630–4.

45 Kupfer MC, Schwimer SR, Lebovic J. Transvaginal sonographic appearance of endometriomata: spectrum of findings. *J Ultrasound Med* 1992;11:129–33.

46 Guerriero S, Mais V, Ajossa S, Paoletti AM, Angiolucci M, Labate F, et al. The role of endovaginal ultrasound in differentiating endometriomas from other ovarian cysts. *Clin Exp Obstet Gynecol* 1995;22:20–2.

47 Patel MD, Feldstein VA, Chen DC, Lipson SD, Filly RA. Endometriomas: diagnostic performance of US. *Radiology* 1999;210:739–45.

48 Chapron C, Dubuisson JB, Pansini V, Vieira M, Fauconnier A, Barakat H, et al. Routine clinical examination is not sufficient for diagnosing and locating deeply infiltrating endometriosis. *J Am Assoc Gynecol Laparosc* 2002;9:115–9.

49 Bazot M, Detchev R, Cortez A, Amouyal P, Uzan S, Daraï E. Transvaginal sonography and rectal endoscopic sonography for the assessment of pelvic endometriosis: a preliminary comparison. *Hum Reprod* 2003;18:1686–92.

50 Bazot M, Thomassin I, Hourani R, Cortez A, Darai E. Diagnostic accuracy of transvaginal sonography for deep pelvic endometriosis. *Ultrasound Obstet Gynecol* 2004; 24:180–5.

51 Bazot M, Malzy P, Cortez A, Roseau G, Amouyal P, Daraï E. Accuracy of transvaginal sonography and rectal endoscopic sonography in the diagnosis of deep infiltrating endometriosis. *Ultrasound Obstet Gynecol* 2007;30:994–1001.

52 Abrao MS, Gonçalves MO, Dias JA Jr, Podgaec S, Chamie LP, Blasbalg R. Comparison between clinical examination, transvaginal sonography and magnetic resonance imaging for the diagnosis of deep endometriosis. *Hum Reprod* 2007; 22:3092–7.

53 Fedele L, Bianchi S, Portuese A, Borruto F, Dorta M. Transrectal ultrasonography in the assessment of rectovaginal endometriosis. *Obstet Gynecol* 1998;91:444–8.

54 Griffiths A, Koutsouridou R, Vaughan S, Penketh R, Roberts SA, Torkington J. Transrectal ultrasound and the diagnosis of rectovaginal endometriosis: a prospective observational study. *Acta Obstet Gynecol Scand* 2008; 87:445–8.

55 Ohba T, Mizutani H, Maeda T, Matsuura K, Okamura H. Evaluation of endometriosis in uterosacral ligaments by transrectal ultrasonography. *Hum Reprod* 1996;11:2014–7.

56 Chapron C, Dumontier I, Dousset B, Fritel X, Tardif D, Roseau G, et al. Results and role of rectal endoscopic ultrasonography for patients with deep pelvic endometriosis. *Hum Reprod* 1998;13:2266–70.

57 Bazot M, Daraï E. Sonography and MR imaging for the assessment of deep pelvic endometriosis. *J Minim Invasive Gynecol* 2005;12:178–85.

58 Ghezzi F, Raio L, Cromi A, Duwe DG, Beretta P, Buttarelli M, et al. 'Kissing ovaries': a sonographic sign of moderate to severe endometriosis. *Fertil Steril* 2005;83:143–7.

59 Hoo W L, Yazbek J, Holland T, Mavrelos D, Tong E N, Jurkovic D. Expectant management of ultrasonically diagnosed ovarian dermoid cysts: is it possible to predict outcome? *Ultrasound Obstet Gynecol* 2010;36:235–40.

60 Caspi B, Appelman Z, Rabinerson D, Zalel Y, Tulandi T, Shoham Z. The growth pattern of ovarian dermoid cysts: a prospective study in permenopausal and postmenopausal women. *Fertil Steril* 1997;68:501–5.

61 Huus M, Lafay-Pillet M C, Lecuru F, Ruscillo M M, Chevalier J M, Vilde F, et al. Granulomatous peritonitis after laparoscopic surgery of an ovarian dermoid cyst. Diagnosis, management, prevention, a case report. *J Gynecol Obstet Biol Reprod* 1996;25:365–72.

62 Coccia M E, Becattini C, Bracco G L, Scarselli G. Acute abdomen following dermoid cyst rupture during transvaginal ultrasonographically guided retrieval of oocytes. *Hum Reprod* 1996;11:1897–9.

63 Remorgida V, Magnasco A, Pizzorno V, Anserini P. Four year experience in laparoscopic dissection of intact ovarian dermoid cysts. *J Am Coll Surg* 1998;187:519–21.

64 Mettler L, Jacobs V, Brandenburg K, Jonat W, Semm K. Laparoscopic management of 641 adnexal tumors in Kiel, Germany. *J Am Assoc Gynecol Laparosc* 2001;8:74–82.

65 Guerriero S, Ajossa S, Lai M P, Mais V, Paoletti A M, Melis G B. Transvaginal ultrasonography in the diagnosis of pelvic adhesions. *Hum Reprod* 1997;12:2649–53.

66 Okaro E, Condous G, Khalid A, Timmerman D, Ameye L, Huffel S V, et al. The use of ultrasound-based 'soft markers' for the prediction of pelvic pathology in women with chronic pelvic pain – can we reduce the need for laparoscopy? *BJOG* 2006;113:251–6.

67 Yazbek J, Helmy S, Ben-Nagi J, Holland T, Sawyer E, Jurkovic D. Value of preoperative ultrasound examination in the selection of women with adnexal masses for laparoscopic surgery. *Ultrasound Obstet Gynecol* 2007;30:883–8.

68 Bhatt S, Kocakoc E, Dogra V S. Endometriosis sonographic spectrum. *Ultrasound Q* 2006;22:273–80.

69 Yazbek J, Raju S K, Ben-Nagi J, Holland T K, Hillaby K, Jurkovic D. Effect of quality of gynaecological ultrasonography on management of patients with suspected ovarian cancer: a randomised controlled trial. *Lancet Oncol* 2008;9:124–31.

70 Jain K A, Friedman D L, Pettinger T W, Alagappan R, Jeffrey R B, Sommer F G. Adnexal masses: comparison of specificity of endovaginal US and pelvic MR imaging. *Radiology* 1993;186:697–704.

71 Melis G B, Ajossa S, Guerriero S. Epidemiology and diagnosis of endometriosis. *Ann NY Acad Sci* 1994; 734:352–7.

72 Kurjak A, Kupesic S. Scoring system for prediction of ovarian endometriosis based on transvaginal color and pulsed Doppler sonography. *Fertil Steril* 1994;62:81–8.

73 Guerriero S, Mais V, Ajossa S, Paoletti A M, Angiolucci M, Melis G B. Transvaginal ultrasonography combined with CA125 plasma levels in the diagnosis of endometriomas. *Fertil Steril* 1996;65:293–8.

74 Guerriero S, Ajossa S, Paoletti A M, Mais V, Angiolucci M, Melis G B. Tumor markers and transvaginal ultrasound in the diagnosis of endometriomas. *Obstet Gynecol* 1996;88:403–7.

75 Alcazar J L, Laparte C, Jurado M, Lopez-Garcia G. The role of transvaginal ultrasonography combined with color velocity imaging and pulsed Doppler in the diagnosis of endometriomas. *Fertil Steril* 1997;67:487–91.

76 Guerriero S, Ajossa S, Mais V, Risalvato A, Lai M P, Melis G B. The diagnosis of endometriomas using colour Doppler energy imaging. *Hum Reprod* 1998;13:1691–5.

4 Instruments and theatre environment

Mohamed Hefni, Simon Edmonds and Mary Gooch

Introduction

The selection of laparoscopic instruments and the operating theatre set-up are essential to the safety of the person undergoing surgery and to theatre efficiency. This chapter addresses the different types of instruments and discusses how combinations of instruments facilitate a surgical intervention. However, we recognise that we cannot mention or discuss all the available instruments as there are simply too many. In addition, as the scope of laparoscopic procedures increases, so does the range of instruments.

We also discuss how the digitalisation of the operating theatre has led to both improved efficiency and a safer environment for staff and patients. Although this chapter addresses instrumentation and theatre environment, we also recognise that without excellent visualisation, the safety of the person undergoing surgery may be compromised.

Essential laparoscopic instruments

The essential laparoscopic instruments are:

- carbon dioxide gas insufflator
- suction/irrigation system
- grasping forceps
- uterine manipulators
- laparoscopic probe
- biopsy forceps
- bipolar diathermy forceps
- clip applicator.

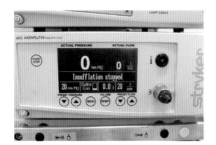

FIGURE 4.1 **High-flow insufflator**

Carbon dioxide gas insufflators

The high-performance suction/irrigation systems used in laparoscopy produce a rapid loss of carbon dioxide gas, which must be replaced by use of a high-flow insufflator (Figure 4.1). The insufflator must clearly show the flow rate, the intra-abdominal pressure, the gas volume used and the amount of gas remaining in the carbon dioxide gas cylinder. Most modern insufflators enable the preselection of pressure and flow rate and will sound an alarm if the pressure exceeds the selected setting (normally 20–25 mmHg) before insertion of the first trocar.[1,2]

Some insufflators have integrated facilities to heat the carbon dioxide gas; this is of particular advantage during prolonged surgery to reduce heat loss and maintain the patient's core temperature.

Suction / irrigation systems

A suction irrigator is one of the most important laparoscopic instruments. To maintain good visualisation in the presence of bleeding, fluids or smoke, it is important to have a functioning and efficient suction irrigator ready to use before starting any laparoscopic surgery. As soon as bleeding commences, even a small

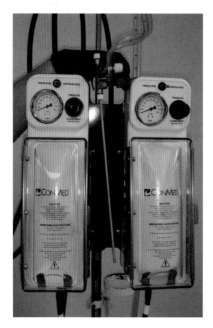

FIGURE 4.2 **Suction / irrigation system**

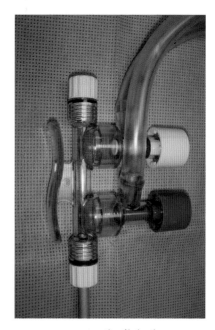

FIGURE 4.3 **5 mm suction / irrigation instrument**

amount of blood can absorb the light, making visualisation difficult. Equally as important as the efficiency of the suction to remove blood, fluid or smoke is a rapid pressurised irrigation with Hartmann's solution or saline. There are many systems available to provide a good powerful stream of irrigation fluid, powered by pressurised carbon dioxide gas (Figure 4.2). It is a waste of resources to use one of the theatre staff to manually squeeze the irrigation fluid. Most suction irrigators are 5 mm instruments with one channel and hand-activated controls (Figure 4.3). This gives the surgeon more control and flexibility to alternate between suction and irrigation and frees the second hand for another instrument to secure any bleeding. Suction irrigators of 10 mm are sometimes useful, particularly with severe bleeding and in the presence of blood clots.

Grasping forceps

The wide range of grasping forceps can be divided into two groups. The first consists of atraumatic graspers, which are designed to handle tissues that are not going to be removed and therefore help to avoid damage to, for example, ovaries, tubes or bowel (Figure 4.4). The second group consists of graspers with toothed, sharp pins or sharp jaws, which give a good grip of the tissue and are useful for tissues that are to be removed (Figure 4.5). Most grasping forceps are available in both 5 mm and 10 mm sizes and are also available with self-closing or ratchet locks.

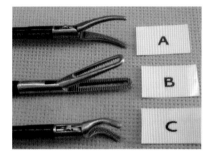

FIGURE 4.4 **Atraumatic forceps:**
(A) Maryland forceps, (B) Johann forceps,
(C) Petelin forceps

In our centre, the essential forceps are:

- atraumatic Johann grasper – blunt-nosed to handle tissues such as the ovary or bowel

- Maryland, Kelly or Petelin dissection forceps – pointed with a curved shape for fine dissection

- alligator/claw or Manhes grasping forceps – for tissue removal.

Most grasping forceps can be connected to monopolar diathermy.

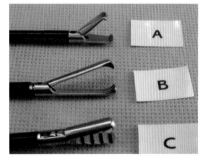

FIGURE 4.5 **Grasping forceps: (A) Manhes forceps, (B) Claw (alligator) forceps, (C) Endo Clinch® (US Surgical Corporation, Norwalk, CT, USA) atraumatic forceps**

Uterine manipulators

Adequate manipulation of the uterus is required in most laparoscopic surgery, including diagnostic laparoscopy. Uterine

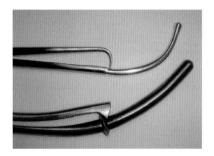

FIGURE 4.6 **Scott's uterine manipulator**

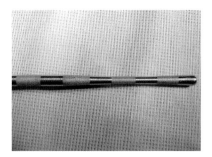

FIGURE 4.7 **Laparoscopic probe**

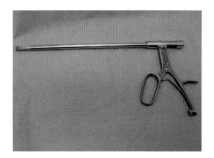

FIGURE 4.8 **Biopsy forceps**

sounds, dilators and/or cannulae can be used. Scott's manipulator (Figure 4.6) is a useful and reusable manipulator in both diagnostic and operative laparoscopy. The Valtchev® (Conkin Surgical Instruments, Toronto, Canada) uterine manipulator with interchangeable tips can also be used for hydrotubation. There are several disposable manipulators available such as the Koh Colpotomizer™ System (Cooper Surgical, Trumbull, CT, USA), designed to simplify total laparoscopic hysterectomy and in particular to prevent the loss of the pneumoperitoneum when the vagina is opened. Similarly, the VCare® (ConMed Endosurgery, Utica, NY, USA) uterine manipulator includes a vaginal cup to define the dissecting plane for the colpotomy incision and prevents any gas leak through the vagina.

Laparoscopic probe

A laparoscopic probe – a metal probe with a centimetre-graded ruler embossed upon it (Figure 4.7) – is useful for measuring cysts or other structures. It is atraumatic and is also useful as a manipulator.

Biopsy forceps

Biopsy forceps are generally used to biopsy suspicious tissue such as ovarian tumours or peritoneal deposits (Figure 4.8).

Bipolar diathermy forceps

Bipolar diathermy forceps are an essential instrument that provides accurate and safe diathermy to secure bleeding points without lateral tissue damage. More detail is given in chapter 5.

Clip applicator

Unfortunately, not many gynaecologists appreciate the value of clips in securing a bleeding vessel such as the ovarian or uterine artery. A clip applicator can be a life-saving instrument, particularly in situations where the artery retracts back into the surrounding tissue and diathermy becomes ineffective and unsafe because the spread of lateral heat causes damage to adjacent organs such as the ureter. It allows accurate, safe and timely occlusion of a bleeding vessel without requiring any energy source. A clip applicator should be available in every theatre as an emergency instrument.

There are 10 mm reusable applicators that apply a single 10 mm titanium clip and require manual reloading outside the abdominal cavity, and disposable 5 mm or 10 mm automated multiclip applicators that contain 20 clips, each of which can be loaded and fired without taking the applicator out of the abdominal cavity (Figure 4.9). The advantages of the disposable automated multiclip applier are obvious.

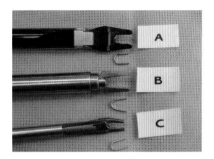

FIGURE 4.9 **(A) 10 mm disposable, (B) 10 mm reusable, (C) 5 mm disposable**

Operative laparoscopic instruments

Operative laparoscopic instruments have a variety of uses and require more specific training and higher skill levels.

Laparoscopic scissors

Sharp scissors are mandatory. Most laparoscopic scissors use a 5 mm port with one tip fixed and the other articulated by opening the hand piece. Reusable scissors may not be as effective because the scissors rapidly become blunt follow-

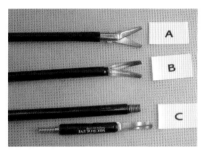

FIGURE 4.10 **Scissors: (A) reusable scissors, (B) disposable scissors, (C) scissors with a disposable tip and reusable handle**

ing the use of diathermy. The combination of a disposable tip and a reusable handle (Figure 4.10) is a good option as the scissors are always sharp and this may be more cost-effective. A very wide range of disposable scissors with a variety of shapes and designs is available. The most commonly used is the curved scissor with a rounded tip, suitable for most gynaecological surgeries. A flat scissor with a rounded end is more suitable for peritoneal or lymph node dissection. Microscissors with needle-shaped points are valuable for more delicate dissection such as that involved during tubal surgery.

Laparoscopic stapling devices

There is little doubt that stapling devices initially played a major role in advancing laparoscopic surgery as they are one of the safest and fastest devices used to secure pedicles in gynaecological surgery, particularly in less experienced hands. It is fair to say that this has created the opportunity for more gynaecologists to perform laparoscopic surgery. However, stapling devices require a 12 mm trocar for insertion and they are expensive disposable instruments. Another disadvantage is that stapling devices are difficult to manipulate in the pelvic cavity. Some devices have both rotation of the shaft and roticulation of the stapler tip to improve application of the staples to tissue lying at an angle to the axis of the device. However, the devices still remain bulky and do not allow any tissue dissection or accurate identification of specific vessels.

The main stapling devices are the Multifire Endo GIA® stapler (US Surgical Corporation, Norwalk, CT, USA) (Figure 4.11) and the Ethicon Endo-Surgery Linear Cutter (Ethicon Endo-Surgery, Cincinnati, OH, USA).

When a stapling device is fired, it delivers two triple-staggered rows of titanium staples into the tissues, followed by advancement of a knife blade between the two rows to divide them (Figure 4.12).

Good haemostasis and pedicle security are usually obtained if the device is correctly applied and the thickness of the tissue is correct; for this reason, the staple cartridge is available in various closure sizes (from 2.5 mm to 5 mm) and also various lengths (from 4.5 cm to 6 cm). Cartridge size selection is important. For example, if the surgeon applies a 2.5 mm staple cartridge to a thick pedicle, haemostasis will fail and to then re-secure such a pedicle would be a challenge. Similarly, if the tissue is too thin, haemostasis will fail because of poor tissue compression.

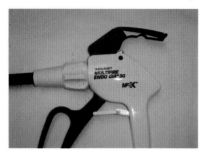

FIGURE 4.11 **Multifire Endo GIA® 30 stapler (US Surgical Corporation, Norwalk, CT, USA)**

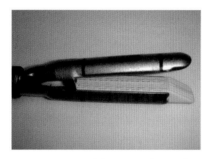

FIGURE 4.12 **Two triple-staggered rows of titanium staples**

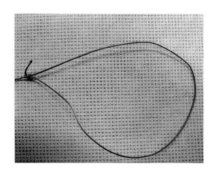

FIGURE 4.13 **Endoloop® system**

Endoloop® system

Semm[3] described the technique of laparoscopic loop ligature (Endoloop®; Ethicon Endo-Surgery, Cincinnati, Ohio USA). This system consists of a pretied Roeder loop attached to a plastic shaft (Figure 4.13). One end of the suture passes up the centre of the shaft and is attached to the proximal 2 cm of the shaft. This can then be broken and pulled to tighten the knot. The Endoloop system may be used to secure haemostasis in pedicles and vessels that have already been divided. It can also be used as a primary method of haemostasis in oophorectomy and salpingectomy for the removal of an ectopic pregnancy, hydrosalpinx or ovary.

Extracorporeal knot pusher

The technique of extracorporeal knot tying was first described by Reich et al.[4] in 1992. This technique has greatly simplified laparoscopic suturing because it is more rapid and easy to perform than the intracorporeal technique. Essentially, following placement of the suture within the abdomen by use of a laparoscopic needle holder and either a curved or a straight needle, the knot is tied outside the abdomen and then pushed down the port with a laparoscopic knot pusher to be tightened at the distal end (the target site). There are several types and designs of knot pusher (Figure 4.14).

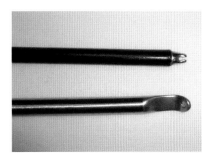

FIGURE 4.14 **Knot pusher**

Surgiwip™ (Autosuture™, Covidien, Mansfield, MA, USA) is another disposable extracorporeal device with a ski-shaped needle, with the suture material attached to a plastic knot pusher similar to the Endoloop; the knot is tied outside the abdomen.

Ligasure™ device

The Ligasure™ (Valleylab, Boulder, CO, USA) device permanently fuses tissue and vessels of up to 7 mm in diameter. It does so by melting the collagen and elastin in the vessel walls and reforming it into a permanent seal in a single application, without dissection. The generator produces a higher current and a much lower voltage than standard diathermy such that the lateral thermal spread is less than 1–2 mm, with minimal risk of damage to other structures surrounding the active device. Through a feedback-controlled response system, the device automatically adjusts the current and power settings to the optimum and stops delivering energy once the seal is complete. Vaporised water is released during activation of the device, which rarely causes a burn (a complication that can arise with the vaginal Ligasure device) because the laparoscopic active jaws grasp smaller pedicles.

The device can also be used to safely grasp tissue and mobilise pelvic organs and is introduced through a 5 mm port.

In gynaecology, the device is most often used for oophorectomy pedicles and for laparoscopically assisted vaginal hysterectomies. Care is required for the larger uterine arteries (over 7 mm) when parallel tissue pedicles should be taken to reduce the risk of bleeding. Repeat sealing of the same tissue should be avoided as this weakens the seal. Initial studies have confirmed that the seal can withstand up to three times the normal systolic blood pressure.[5]

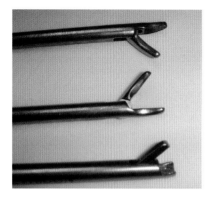

FIGURE 4.15 **Two types of needle holder**

The lower needle holder has the advantage that it automatically rotates the needle to a position where it is ready to be used with high accuracy to ensure precise and reliable control of the needle.

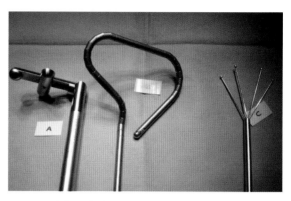

FIGURE 4.16 **Intestinal retractors**

Newer devices include a central blade that cuts the sealed tissue, thereby avoiding the need for multiple reinsertions of scissors, and a monopolar diathermy tip for small vessel coagulation.

Limitations of the device include the lack of a roticulated distal end (as in the stapler), although rotation of the head through 180° is possible. More detailed dissection is not possible with the device and other energy sources are required if endometriosis or complex adhesions are present.

Helica thermal coagulator

The Helica thermal coagulator (Helica Instruments; Riccarton, Edinburgh, UK) has been available since 1993. It delivers a stream of helium gas through the tip of the probe, through which electrons pass to fulgurate the tissue, to a depth of 1 mm in healthy tissue. The depth and speed of penetration can be varied by adjusting the power setting, which runs at 2–33 W (considerably less than conventional diathermy, which runs at 50–200 W).

It has been shown to be safe in the treatment of early-stage superficial endometriosis,[6] but further evidence is required for its use in excising deeper deposits.

Diathermy, laser and ultrasound instruments

The details, risks and benefits of these devices are discussed in chapter 5.

Laparoscopic needle holder

There are several types of needle holder; some have the traditional jaws of the regular needle holders, whereas others have special jaws that rotate and hold the needle very firmly in the suture position and resist twisting (Figure

4.15). The needle holder is usually a 5 mm instrument. To perform intracorporeal sutures, it is necessary to have two needle holders or a needle holder and a closed jaw grasper. The challenge of the intracorporeal suture technique is to be able to tie surgical knots inside the abdomen that provide the same security as that acceptable at open surgery.

Intestinal probe

The intestinal probe is mainly used as a retractor to keep the bowels out of the operating field, particularly with electrosurgical instruments (Figure 4.16).

Puncture needle

The puncture needle is used to aspirate ovarian cysts (Figure 4.17).

Instruments for port closure

The incidence of herniation increases with larger ports,[7] although some of the newer trocars may cause less tissue damage at insertion. Predisposing factors include obesity, chronic cough, excessive manipulation and extension of the puncture site to retrieve tissue specimens. Suturing of the sheath is mandatory following a Hasson entry and should be considered for 10 mm ports and above.

The simplest and cheapest way of closing the sheath under direct vision laparoscopically is a reusable J needle (Figure 4.18A). Other reusable devices include EndoClaws™ (Elemental Healthcare, Berkshire, UK) (Figure 4.18B). A single-use device (Endoclose™; Autosuture™, Covidien, Mansfield, MA, USA) is also available.

Tissue retrieval systems

Bags

Extraction of large, potentially malignant specimens risks spillage of malignant cells within the peritoneal cavity and seedling implantation at the access wounds.

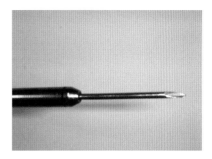

FIGURE 4.17 **Puncture needle**

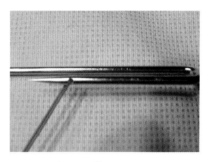

FIGURE 4.18A **J needle**

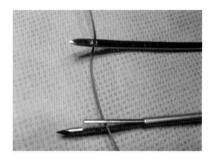

FIGURE 4.18B **EndoClaws™**
(Elemental Healthcare, Berkshire, UK)

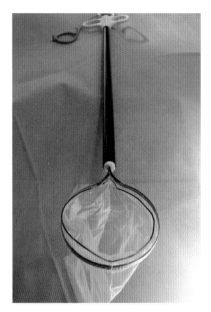

FIGURE 4.19 **Tissue retrieval bag EndoCatch™ (Autosuture™, Covidien, Mansfield, MA, USA)**

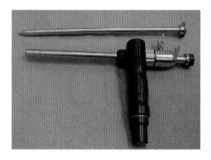

FIGURE 4.20 **Reusable morcellator**

Similarly, removal of dermoid cysts without spillage of the contents can present a challenge if retrieval bags are not used; spillage of the contents may lead to a chemical peritonitis. Therefore, extraction is best conducted through a rip-proof sleeve retrieval system that creates a 'third space' in which the specimen can be sliced under direct vision or removed intact. In fact, most ovarian cystectomies for dermoid cysts or suspicious malignant cysts can be performed inside the bag by placing the ovary over or in the bag before commencing the first ovarian incision. Thus, if contents leak, they can be safely aspirated from within the bag.

Tissue retrieval bags can also be useful for the removal of ectopic pregnancies, large blood clots or endometriotic tissues.[8]

A variety of tissue retrieval bags are available on the market, but they should be rip-proof, transparent and easy to keep open. The EndoCatch™ (Autosuture™, Covidien, Mansfield, MA, USA) bag (Figure 4.19) is easy to use since it has a spring action to keep the mouth of the bag open at all times. Others, such as the Nubert™ (Synergy Health, Swindon, UK) retrieval bag, have a stronger, tear-resistant, X-ray-detectable fabric-walled bag that requires manipulation within the pelvis with at least two graspers to keep the mouth of the bag open.

Morcellators

A morcellator is used to cut up masses or tissue specimens for removal, including the uterus, benign ovarian cysts and fibroids during laparoscopic procedures.[9] The first hand-activated morcellator was developed by Semm in 1973, but the destruction of even small fibroids was found to be time consuming. Development of the device has now produced an instrument with a 10–25 mm shaft and a central grasper surrounded by a cylindrical cutting blade that is rotated by electromechanical energy produced from the control box (Figure 4.20). Most are foot-pedal-activated and contain a retractable blade guard at the tip, which should be used whenever the device is not in use. The potential of trauma to other surrounding tissues and vessels is high, so any surgeon using this device must have received appropriate training and must keep the tip of the device under constant vision at all times within the abdomen and pelvis. Complications are rare and not often reported in the literature, but they can be fatal, particularly if unrecognised bowel injury or major vascular injury occurs.[10]

Retraction of the grasped specimen while the device is activated allows an 'apple-coring' effect and removal of large tissue masses down the port. This technique has been applied to laparoscopic supracervical/subtotal hysterectomy for the removal of the uterine body with fibroids.[11]

Reusable and single-use devices are available (Figure 4.21), although with repeated use the reusable blade of the device may become blunt and resterilisation can prove difficult as tissue becomes trapped between the blade and outer shaft. However, on single-use devices the power cable can become twisted, whereas newer reusable designs developed by Karl Storz (Tuttlingen, Germany) have a direct drive motor to transmit the rotational energy to the blade, giving variable speed and a faster blade rotation without the cable twisting.

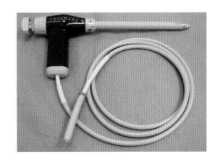

FIGURE 4.21 **Disposable morcellator**

Reusable versus disposable laparoscopic instruments

Any laparoscopic instrument or medical device has to be fit for purpose. There are advantages and disadvantages for both disposable and reusable instruments.

By the very nature of the size and length of laparoscopic instruments, it is even more important to be aware of the issues set out in the following section of this chapter.

Disadvantages of reusable instruments

Despite extensive research investigating both bovine spongiform encephalopathy in animals and variant Creutzfeldt–Jakob disease in humans, there is still no hard evidence regarding their transmission or the potential for any curative treatment. Sterile Services Department procedures have been implemented to minimise the spread of any infections.[12] Guidelines issued by the Department of Health[13] recommend that each medical device is marked with the Conformité Européenne (CE) mark and medical device companies are obliged to supply clear guidance on the decontamination process required for each of their products. If there are concerns that a medical device cannot be decontaminated and sterilised effectively, it should not be used. This problem has been known to occur when processing laparoscopic devices with a small lumen and a long shaft. Fengler et al.[14] highlight the need for the dismantling of laparoscopic instruments so that the decontaminating and sterilisation process can be effectively applied.

According to guidance from the Institute of Decontamination Sciences,[15] the process of decontamination and sterilisation of medical devices may take in excess of 3 hours before the device can be returned to theatre for use. This requires forward planning and consideration of the financial burden of excess equipment, to allow for adequate availability of instruments for emergencies and accidental desterilisation.

Advantages of reusable instruments

The purchase, reprocessing and maintenance of reusable devices is, at present, more economically viable than the purchase of single-use devices.[16] Although the initial purchase of reusable devices may be more expensive, the design and materials used in their construction tend to be of a higher quality compared with the cheaper disposable devices.

Disadvantages of single-use instruments

All instruments have to be CE-marked and have a symbol indicating that the item is single-use only and must not be reprocessed for reuse.[13] To comply with traceability, the device must have a removable sticker with details of how it was sterilised, including the date, so this may be attached to the operated woman's documentation.

The quality of an instrument will depend on the design, materials used and price of sale.

Advantages of single-use instruments

Single-use devices are available off the shelf as and when required. There is no risk associated with decontamination or sterilisation.

Theatre environment

Theatre team

The theatre team, including the team leader, is of paramount importance to the smooth running of the operating list. Powell et al.[17] liken nurse teams to football teams, where the coach or manager should be able to provide support and structure in a team without creating dependence. The theatre team facilitates and supports both the anaesthetist and the operating surgeon in their duty of care to the woman undergoing surgery.

The Association for Perioperative Practice[18] provides recommendations for the optimum numbers of personnel required to ensure the safety and quality of care for the woman while in the theatre. The Association for Perioperative Practice states that organisational staffing establishments must be developed with regard to clinical governance frameworks. Berguer[19] also emphasises the importance of a 'well-rehearsed operating theatre team' that may contribute to reducing the length of the operating time.

Each operating theatre should have a team leader organising the theatre, a minimum of two scrub practitioners who prepare the sterile trolleys and one circulating assistant. The circulating assistant is integral in anticipating the needs of the scrub team. If there is an emergency situation, a minimum amount of time is wasted. On the surgical team, there will be the need for the operating surgeon and a minimum of one or, occasionally, two assistants. One of the assistants will be required to hold the laparoscopic camera and 'follow' the surgeon's working area, constantly keeping the operating field centralised on the monitors. This can prove to be difficult and requires experience.

Positioning of the equipment and theatre staff

One of the great advantages of laparoscopic surgery is that all staff in theatre are able to continuously see the surgical procedure and be alert to any problems or complications as they occur. This is quite different from all other open gynaecological surgeries, where vision of the surgical field is usually limited to the operating surgeon and the assistant. Therefore, the positioning of the equipment and theatre staff is very important as it helps to provide the best view for all members of the team.

Laparoscopic surgery requires a large amount of equipment. This may have an effect on the ergonomics of the theatre, including some potential hazards, such as cables across the floor and lack of space. There is also the potential for the desterilisation of equipment or trips, slips and falls. This can be exacerbated when the majority of the surgery is performed in the dark. To some extent, this can be overcome by the use of a diffused 'green light', which does not compromise the surgeon's view but allows the theatre team to work in a more suitable environment. However, reducing movement and unnecessary traffic in and out of the operating theatre is still of significant importance when organising the area.[20]

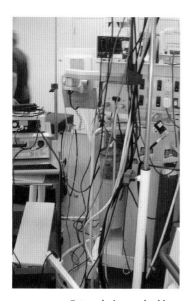

FIGURE 4.22 **External wires and cable are avoided in digital theatres**

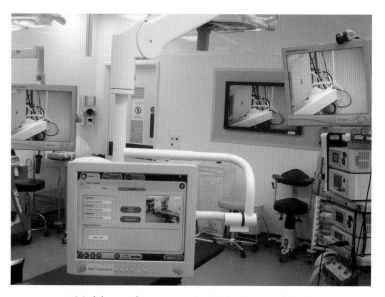

FIGURE 4.23 **Digital theatre; the centre monitor is also the control panel**

The digital theatre

A digital operating theatre may be defined as 'an integrated system consisting of electrical power, insufflations gas and video connections through central channels. Monitors, light sources, insufflators and electrosurgical generators are moved from mobile carts onto ceiling-mounted pendants. To be able to achieve this at a high standard, all of the equipment within the theatre is positioned and fitted to the requirements of all the personnel working in the theatre. The technology of Digital Theatre creates one point of contact to integrate multiple technologies, brings to life patient critical information within the operating theatre, and provides interactive connectivity to the rest of the hospital and the outside world.'[21]

The requirements for a digital theatre include that the equipment may be moved easily depending on the individual surgical procedure and that the surgeon is able to view and control the equipment when scrubbed at the operating table.[22] Also, the support personnel must be able to move safely around the theatre, providing support when required with minimal intrusion. There should be the possibility to teach procedures or to disseminate information for the training of medical, paramedical and nursing personnel without those individuals being physically present.

To be able to achieve some of these requirements, the design of the digital operating theatre is of paramount importance.

Most of the digital equipment can be suspended from the ceiling with the use of pendant arms, with cabling being attached to the pendants, thereby avoiding trailing cables (Figure 4.22).

An operating theatre is considered to be one of the most costly areas within the healthcare setting to renovate, construct or run,[23] so it is important to consider all areas that affect the efficiency of theatre use, including benefits to the hospital, women undergoing surgery, surgeons and theatre personnel, and the capacity to offer educational opportunities (Figure 4.23).

References

1 Phillips G, Garry R, Kumar C, Reich H. How much gas is required for initial insufflation at laparoscopy? *Gynaecol Endosc* 1999;8:369–74.

2 Tsaltas J, Pearce S, Lawrence A, Meads A, Mezzatesta J, Nicolson S. Safer laparoscopic trocar entry: it's all about pressure. *Aust N Z J Obstet Gynaecol* 2004;44:349–50.

3 Semm K. Operative pelviscopy. *Br Med Bull* 1986;42: 284–95.

4 Reich H, Clarke H C, Sekel L. A simple method for ligating with straight and curved needles in operative laparoscopy. *Obstet Gynecol* 1992;79:143–7.

5 Kennedy J S, Stranahan P L, Taylor K D, Chandler J G. High-burst-strength, feedback-controlled bipolar vessel sealing. *Surg Endosc* 1998;12:876–8.

6 Hill N C, El-Toukhy T, Chandakas S, Grigoriades T, Erian J. Safety of the Helica Thermal Coagulator in treatment of early stage endometriosis. *J Obstetric Gynaecol* 2005;25:52–4.

7 Nezhat C, Nezhat F, Seidman D S, Nezhat C. Incisional hernias after operative laparoscopy. *J Laparoendosc Adv Surg Tech A* 1997;7;111–5.

8 Cuschieri A, Frank T. Slicer and tissue retrieval system for excisional endoscopic surgery. *Surg Endosc* 1994;8:1246–9.

9 Segen J C. *Concise Dictionary of Modern Medicine*. New York: McGraw-Hill; 2006.

10 Milad M P, Sokol E. Laparoscopic morcellator-related injuries. *J Am Assoc Gynecol Laparosc* 2003;10:383–5.

11 Erian J, Hassan M, Pachydakis A, Chandakas S, Wissa I, Hill N. Efficacy of laparoscopic subtotal hysterectomy in the management of menorrhagia: 400 consecutive cases. *BJOG* 2008;115:742–8.

12 Department of Health. *Controls Assurance in Infection Control: Decontamination of Medical Devices*. Health Services Circular 1999/179. London: DoH; 1999.

13 Department of Health [www.dh.gov.uk].

14 Fengler T W, Pahlke H, Kraas E. Sterile and economic instrumentation in laparosopic surgery. Experiences with 6,000 surgical laparoscopies, 1990–1996. *Surg Endosc* 1998;12:1275–9.

15 Institute of Decontamination Sciences. *Standards and Practice for Medical Device Decontamination*. West Lothian: IDSc; 2007.

16 Yung E, Gagner M, Pomp A, Dakin G, Milone L, Strain G. Cost comparison of reusable and single-use ultrasonic shears for laparoscopic bariatric surgery. *Obes Surg* 2010;20:512–8.

17 Powell H, Kwiatek E, Murray G. The ward manager's premier league. *Nurs Manage* 2005;12:12–5.

18 Association for Perioperative Practice. *Standards and Recommendations for Safe Perioperative Practice*. Harrogate: AfPP; 2007.

19 Berguer R. Surgery and ergonomics. *Arch Surg* 1999;134:1011–6.

20 Brogmus G, Leone W, Butler L, Hernandez E. Best practices in OR suite layout and equipment choices to reduce slips, trips, and falls. *AORN J* 2007;86:384–94.

21 Kenyon T A, Urbach D R, Speer J B, Waterman-Hukari B, Foraker G F, Hansen P D, et al. Dedicated minimally invasive surgery suites increase operating room efficiency. *Surg Endosc* 2001;15:1140–3.

22 van Det M J, Meijerink W J, Hoff C, van Veelen M A, Pierie J P. Ergonomic assessment of neck posture in the minimally invasive surgery suite during laparoscopic cholecystectomy. *Surg Endosc* 2008;22:2421–7.

23 Riedl S. [Modern operating room management in the workflow of surgery. Spectrum of tasks and challenges of the future]. *Anaesthesist* 2003;52:957–63. Article in German.

5

Energy sources and laparoscopy

Andrew Kent and Natasha Waters

Introduction

This chapter is a practical guide to the use of energy sources in laparoscopic gynaecology. There are three main categories of energy:

- electromagnetic energy (light or laser energy)

- mechanical energy

- electrical energy.

An understanding of the basic science and physics behind these modalities will enable a full appreciation of their individual qualities and result in using them to their full potential. Apart from lasers, none of these energy sources requires any formal training or certification.

We initially summarise the specific challenges in relation to the use of energy in the laparoscopic environment and then approach each category of energy modality in terms of its underlying science and practical application in laparoscopic surgery. We have avoided the discussion of specific instruments and concentrated on the understanding and use of each generic energy source wherever possible.

Challenges of the laparoscopic environment

Dissection and haemostasis are of particular importance in laparoscopic surgery, which explains the medical industry's continual efforts to produce better instruments by investing in new technologies. Laparoscopic surgery is different from the open approach and has the following specific features and limitations with regard to the use of different energy sources.

Limited space

The physical space is accessed by small ports, which can in turn restrict the range of movement. Most surgeons still rely on a two-dimensional image on screen, which reduces depth perception. Three-dimensional optics, for example in the *da Vinci®* (Intuitive Surgical, Sunnyvale, CA, USA) system or the new cinematographic three-dimensional systems that integrate into existing theatre environments, recover the perception of depth. With the robot, this comes at the cost of reducing the surgeon's perception of the overall operating environment, particularly outside of the patient, and the loss of tactile feedback, which helps to assess the grip force applied to tissues and to avoid the clashing of instruments.

Surgical exposure

The exposure of the surgical field is enhanced by laparoscopy, but the view can be compromised by blood, which absorbs white light. Areas of the abdomen behind the telescope's objective are not within the field of view. Energy may stray unseen into tissues out of the field of view, unintentionally causing damage. New developments in telescope technology such as the EndoCAMeleon® (Karl Storz, Tuttlingen, Germany) laparoscope, which has a variable angle of view (0–120°), may help to overcome these problems.

Smoke

Plume, or surgical smoke, is produced by both electrosurgery and laser. It is created by heating target cells to the point of boiling, which causes cell membranes to rupture. In addition to limiting the laparoscopic view, it contains chemicals and cellular contents, including virus and tumour particles, dispersing them into the peritoneal cavity.[1,2] If a port is opened or leaking, the high intra-abdominal pressure can create a 'chimney' effect, where smoke is released in a high-velocity jet with potential risk to the theatre team. This can also potentiate the risk of port site metastasis.[3–5]

With ultrasonically activated devices, an aerosol or vapour is generated, creating a fine mist of water or fat droplets, but no boiling occurs.[6]

Smoke can be extracted by a variety of vacuum or suction devices, but this active extraction can compromise the pneumoperitoneum. The alternative is passive extraction, whereby filters can be attached to a one-way valve to allow continuous filtration and ventilation of the pneumoperitoneum.[7]

Instrument functionality

Ideally, laparoscopic procedures should be carried out through as few small incisions as possible, as dictated by the procedure. Port planning and placement are crucial. Getting it wrong requires a further incision. Thus, multifunctional instruments combining coagulation, dissection, grasping and cutting give the advantage of fewer instrument changes.

Power density

The surface area of the operating tip of laparoscopic instruments can be small, with a consequential increase in the density of energy at the tissue. This can be an advantage, but in some circumstances the power level for laparoscopic surgery may have to be adjusted.

Thermal spread

Dissipation of heat is not as fast as in open surgery. Moreover, it is difficult to predict the degree of heating and spread of thermal energy in the tissues and its dissipation particularly in a multifunctional instrument.

Stray energy

Energy always travels the path of least resistance. This is particularly true of electrical energy. Inappropriate use of return plates can result in burns well away from the operating field. If an instrument is activated on the wrong target or without touching tissues, this can cause unintentional injury. Instruments are often not seen in full view. Insulation failure and failure to identify this before surgery, particularly in the case of reusable electrosurgical instruments, can result in unrecognised injury.

Laser energy

Lasers are a very safe energy source when they are used correctly. There can be a high set-up cost, although running costs for some lasers such as the carbon dioxide laser are relatively low. To put this into perspective, the use of lasers is much cheaper than purchasing or running a robot. Packaged with a laser comes a huge amount of legislation, far greater than that in place for any other surgical instrument. This often results in a perceived barrier to implementation.

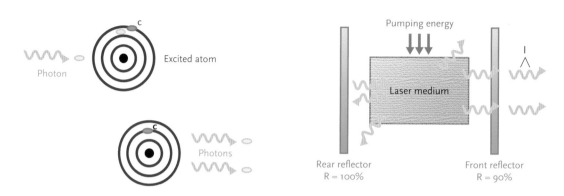

FIGURE 5.1 **Laser-stimulated emission**   FIGURE 5.2 **Laser schematic**

Laser energy: science

Light amplification by the stimulated emission of radiation (LASER) is a means whereby electromagnetic radiation is emitted via the process of stimulated emission. Photons are pumped into excited atoms in a laser medium, causing the ejection of additional photons (Figure 5.1). Eventually, the amount of stimulated emission owing to light that passes through the medium is larger than the amount of absorption (population inversion). Hence, the light is amplified. When such an optical amplifier is placed inside a reflective optical cavity and a certain wavelength is allowed to escape in a controlled fashion, one obtains a laser (Figure 5.2). The resulting laser beam is monochromatic (single wavelength), coherent (photons in phase), collimated (low divergence angle) and bright (high power density).

Lasers range right across the entire electromagnetic spectrum (Figure 5.3), but there are a few commonly used in gynaecology:

- carbon dioxide laser: an invisible infrared gas laser

- neodymium:yttrium–aluminium–garnet laser (Nd:YAG) laser: an invisible solid-state laser

- potassium–titanyl–phosphate (KTP) laser: a visible, bright emerald green solid-state laser

- helium–neon (HeNe) laser: a visible red gas laser often used as an aiming beam for the carbon dioxide and Nd:YAG lasers.

Laser spectrum		
Laser	Colour	Wavelength nm
Excimers	Ultraviolet	200–400
Argon	Blue	488
Argon	Green	515
KTP	Emerald green	532
Krypton	Green	531
Krypton	Yellow	568
Dye laser	Yellow/green	577
Dye laser	Red	630
Helium neon	Red	630
Gold vapour	Red	630
Krypton	Red	647
Ruby	Deep red	694
NdYAG	Infrared	1064
	Infrared	1318
CO$_2$	Infrared	10 600

FIGURE 5.3 **Laser spectrum**

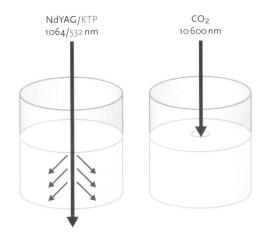

FIGURE 5.4 **Absorption of laser energy in water**

Gas lasers

Gas lasers using many different gases have been built and used for many purposes.

Carbon dioxide lasers operate in the infrared spectrum at 9600–10 600 nm and are incredibly versatile. Industrial carbon dioxide lasers can deliver outputs of several kilowatts and are often used in industry for cutting and welding. Medical lasers have a power output range of 10–100 W.

Medical carbon dioxide lasers can be incredibly precise ('what you see is what you get') and are completely absorbed by substances such as glass, water and other fluids (Figure 5.4). This means that they are theoretically 'safe' in the laparoscopic environment and are stopped by body fluids or fluid placed in the pelvis to act as a backstop during treatment.

The carbon dioxide laser, being a true beam laser, is delivered into the operative field via an articulated arm containing a series of mirrors (Figure 5.5). Being in the invisible infrared spectrum, it requires an aiming beam such as the red HeNe. It is important that the two are exactly aligned. This can be checked before surgery by firing the laser at an inert target and ensuring the treatment carbon dioxide laser hits the correct spot.

The HeNe laser emits at a variety of wavelengths and is ideal as an inert aiming beam for the invisible therapeutic lasers. Lasers operating at 633 nm with a power output of less than 1 mW are also very common in education as laser pointers.

Solid-state lasers

Solid-state laser materials are commonly made by contaminating ('doping') a pure crystalline solid with ions that create the appropriate energy state. For example, the first working laser was a ruby laser, made from a ruby (aluminium oxide) crystal where some of the aluminium atoms had been replaced with chromium atoms. Chromium absorbs blue and green light and reflects/emits only red light, hence the colour of the laser.

Neodymium is a 'dopant' in various solid-state laser crystals, including yttrium–aluminium–garnet. As with the carbon dioxide laser, Nd:YAG lasers have tissue effects at low power outputs of 10–100 W in the infrared spectrum at 1064 nm. At higher powers, they can also be used for cutting, welding and marking of metals and other materials, as well as in spectroscopy and for pumping dye lasers. These lasers are often frequency-doubled, frequency-tripled or frequency-quadrupled to produce the 532 nm (green, visible), 355 nm (ultraviolet) and 266 nm (ultraviolet) light, respectively. In the case of the KTP-532 laser, this is achieved by passing an Nd:YAG beam through a KTP crystal.

KTP and Nd:YAG lasers are delivered via semiflexible coated fibres (Figure 5.6). The Nd:YAG laser, being invisible, requires a red HeNe aiming beam, but the KTP laser appears as a visible bright green spot. The KTP laser is preferentially absorbed by red and brown pigments but can be used in clear fluids. The Nd:YAG laser passes through both.

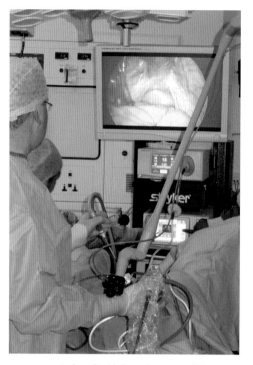

FIGURE 5.5 **Carbon dioxide laser (courtesy of Sigmacon)**

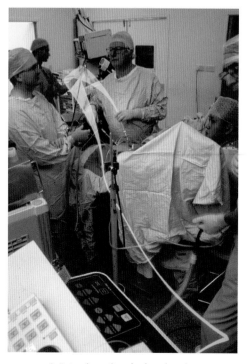

FIGURE 5.6 **Potassium–titanyl–phosphate laser**

Laparoscopic surgery and lasers

In the laparoscopic situation, lasers vaporise tissue, in effect sending it up in smoke. As a consequence, lasers can be used as a laser scalpel to excise tissue or to remove tissue en bloc, often referred to as laser ablation. To ablate means to remove and should not be confused with 'ablation' with bipolar diathermy, which is a technically incorrect use of the term because with bipolar electrosurgery tissue is desiccated and not removed.

The penetration, and therefore the surgical effect, of each laser is proportional to the relative scatter of laser light, which is a function of its wavelength and the type of target tissue. With regard to the type of target tissue, the important factors are the property and behaviour of the tissue surface – for example colour, reflectivity, density, water content and surface wetness – at the impact point of the laser.

The Nd:YAG laser has the highest penetration, particularly when used in bare fibre mode. As a consequence, some efforts have been made to control the energy penetration by adding a sapphire tip to the end of the laser fibre. This creates a wand with a hot tip, which rather negates the benefits of laser energy in laparoscopic surgery in that contact with the tissue is required for effect. The HeNe laser has no therapeutic effect of note and is used only as an aiming beam for the carbon dioxide laser.

From a practical point of view, we will therefore only discuss and compare the carbon dioxide and KTP lasers in terms of their use in laparoscopic surgery. Both are Class 4 lasers.

Before such lasers are used in any setting, all the safety boxes have to be ticked. The dangers are real but easy to protect against. Lasers are governed by a raft of legislation, but the key guidance is the Control of Artificial Optical Radiation at Work Regulations 2010.[8] Overseeing the safety issues are the laser protection advisor and laser protection supervisor, who usual work closely with a clinical laser expert (usually a clinician). Surgeons and laser operators must be authorised users.

Laparoscopic surgery and the carbon dioxide laser

Once down the articulated arm, the carbon dioxide laser beam is delivered into the abdomen via an operating laparoscope or a second side port. The former allows one fewer port and means that the laser beam and laparoscope are in the control of the surgeon and the laser is therefore always in view. It is usually activated by a foot switch.

The laser arm can be directly coupled to the laparoscope via a lens (Figure 5.7) (300 mm for an operating laparoscope, 200 mm for the shorter side tube),

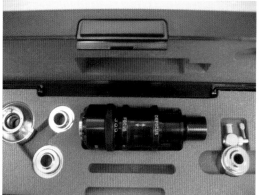

FIGURE 5.7 **Laparoscopic lens and couplers**

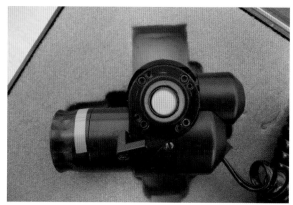

FIGURE 5.8 **SurgiTouch™ (Sharplan Lasers, London, UK)**

which allows focus and defocus of the laser beam. One can also interpose devices containing rotating mirrors between the lens and articulated arm. These mirrors spin the laser beam in a circle, the diameter of which can be varied (1–3 mm) (Figure 5.8). This increases the fluence of the laser over the target, allowing the use of higher power settings (30–50 W). This gives greater precision and more control to the surgeon. The higher power also enables the surgeon to overcome a wet surface, which would normally block any laser effect. Water will be vaporised by the laser, but this is dependent on time and the power density at the point of impact (POI).

Once connected for laparoscopic use, it is effectively a sealed system and the only way laser energy can escape is if the laser is disconnected or the telescope is removed from the abdomen.

The carbon dioxide laser is perfect for adhesiolysis and vaporising superficial and deep infiltrating endometriosis down to normal tissue. With care, it can be used over the bowel, ureters and bladder. As a general rule, there is very little tissue damage beyond the POI (50 nm). This laser has the advantages of speed, precision and control. As the beam stays focused over long distances, it can be aimed at some distance from the target, so allowing an excellent view of the surgical field. However, this can be a disadvantage if the laser overshoots. Fluid or nonreflective instruments can be used as a backstop to prevent overshoot and collateral damage.

The carbon dioxide laser can also be used as a laser scalpel to excise larger areas of deep endometriosis (Video 5.1) and, in conjunction with a haemostatic instrument such as bipolar diathermy, to divide vascular pedicles. At higher power, the carbon dioxide laser vaporises the fluid in the wet field associated with endometriomas by rapid heating, allowing destruction of the endometriotic tissue underneath. Activation at low power with a defocused beam can be used to coagulate bleeding points by desiccating tissue. This effect is also useful for fenestrating ovarian cysts or peeling back the petals of a salpingostomy in tubal surgery. Smoke can be a problem unless some form of extraction is used.

Laparoscopic surgery and the potassium–titanyl–phosphate laser

The KTP laser is delivered down a semiflexible fibre and is characterised by its bright green emerald light. The coated fibres, which are 1–1.5 mm in diameter, can be introduced down an irrigator or any instrument with a suitable operating channel. The laser energy is released by removing (stripping) the coating at the end of the fibre. With use, the end of the fibre can get burnt out, losing effectiveness and spot definition. This can then be cleaved or cut and re-stripped by the surgeon to restore function. Fibres can be reused many times by autoclaving the fibre coil, a practice followed for many years without any problems. However, some fibres are now often labelled as single-use, which increases the cost dramatically. The laser is usually foot-switch-activated.

The wavelength of the KTP-532 laser is ideally suited to the vaporisation of endometriotic deposits because it is preferentially absorbed by red and brown pigments. This means that when the KTP laser is used to treat endometriosis on the surface of the ovary, for example, the dark-pigmented deposits are rapidly vaporised, leaving the white surface of the ovarian cortex relatively untouched (Video 5.2). As it is not absorbed by water, the laser can be activated through irrigation and is particularly useful for ablating the lining of endometriomas.

As the energy is more penetrative, this laser is less suited for use over delicate structures such as the bowel or ureters compared with the carbon dioxide laser. Unlike the beam of the carbon dioxide laser, the beam of the KTP laser starts to spread (defocus) immediately after leaving the end of the fibre, so the further the tip of the fibre is away from the POI, the lower the tissue effect because the same energy is spread over a greater target area. This can be useful if ablating large areas but does result in less precision and control.

Ultrasonic energy

Laparoscopic surgery requires instruments that can cut and coagulate while minimising collateral damage and complications. Traditional techniques such as suturing and unipolar and bipolar diathermy were perceived as being potentially problematic or requiring a high skill set when used laparoscopically. Integration of ultrasonic energy into a usable surgical hand piece began

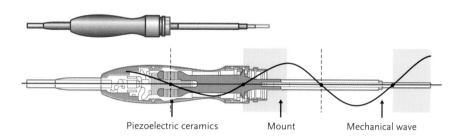

FIGURE 5.9 **Ultrasonic technology (courtesy of Ethicon Endo-Surgery, a division of Johnson & Johnson Medical Ltd)**

Piezoelectric ceramics   Mount   Mechanical wave

in the early 1990s in the USA and Japan. The first instruments were fairly rudimentary and available only for open use. They quickly developed into usable laparoscopic instruments that provided precise cutting and coagulation in one action and one instrument with little collateral tissue damage.

Ultrasonic energy: science

Ultrasonic instruments are piezoelectric devices that convert electrical energy into mechanical energy (ultrasound vibration) (Figure 5.9). This conversion invariably takes place in a reusable hand piece, which in turn is transferred to the blade tip via a disposable or limited-life reusable instrument.

There are four key tissue effects, all of which occur at the same time: coaptation, coagulation, cavitation and cutting. The relative impact of these tissue effects can be modified by the surgeon to enhance dissection, cutting or coagulation.

Coaptation

The vibration of the active blade causes defragmentation of proteins by breaking tertiary hydrogen bonds. The tissue protein is transformed into a sticky coaptate that seals smaller vessels.

Coagulation

Secondary heat from friction causes protein denaturation, sealing larger vessels. In practice, there is a fluent transition between coaptation and coagulation (Figure 5.10).

Cavitation

The vibrating tip of the active blade produces transient pressure changes in the tissue, which cause extracellular and intracellular water to vaporise at low

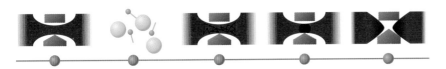

| Coagulation with Harmonic requires collapsing of the blood vessel | H+ bonds are broken; protein in the cells is denatured | Denatured protein forms a sticky coagulum | Internal tissue heat generated from friction then seals or welds vessel walls | Simultaneous cutting and coagulation takes place at a lower temperature than electrosurgery with minimal lateral thermal spread |

FIGURE 5.10 **Ultrasonic coagulation (courtesy of Ethicon Endo-Surgery, a division of Johnson & Johnson Medical Ltd)**

temperatures. This agitated water vapour (it is not steam) expands the tissue planes, causing separation along the natural planes of cleavage. This enhances anatomical dissection, which in turn aids surgery.

Cutting

In the majority of instruments, the active blade vibrates back and forth (50–100 micrometres) at around 55 000 Hz. The alternative is an active blade that rocks from side to side. The vibrating blade edge cuts tissue by stretching it beyond its elastic limit. In effect, this is a hot saw. As a consequence, this energy not only cuts tissue but can divide sutures and mesh, which can be very useful in repeat surgery.

Laparoscopic surgery and ultrasonic energy

There are various factors that allow the surgeon to control the balance of the above tissue effects. For simplicity, these are described in relation to instruments with longitudinal action as opposed to rocking action.

Power

Variance in 'power' is in effect achieved by altering the range of movement of the active blade. A low power setting (settings 1–3) causes the blade to move in and out by 50 micrometres, which in turn increases coagulation and decreases the speed of cutting. A higher power setting causes the blade to move by 80–100 micrometres, resulting in higher stretching forces, which causes faster cutting with less coagulation. A simple analogy is a tenon saw; the longer the stroke, the faster the cutting action. Occasionally, the power may need to be modified by the surgeon in reaction to changing tissue characteristics.

Sharpness

The sharper the active edge that is in contact with the tissue, the faster the cut. This depends on the configuration of the active blade. Some instruments have different edges, which can be brought into contact with the tissue as required.

Tissue tension

Tissue tension is probably the main factor that can be controlled by the surgeon and that can be varied on a continuous basis to achieve the desired surgical effect (the balance between cutting and coagulation). The higher the tissue tension, the faster the cutting action. The lower the tissue tension, the higher the coagulation and coaptation effect.

Blade pressure

Blade pressure can be controlled in two ways. Firstly, grip force is controlled with the shears themselves. The higher the pressure, the faster the cut. The second factor is actual pressure of the active blade in contact with the tissue. Even with the shears closed to maximal grip force, if the tissue is levered against the inactive blade, the cut will be slower with increased coagulation. Opposite leverage against the active blade will allow the instrument to pass through the tissue much faster.

Time

The longer the application time, the higher the transfer of energy. This can be particularly useful if coagulation is required without cutting, in which case 5–7 beats of energy will usually suffice, depending on the diameter and type of vessel.

Appreciation of tissue characteristics

Together with tissue tension, it is important to appreciate the type of tissue and its actual characteristics. A nodule of deep infiltrating endometriosis is denser than fat, for example. A tissue with higher water content takes longer to cut and coagulate. Likewise, if there is blood or fluid flowing over the active blade, a higher power setting may be required to achieve the desired tissue effect so as to overcome the cooling effect of the fluid on the active blade.

    The advantage of ultrasonic devices (Video 5.3) is that cutting, coagulation and cavitation all happen at the same time in one instrument. This allows for seamless surgery with minimal need for instrument change. The end result is a quicker operation, even though the tissue effect itself seems slower. The instruments also require fewer actual movements to achieve dissection and haemostatic division of tissue compared with equivalent bipolar devices. Activation is usually either by hand on the instrument itself or via a foot pedal.

Rapid dissection can be achieved in normal tissue using shears in an almost scissor-like action. This is aided by the cavitation wave opening up the normal tissue planes. This can also be achieved in avascular tissue by use of the back of the shears or a hook as a true ultrasonic scalpel. This scalpel effect is also very useful in subtotal hysterectomies, when it can be used to divide the uterocervical junction. There is no requirement for unipolar diathermy or loops. Consequently, just one operating port is often sufficient to complete the operation.

The division of vascular pedicles is simple and straightforward. Various manufacturers quote a maximum vessel diameter of 5 mm for 100% haemostasis every time, but in reality this is conservative. However, one must also take into account extra perivascular tissue in this measurement. In essence, this means that the greater the preparation of the pedicle, the greater the diameter of the vessel that can be taken securely.

One of the greatest benefits of this energy source is its mechanical nature and its inherent safety. There is no chance of stray mechanical energy. If energy ends up in the wrong target, it is put there by the surgeon. A by-product of the mechanical energy is thermal energy, which is harnessed by the surgeon. Thermal spread or blanching is said to be less than 1 mm, most of which is reversible damage as actual tissue temperatures remain low. However, heat is temporarily retained in the active blade, so care should be taken when using it as a dissector immediately after heavy usage.

These properties highlight the multifunctional capability of ultrasonic energy, which in turn gives an enviable versatility in laparoscopic surgery that cannot be matched by any of the other energy sources. The real benefit for the woman undergoing the operation is quicker, safer surgery with minimal collateral damage to remaining tissue and a requirement for fewer ports.

Electrosurgical energy

Since electrosurgery was introduced into surgical practice in the 1920s, it has broadened the range and complexity of operations that can be performed safely, with better haemostasis and fewer complications. It is still the energy most commonly used by surgeons in both open and laparoscopic surgery for achieving haemostasis and tissue effects such as cutting, coagulation and their combination.

Basic knowledge of physics and the principles of electricity among surgeons remains poor. A survey[9] of trainees in the UK revealed that 69% did not know the difference between cutting and coagulation and 45% did not know the difference between bipolar and monopolar diathermy. Some 10% did not

Monopolar circuit
- Current flows from an electrode through the patient to a ground electrode/pad
- The patient is vital to completing the circuit

Bipolar circuit
- Current is applied to the patient using two closely approximated electrodes
- Electrical current flows from one electrode to the other through the intervening tissue only

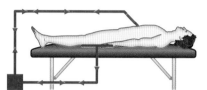
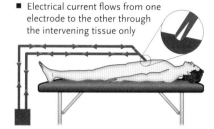

FIGURE 5.11 **Electrical circuits (courtesy of Ethicon Endo-Surgery, a division of Johnson and Johnson Medical Ltd)**

correctly identify the 'coag' pedal as the blue pedal. Interestingly, attending a basic surgical skills course did not seem to improve the answers significantly. There is currently no standardised teaching on this subject in the gynaecological curriculum.

Unipolar electrosurgery: science

A closed radiofrequency current is converted from the mains electricity supply by a generator. An alternating domestic electrical current with a frequency of 50 Hz is converted to a current with a frequency of 400 000–600 000 Hz. Because of the frequency increase, the passage of electrons occurs only at the external surface of the conductor (tissue) and therefore neuromuscular stimulation and tetany are avoided (faradic effect). The current passes through the body and returns to the generator via a return electrode to complete a closed circuit (Figure 5.11). The current will, however, always follow the path of least resistance. When used on the tissues, the electrical current is converted into thermal energy and causes three biological effects (dissection and coagulation, which is divided into fulguration and desiccation).

Two types of current are used: cutting and coagulation. Dissection and desiccation can be achieved with both currents but with different application techniques, whereas fulguration can be produced only by use of the coagulation current.

The cutting current is an alternating high-frequency, low-voltage current that is on all the time (Figure 5.12). The effect of dissecting or cutting tissues is achieved by the cutting current, which rapidly heats up intracellular water to 100°C. The intracellular water boils, the cell membrane ruptures causing explosive vaporisation and the division of tissues ensues, causing dissection or cutting. The lateral thermal spread is minimal and so is the depth of necrosis (Video 5.4).

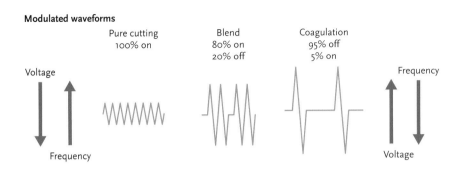

Modulated waveforms

FIGURE 5.12 **Modulated unipolar electrosurgical waveforms**

The coagulating current uses a high-voltage interrupted current (Figure 5.12). It is on only 5% of the time, which allows cooling periods that permit slow dehydration of the cellular fluid and protein. Protein denaturation starts at around 50–80°C, with blanching of tissue as a visible external change. The trihelical structure of collagen is disrupted, which results in shrinkage. When cells heat up to 200–300°C, tissue will carbonise from dehydration. With continued heating of the tissue, the hydrocarbons combust, resulting in vaporisation. Desiccation ensues by making contact with the active electrode to the tissue. This produces a deep necrosis and a sticking eschar. If the coagulation mode is used in noncontact mode with the tissue, a fulguration effect is produced. It sprays electric sparks to the tissue, producing a superficial eschar with minimal tissue necrosis. The accuracy of fulguration can be difficult to control with standard electrodes.

To a certain degree, the accuracy of fulguration can be controlled and focused by use of an inert gas jet as used in some argon or helium beam coagulators. This allows the spark to travel down the jet of gas, focusing the energy at the POI and giving greater accuracy. The tissue effect is superficial with little control over depth. This technology is therefore of limited use with deep infiltrating endometriosis and is not designed for the division of vascular pedicles.

A variation on this theme is plasma jet technology. Plasma is defined as a gas in which a certain proportion of the particles are ionised resulting in an electrically neutral medium of positive and negative particles. It has been popularised in the form of novelty plasma lamps and globes. A jet of argon gas is excited into the plasma state by use of a low direct electrosurgical current passing across a series of electrodes. The 'plasma' emerges from the tip of the hand piece as a precise pale blue plume. Its surgical effect is brought about by heat, resulting in surface coagulation of tissue and a degree of kinetic energy, which disperses the tissue fragments. In essence, it resembles a mini-blowtorch. Again, control of the depth of the effect is limited and there may be concern regarding the uncontrolled spread of particles within the laparoscopic environment. Coagulation and haemostasis are superficial. This technology is not designed for dividing pedicles.

Both inert gas coagulators and plasma jets have the theoretical risk of vascular embolism if inadvertently directed into an open vessel.

The main problem with unipolar electrosurgical energy is the risk of stray electrical and thermal energy both inside and outside the woman. Failure to apply a return plate, or applying it incorrectly, can result in skin burns if the skin comes into contact with a grounded conductor. This risk can be significantly reduced with the use of adherent gel return plates with integrated monitors and alarms built into the electrosurgical generators.

Inside the woman, energy can also escape through damaged insulation on laparoscopic instruments, resulting in unintentional burns on tissue out of the line of sight. There is also the very rare capacitance effect, which is unique to laparoscopic surgery. This can result in a high-power energy discharge (spark) when hybrid plastic and metal ports are used. These types of port are no longer available.

Energy tracking can cause inadvertent collateral damage. For example, if an ovary is lifted away from the sidewall and unipolar diathermy is applied to treat endometriosis or 'drill' the ovary, the current will take the easiest route back to the return plate, which is often up the ovarian pedicle or down the ovarian ligament. The energy is concentrated in the pedicle track and may coagulate the vessels unintentionally. Providing the ovary with a broad contact base against the sidewall or uterus avoids this, allowing the energy to flow from the ovary into the body and back to the return plate, so completing the circuit.

Bipolar electrosurgical energy: science

Bipolar electrosurgery (Video 5.5) overcomes many of these problems by incorporating both electrodes into the surgical instrument (Figure 5.11, page 84). The current passes between the two electrodes so that only the tissue in between is desiccated. As with unipolar diathermy, the electrical energy is converted into thermal energy on passage through the tissue with subsequent biological effects. Most bipolar electrosurgical energy devices used in laparoscopic surgery can only be used in coagulation mode. Bipolar devices that cut are more commonly used in hysteroscopic surgery. They are ideally suited for the coagulation and haemostasis of vascular pedicles, but additional devices are required for division. These can be incorporated into the bipolar device (sliding blades) or remain separate (scissors).

As a consequence, the usefulness of bipolar devices for dissection and the division of nonvascular tissue is limited. There also remains the problem of lateral thermal and electrical spread, which, although less than with unipolar coagulation, is still a significant factor that can result in collateral damage to delicate structures such as the ureter and bowel.

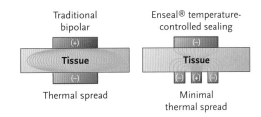

FIGURE 5.13 **Offset electrode configuration (courtesy of Ethicon Endo-Surgery, a division of Johnson & Johnson Medical Ltd)**

Minimising the thermal effect of bipolar devices

A variety of novel systems have been developed to deliver clever bipolar electrosurgical energy to the tissues in as safe and effective ways as possible while minimising the lateral thermal spread. Various instruments are available, all working in slightly different ways to achieve a similar effect. They are all designed for taking pedicles and do not have the multifunctional capability associated with other energy delivery systems.

EnSeal® system

The EnSeal® (Ethicon Endo-Surgery, Cincinnati, OH, USA) system employs temperature-controlled tissue-sealing technology. The instrument's jaws are configured in such a way that the electrosurgical energy is held close to the instrument tip (Figure 5.13). The lower jaw is a bipolar instrument in its own right with the two electrodes separated by a thin layer of zircon. The upper jaw is a second return electrode. The surfaces of the electrodes are coated in a polymer that in its cool state allows the flow of electrons down the contiguous carbon chains. As it heats up, these chains are broken up, disrupting the flow of energy to those areas that have reached operating temperature. This micromanages the flow of energy throughout the instrument jaws, allowing vessel sealing at lower overall temperatures with a consequent reduction in thermal spread (Figures 5.13 and 5.14).

The technology can reliably seal vessels of up to 7 mm in diameter. Tissue is divided by a cutting blade that is I-shaped in cross-section. This passes down between the jaws in a single movement as the jaws are closed, compressing the tissue in between even further. Energy activation is via a trigger on the front of the handle. It can be used to cut tissue other than pedicles but is not designed as a dissector or scalpel. The new generator is housed in the same unit as that used for the Harmonic ACE® (Ethicon Endo-Surgery, Cincinnati, OH, USA) device.

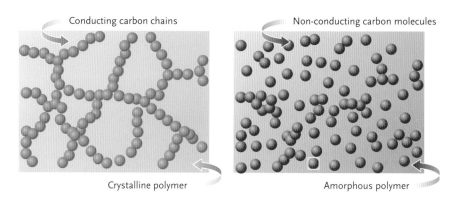

FIGURE 5.14 **Carbon polymer blade coating (courtesy of Ethicon Endo-Surgery, a division of Johnson & Johnson Medical Ltd)**

Vapour pulse coagulation

Vapour pulse coagulation is used by the PlasmaKinetic® system (Gyrus Medical, Maple Grove, MN, USA) and delivers energy in a pulsed manner, with the dedicated generator controlling the on/off cycle. During the off phase, the tissue cools, which reduces hot spots. This in turn allows uniform vessel sealing and reduces thermal spread. Again, tissue division is via a blade passed between the jaws, requiring a separate movement once the generator has indicated tissue desiccation is complete.

This instrument is designed for taking pedicles and is limited in terms of dissection and other tissue division.

Ligasure™ system

The Ligasure™ (Valleylab, Boulder, CO, USA) system uses energy and pressure to create vessel fusion, melting the collagen and elastin in the vessel wall to create a seal across the pedicle, which is then divided by a blade that passes between the jaws in a separate movement once sealing is complete. This is controlled by the dedicated electrosurgical unit.

This system is designed for pedicles with a maximum vessel diameter of 7 mm, but has limited use on other tissues such as the uterosacral ligaments or uterocervical junction in subtotal hysterectomy.

Laparoscopic surgery and electrosurgical energy

The effect of electrosurgical energy on tissues is multifactorial. It depends on the waveform chosen (cutting, coagulation or blended current) and the circuit type (monopolar or bipolar). The size of the electrode is of particular importance in laparoscopy, where the surface areas on the tips of the instruments are generally smaller than those in open surgery. The smaller the contact with the tissue, the higher the current density, which results in a more rapid thermal effect, exploding cells. This in turn results in vaporisation with little collateral damage. Tissue effect is also dependent on power settings. Generally, lower power settings are required compared with open surgery. Time of exposure and surgical technique of application (contact/noncontact mode), tissue type (adipose tissue has a higher resistance than vessels) and eschar formation are important. Once eschar coats a tip of the electrode, resistance rises and voltage (current flow) increases significantly for the same amount of power. This could lead to stray energy travelling to structures in close proximity.

Conclusion

Energy is just like any other surgical tool. It is only by understanding the science behind it and knowing how it works that one can truly use it safely, to optimum effect.

References

1 Ott D. Smoke production and smoke reduction in endoscopic surgery: preliminary report. *Endosc Surg Allied Technol* 1993;1:230–2.

2 Hensman C, Baty D, Willis R G, Cuschieri A. Chemical composition of smoke produced by high-frequency electrosurgery in a closed gaseous environment. An in vitro study. *Surg Endosc* 1998;12:1017–9.

3 Tseng L N, Berends F J, Wittich P, Bouvy N D, Marquet R L, Kazemier G, et al. Port-site metastases. Impact of local tissue trauma and gas leakage. *Surg Endosc* 1998;12:1377–80.

4 Wang P H, Yen M S, Yuan C C, Chao K C, Ng H T, Lee W L, et al. Port site metastasis after laparoscopic-assisted vaginal hysterectomy for endometrial cancer: possible mechanisms and prevention. *Gynecol Oncol* 1997;66:151–5.

5 Wang P H, Yuan C C, Lin G, Ng H T, Chao H T. Risk factors contributing to early occurrence of port site metastases of laparoscopic surgery for malignancy. *Gynecol Oncol* 1999;72:38–44.

6 Ott D E, Moss E, Martinez K. Aerosol exposure from an ultrasonically activated (Harmonic) device. *J Am Assoc Gynecol Laparosc* 1998;5:29–32.

7 Barrett W L, Garber S M. Surgical smoke: a review of the literature. Is this just a lot of hot air? *Surg Endosc* 2003;17:979–87.

8 Control of Artificial Optical Radiation at Work Regulations 2010 [www.legislation.gov.uk/uksi/2010/1140/contents/made].

9 Pandey U, Killick S R, Lindow S W. Obstetrics and gynaecology trainees' knowledge of electrosurgical equipment. *J Obstet Gynaecol* 2007;27:721–2.

6 Training

Jeremy Wright and Karen Ballard

Introduction

The acquisition of skills, especially laparoscopic skills, in surgical training has moved from a time-based to a competency-based training programme, with predetermined levels of skill acquisition needing to be achieved. The formulaic approach to this competency-based training aims to provide more objective forms of assessment. This shift in training has been driven in part by the European Working Time Directive, competing needs of the service and frequent rotation of doctors in training from hospital to hospital and, within the hospital, from service to service. Against this background, there is now strong evidence[1] that all adnexal surgery for benign gynaecological pathology and the management of ectopic pregnancy is best performed using minimal access techniques as it results in significantly reduced short-term and long-term morbidity.[2] The evidence for the use of minimal access techniques for hysterectomy is less clear,[3] although laparoscopic hysterectomy and vaginal hysterectomy have been shown to significantly reduce complications compared with abdominal hysterectomy.[4] Despite this evidence, the majority of hysterectomies are still carried out using the abdominal route, possibly because this is the procedure that most gynaecologists feel comfortable with. This is in part because they have not had the opportunity to train in minimal access techniques.

The European Society of Human Reproduction and Embryology[5] and the Royal College of Obstetricians and Gynaecologists (RCOG)[6] recommend that endometriosis is best managed surgically in specialist centres. As yet, in the UK these specialist centres have not been established, although various groups with the necessary expertise are beginning to offer this surgery and publish their audited results. Currently, however, it is not known how many women with deep infiltrating endometriosis are offered the appropriate recommended treatment, or whether this is being carried out by groups with the necessary endoscopic skill. It is likely that many women are denied surgery or have extensive surgery at laparotomy carried out by those without the appropriate understanding of the disease or the requisite surgical skill. It

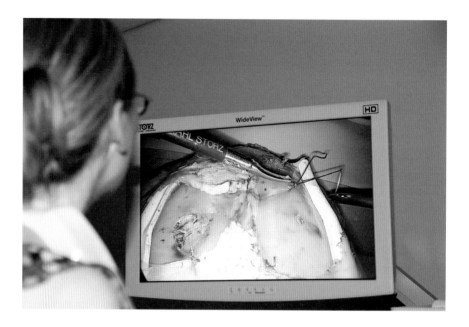

is thus apparent that there is a requirement to address these training needs to help ensure that women are offered the appropriate surgery by the appropriately trained and skilled specialists. Currently, the RCOG offers two Advanced Training Skills Modules (ATSMs) in operative laparoscopy. Diagnostic laparoscopy is taught as a core skill. Individuals who have completed the ATSM covering laparoscopy for benign gynaecological conditions will be:[7]

- able to select and counsel woman appropriate for laparoscopic surgery

- familiar with the instruments, equipment and energy sources used in laparoscopic surgery

- competent at intermediate-level laparoscopic surgery

- aware of the limits of their skills in laparoscopic surgery and refer women to appropriate colleagues for advanced laparoscopic surgery.

Attendance at an RCOG/British Society for Gynaecological Endoscopy (BSGE) theory course on laparoscopic surgery is also required during this training module.

The RCOG and BSGE have more recently agreed an advanced ATSM for those wishing to train in the advanced techniques required for managing such conditions as hysterectomy, deep infiltrating endometriosis and myomectomy. Other areas of expertise are advanced laparoscopic techniques in oncology, but these are assessed in the oncology subspecialist training module because laparoscopy is not considered a special skill. If, as was suggested at the beginning of this chapter, the majority of benign gynaecology operations were to be carried out either vaginally or laparoscopically, possibly by accredited gynaecological surgeons, this would further emphasise the need to ensure that these surgeons are appropriately trained and assessed to undertake such surgery.

The issues that we face then are not only the delivery of high-quality skills training both for gynaecologists in training and for those who already hold their Certificate of Completion of Training, but also the implementation of a mechanism for assessing competence in these skills. To do this, we need to understand how adults learn skills, how these skills are best taught and maintained while preserving the highest standards of patient safety, and how these skills are assessed and reassessed as appropriate. There are only a few units offering skills training in the UK. These units offer either 'dry lab' training, in which manip-

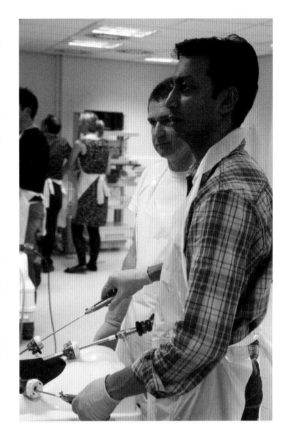

ulative skills are taught using simple equipment (for example, piling sugar lumps, placing dried peas into containers or removing boiled sweets from their wrappers) or training in more advanced skills, for example intracorporeal suturing taught on rubber models in pelvic trainers (Video 6.1). As discussed later in the chapter, there is evidence[8] to suggest that these techniques are perfectly adequate to teach these early skills.

Further skills using energy sources such as diathermy, ultrasonic dissectors and various forms of laser energy can be taught using 'wet' preparations such as porcine bowel and chicken pieces with the skin left on. Much ingenuity has gone into developing suitable models for teaching laparoscopic surgery, such as tomatoes placed in porcine bowel representing ectopic pregnancy and ox tongue to teach morcellation techniques. There is continuous development of many of these models to improve technical skills. Since re-examination of the Human Tissues Act, fresh or fresh/frozen cadaver specimens are increasingly being used to teach laparoscopic anatomy and dissection.

The manufacturers of laparoscopic equipment have also developed teaching laboratories allowing the use of live porcine models under very strict conditions to teach laparoscopic surgical techniques. There are few of these laboratories in Europe and it is illegal to train on live animals in the UK. A possible limitation exists in that teaching in these laboratories is often directed towards the use of specific equipment. Much of the development of, and training in, the use of new energy sources and equipment is thus led, promoted and paid for by the manufacturers of this equipment and as such is directed at those who are most likely to be in a position to advise the National Health Service on the purchase of the equipment. There are relatively few opportunities for doctors in training to have exposure to this advanced-level training. There is also evidence to show that this advanced-level training has limited value for surgeons with little more than basic surgical skills training.

In this chapter, we consider the evidence to support the need for a structured laparoscopic skills training programme. We then consider the educational literature on the principles underpinning effective learning of clinical skills. Finally, we use the evidence to discuss different ways in which laparoscopic skills can be taught and offer suggestions on how competence may be assessed effectively.

The photographs in this chapter illustrate some of the training techniques that can be used in laparoscopic surgery.

The need for training in laparoscopic skills

There seems to be little doubt from the available published literature that the complication rate in laparoscopic surgery, of whatever specialty, decreases with increasing experience. A prospective multicentre observational study[9] of nearly 26 000 laparoscopic procedures showed (using a step-wise logistic regression analysis) that with increasing experience, particularly in operative laparoscopy, the risk of complications decreased. In their discussion, the authors argue that training in diagnostic procedures and simple operative procedures such as laparoscopic sterilisation increases the skills of residents and doctors in training so that when they came to undertake more complex procedures, they are able to quickly build on their basic skills and their complication rate is decreased.

Similarly, a multicentre study[10] of some 7500 diagnostic and laparoscopic operations demonstrated that increased experience by the surgeons significantly reduced the number of bowel injuries and complications requiring laparotomy, and increased the ability to deal with any complications laparoscopically.

These data from gynaecological surgery reflect the findings in upper gastrointestinal surgery, colorectal surgery and laparoscopic urology. In a study[11]

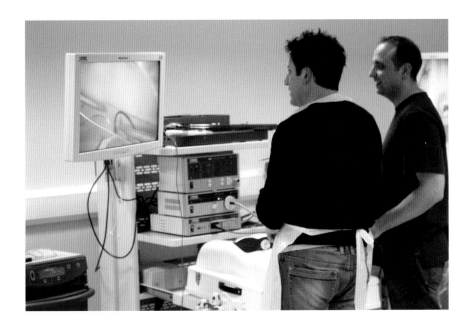

looking at laparoscopic jejunogastric bypass, with 150 consecutive people split into three historical 50-person cohorts, operating time and technically related complications decreased with time, even though the last cohort had a greater body mass index and had had prior abdominal surgery or received a second operative procedure at the same time.

In colorectal surgery, Schlachta et al.[12] reported on 461 consecutive people undergoing colorectal resection and showed that the rates of intraoperative complications and conversion to open surgery, and the operating time in people who required conversion, declined with increasing experience of the surgeon. Similarly, Ahlering et al.[13] showed that proficiency with laparoscopic radical prostatectomy could be achieved by an experienced laparoscopic surgeon after 40–60 procedures and by a skilled surgeon without laparoscopic experience after 80–100 procedures.

From this literature, it would seem that for skilled and experienced laparoscopic surgeons, approximately 50 procedures are required to become competent in complex procedures. For laparoscopically naïve surgeons, it may be between 80 and 100 procedures, provided they have sufficient competence at open surgery.

A survey[14] of 181 participants undertaking a laparoscopic urological surgery course showed that surgeons who were in single-handed practice and performed procedures with different, rather than regular, assistants each time were four times more likely to have complications than surgeons who sought additional training. Of particular interest in this survey was that surgeons

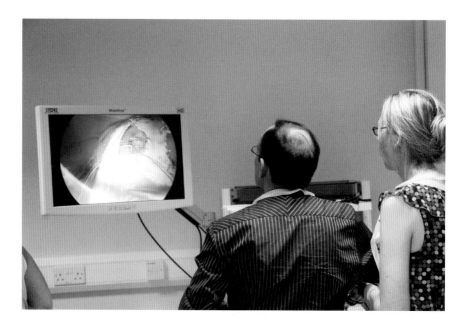

who operated with the same assistant or in a group practice and whose partners had attended the same course had a significantly reduced complication
rate, showing the importance of team training and team working. Similarly,
Menon et al.[15] showed that a structured laparoscopic radical prostatectomy
programme dramatically improved performance in both laparoscopic radical
prostatectomies and robot-assisted prostatectomies. The authors also found
that participation in a longer programme of training, as opposed to attendance at a single training session, significantly improved patient outcome and
reduced morbidity. Concerns arise, however, in whether the skills acquired
in the laboratory setting are retained. There is considerable evidence[16] that
practice on a simulator improves the ability to perform the functions set on
that simulator quickly over a very short period of time, but it is not known
whether these skills are lost again if procedures are not practised frequently.

These studies suggest that short courses are of little value in improving
laparoscopic skills or increasing patient safety. It would thus seem apparent
that a consistent training programme, training as a team and experience in
the laboratory help with gaining proficiency and reducing complications.

Having established that training programmes, when delivered over a
period of time, reduce the complication rate associated with laparoscopic surgery, we now consider the principles underpinning effective learning within a
clinical skills training programme.

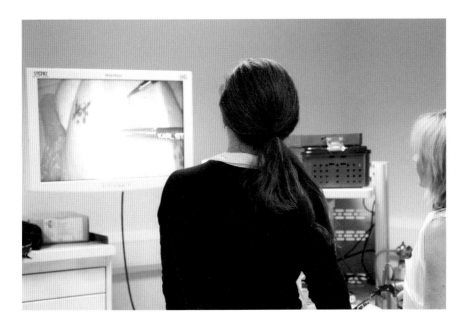

Principles underpinning effective learning of clinical skills

Most people will recall being taught by someone who really inspired them to learn. This person will have been able to explain new concepts or skills clearly and will generally have been doing so with enthusiasm. They will often display self-confidence and, by respecting and believing in the learner, they instil this confidence in the learner. The good teacher will also find ways to engage the learner in the new activity, providing intellectual challenges but also fostering a sense of student control in learning. Most people, however, will also recall being taught by someone who was unable to explain new information and who, by conveying a distinct uncertainty about the subject matter, reduced the quality of the learning experience. While some people do appear to have a natural teaching ability, it is possible for everyone to enhance their teaching skills by understanding the process by which people learn new knowledge and skills. In the following section, we outline two key learning theories that are useful for understanding how gynaecologists develop laparoscopic skills. We then consider the value of different learning environments and discuss how effective they are for training in laparoscopic gynaecology.

Learning theories

There are two key learning theories – behaviourism or association and cognitive development – that are useful for understanding the ways in which laparoscopic skills may be best taught.

Theories of behaviourism or association involve learning by association with previous understanding or learning (for example Skinner, Piaget; cited by Mazur[17]). Here, the student will learn through a series of small steps or stages, using learning from different stages to build a composite skill. Learning occurs when rewards are received for correct learning and therefore it is essential that the teacher provides immediate feedback on good and poor performance. The theory relies on a sequential model of learning and therefore the learner needs to master the basic skills before they can move on to higher-level skills. Learning relies on the student being able to associate the skills learnt at one level with those required at a higher level and on the teacher being able to break down the training into small manageable chunks that link to each other.

Theories of learning through cognitive development, on the other hand, involve active understanding and problem solving (for example Piaget, Bruner; cited by Bereiter[18]). Here, the student will learn from active discovery and experimentation, often through problem solving. The 'active' learner is encouraged to interact and engage with the learning task to allow them to find their own individual ways of understanding the problem. The teacher provides feedback on the learning and, through reflection on this, the student develops further understanding. Influenced by this approach to learning, contemporary teaching has shifted away from a series of traditional didactic lectures, where the teacher imparts new knowledge to the rows of passive students, eagerly waiting to absorb the teacher's wisdom. This active approach to learning is now widely adopted in the undergraduate medical teaching programme, so will not be new to students, but it may not be easily understood by those whose undergraduate education was predominately didactic in nature.

The idea of learning through participation is emphasised in other learning theories, for example experiential learning,[19] which is based on the premise that prior experiences are used within learning situations and are built upon in the search of new understanding. This focus on participative learning stems from the idea that students will adopt a deeper approach to learning, which, in turn, enables different aspects of knowledge to be related in the process of understanding a concept.[20] This is in contrast to a surface approach to learning, whereby numerous 'facts' are learnt but rarely seen as part of a whole concept.

In both the behaviourism learning theory and the cognitive development learning theory, the feedback provided by the teacher or the trainer is imperative, facilitating the movement to the next stage of skill development or helping the learner to reflect on their performance and develop further skills based on this reflection.

Teaching laparoscopic skills

Traditionally, the apprenticeship model of teaching clinical skills has been adopted, with the apprentice observing and assisting the 'master' to imitate these skills. The apprentice adopts any actions that are seen to result in rewards or success and rejects those that result in failure. Although this approach to training has, in the past, been popular, its reliance on passive learning encourages surface rather than deep learning. It works best in practice when the apprentice is allowed to undertake the procedure assisted by, and under the direct supervision of, the 'master'. Master classes in which attendees observe surgery on video links distant from the surgery have limited learning opportunity unless they are facilitated by skilled teachers, with interactive discussion. Their value lies in the ability of the student to observe how technical difficulties are dealt with when they are encountered in these live conditions. The apprenticeship model has, however, largely broken down, with reduced working hours and accelerated training requiring new methods of ensuring competency in a shorter time.

To move towards a more participative approach to training and to gain maximum benefit from training in the operative theatre environment, the trainee requires some basic laparoscopic manipulative skills. This, coupled with the more limited time that trainees spend in the operating theatre, means that it is essential that the trainee arrives in theatre armed with a basic level of training. Physical simulators such as pelvic training boxes provide an ideal and relatively inexpensive opportunity for the trainee to gain these initial laparoscopic skills, and have been shown in small randomised controlled trials to be effective in improving suturing skills[21] and time and accuracy of laparoscopic tasks[22,23] when compared with no training. These skills learnt on physical simulators have also been found to translate to improved competence within the operating theatre.[24]

Further training opportunities exist with the use of virtual reality surgical simulation, although the costs prohibit this from being as widely available as the physical simulators. Again, relatively small randomised controlled trials have found virtual reality simulators to be effective in improving laparoscopic skills, both when tested within the laboratory[8] and when tested within the operating theatre.[25,26]

Although virtual reality trainers have gained popularity, there is no conclusive evidence to show that they are more effective in laparoscopic skills training than simple physical reality trainers. For example, two randomised controlled trials[27,28] showed no difference in skills gained with a virtual reality trainer compared with a physical reality trainer, whereas another two randomised controlled trials[23,29] showed the virtual reality simulator to be more effective than the physical reality trainer. A key difficulty in interpreting this evidence lies in the study design, with small sample sizes (between 20 and 46 in total), absence of power calculations, differences in the types of outcome measured and differences in the amount of training provided.

While both physical and virtual reality trainers clearly have a role in training in laparoscopic gynaecology, we suggest that they are an adjunct to the more traditional training that takes place within the operating theatre. Indeed, we were able to find only two randomised controlled trials that compared the standard operating theatre training with simulated training: one study[30] reported that surgeons who had virtual reality training performed better than those who had traditional training; the other[31] reported equal performance in both virtual-reality- and traditionally trained surgeons.

Development of a laparoscopic training programme

While we have discussed the potential learning opportunities associated with reality trainers, this is dependent upon the type of training that is provided. Although there are no validated structured training programmes that specify the tasks to be completed and the level of competence to be achieved,[32,33] evidence from studies can be used to draw some guidelines about training in laparoscopic gynaecology. It has been shown that the learning curve of inexperienced surgeons plateaus once the procedure has been performed between five[34] and seven[33] times.

Studies have shown that the development of clinical skills is enhanced by the integration of a cognitive component to the training programme,[35] with pathophysiological explanations, visual demonstration and case studies providing variation in the learning experience and engaging the trainee in active learning. The use of computer-assisted instruction, with tutorials delivered by a CD-ROM, provides easily accessible learning opportunities that can be undertaken at a pace that is appropriate to the trainee. The use of CD-ROM tutorials in the development of laparoscopic skills has been shown to be as effective as tutorials delivered by a live instructor[36] and such tutorials have been developed for many specific skills such as laparoscopic suturing.

While we support the use of multimedia tutorials and recognise their role in providing easily accessible and relatively inexpensive teaching in cognitive skills, it is also important to recognise the need for learner feedback, which has been shown to be invaluable in the enhancement and retention of clinical skills.[37,38] Similarly, cognitive knowledge is enhanced when the learner has the opportunity to talk through the concepts that they are engaging with via computer-assisted instruction. The computer-generated feedback obtained from the virtual reality simulators, however, does not appear to be adequate, with studies demonstrating no difference in skill acquisition in a group receiving computer feedback compared with those who did not receive feedback.[39] Feedback received from an expert instructor about performance in suturing and knot-tying skills, however, has been shown to be effective in skill acquisition.[40] In this small randomised controlled

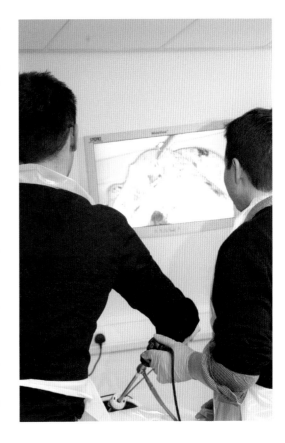

trial of medical students, those receiving verbal feedback, including answering of questions, from an expert instructor retained their skills after 1 month, whereas those receiving computer-generated feedback about economy of movement did not retain their skills.[41]

Trainees learn at different rates,[42] with some trainees having prior experience in activities such as playing computer games which appear to be transferred to the development of laparoscopic skills.[43] Since differences in learning rates are inevitable, the use of time-based training should be avoided. To do this, however, we need to have firmer agreement over what we consider to represent 'competence', with appropriate metrics to measure it. Traditional metrics of speed and accuracy fail to provide a true picture of high-quality skills performance with absolutely no recognition of the skills required in complex situations.

Although virtual reality simulators have been used extensively in the aeronautical industry to explore emergency scenarios and to model appropriate responses before teaching these to trainees, this approach has not been adopted in laparoscopic training. This is despite the well-recognised hazards of immediate bowel and vascular injury, the latter having a high intraopera-

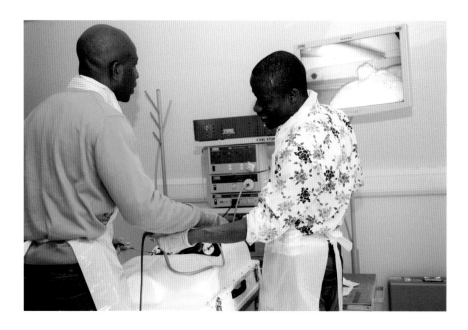

tive mortality rate. This is in marked contradistinction to obstetric practice, where emergency drills are now a requirement of good practice. The rate of serious complications reported in multicentre studies is much lower than that reported in smaller single-centre studies.[44] Each unit should develop and practise drills to respond to emergency situations. This was highlighted by Sandadi et al.[45] These drills can and should be practised using virtual reality trainers and training boxes. Deliberately injured porcine bowel can be identified and repaired and scenarios for the repair of both large and small bowel discussed and practised. As live porcine models are sacrificed after use, they could and should be used for practising management of great vessel injuries. Although intraoperative laparoscopic deaths from vascular damage are rare, these are universally associated with both delayed recognition and inadequate management; training needs to ensure that all trainees are equipped to deal with these emergencies promptly and control the situation until appropriate help arrives. Similarly, there is a need to train to respond to intraoperative medical emergencies – grave ones such as gas embolus and more self-limiting ones such as vagal bradycardia. Training so far has concentrated on teaching operative technique, but it also needs to be developed to deal with intraoperative complications and emergencies so that surgery is carried out with the minimum risk to those undergoing it.

In summary, based on the available evidence, we suggest that to develop more 'active' and 'participative' learners, initial laparoscopic training should commence within the laboratory, using either physical or virtual reality trainers, depending on availability. An accompanying cognitive component should be built into a programme of skills training, with the trainee receiving regular feedback and discussions surrounding their performance. Once the trainee has gained the basic manipulation skills, they will be in a position to gain from participative training within the operating theatre. Using this active approach to the training of clinical skills will not only facilitate a deep rather than a surface approach to learning but will also allow trainees to critically reflect upon their own surgical progress and tailor their training to their own individual needs.

Assessment of competence

One of the difficulties, of course, is how these assessments are carried out, as objective assessment can be difficult and this can result in the time taken to complete the task being regarded as an important parameter because of its relative ease of measurement. Computer scientists are trying to develop a standardised global scoring system that is usable across different laparoscopic trainers and tasks.[46] The development of software should allow real-time information feedback, which may reflect a technically sound approach that allows computerised training for any laparoscopic task.

The Royal College of Surgeons has produced an appropriate assessment tool for open surgery (Table 6.1).[47] They have suggested this assessment tool is used regularly to assess progress in surgery; however, it tends to be used as an exit assessment. The marking scheme, however, is not really directly referable to laparoscopic surgery. Other assessment tools include prepared and edited video recordings of procedures undertaken by the surgeon. Although these have not been validated, a qualitative assessment of doctors producing videos has shown that self-editing allows surgeons to become much more critical of their surgical technique as they closely observe their use of instruments and dissection. Equally, an apparently important 'rite of passage' for doctors in training is the feeling that their mentor or preceptor feels sufficiently confident in their skills to allow them to undertake surgery without direct supervision, which for them is the recognition that they are competent surgeons. There has been development of computer simulation of operations; however, this has yet to reach the advanced level of the aeronautic industry, and the models are relatively crude and lack tactile feedback. However, they may well be developed to allow appropriate surgical training and training in the management of surgical complications while preventing risk to the women on whom the operations are performed.

TABLE 6.1 **Objective structured assessment of technical skills (OSATS)**[47]

| Variable | Rating | | | | |
	1	2	3	4	5
Respect for tissue	Often used unnecessary force on tissue or caused damage by inappropriate use of instruments		Careful handling of tissue but occasionally caused inadvertent damage		Consistently handled tissues appropriately, with minimal damage
Time and motion	Many unnecessary moves		Efficient time and motion, but some unnecessary moves		Economy of movement and maximum efficiency
Instrument handling	Repeatedly makes tentative or awkward moves with instruments		Competent use of instruments, although occasionally appeared stiff or awkward		Fluid moves with instruments and no awkwardness
Knowledge of instruments	Frequently asked for the wrong instrument or used an inappropriate instrument		Knew the names of most instruments and used appropriate instrument for the task		Obviously familiar with the instruments required and their names
Use of assistants	Consistently placed assistants poorly or failed to use assistants		Good use of assistants most of the time		Strategically used assistant to the best advantage at all times
Flow of operation and forward planning	Frequently stopped operating or needed to discuss next move		Demonstrated ability for forward planning with steady progression of operative procedure		Obviously planned course of operation with effortless flow from one move to the next
Knowledge of specific procedure	Deficient knowledge; needed specific instruction at most operative steps		Knew all important aspects of the operation		Demonstrated familiarity with all aspects of the operation

References

1 Medeiros L R, Fachel J M, Garry R, Stein A T, Furness S. Laparoscopy versus laparotomy for benign ovarian tumours. *Cochrane Database Syst Rev* 2005;(3):CD004751.

2 Hajenius P J, Mol F, Mol B W, Bossuyt P M, Ankum W M, van der Veen F. Interventions for tubal ectopic pregnancy. *Cochrane Database Syst Rev* 2007;(1):CD000324.

3 National Institute for Health and Clinical Excellence. *Laparoscopic Techniques for Hysterectomy.* Interventional Procedure Guidance 239. London: NICE; 2007 [www.egap. evidence.nhs.uk/IPG239].

4 Johnson N, Barlow D, Lethaby A, Tavender E, Curr L, Garry R. Methods of hysterectomy: systematic review and meta-analysis of randomised controlled trials. *BMJ* 2005;330:1478.

5 Kennedy S, Bergqvist A, Chapron C, D'Hooghe T, Dunselman G, Greb R, et al. ESHRE guideline for the diagnosis and treatment of endometriosis. *Hum Reprod* 2005;20:2698–704.

6 Royal College of Obstetricians and Gynaecologists. *The Investigation and Management of Endometriosis.* Green-top Guideline No. 24. London: RCOG; 2008 [www.rcog.org. uk/womens-health/clinical-guidance/investigation-and-management-endometriosis-green-top-24].

7 Royal College of Obstetricians and Gynaecologists. *Benign Gynaecological Surgery: Laparoscopy. Advanced Training Skills Module.* London: RCOG; 2010 [www.rcog.org.uk/curriculum-module/atsm-benign-gynaecological-surgery-laparoscopy-0].

8 Harold K L, Matthews B D, Backus C L, Pratt B L, Heniford B T. Prospective randomized evaluation of surgical resident proficiency with laparoscopic suturing after course instruction. *Surg Endosc* 2002;16:1729–31.

9 Jansen F W, Kapiteyn K, Trimbos-Kemper T, Hermans J, Trimbos J B. Complications of laparoscopy: a prospective multicentre observational study. *Br J Obstet Gynaecol* 1997;104:595–600.

10 Chapron C, Querleu D, Mage G, Madelenat P, Dubuisson J B, Audebert A, et al. [Complications of gynecologic laparoscopy. Multicentric study of 7,604 laparoscopies]. *J Gynecol Obstet Biol Reprod (Paris)* 1992;21:207–13. Article in French.

11 Schauer P, Ikramuddin S, Hamad G, Gourash W. The learning curve for laparoscopic Roux-en-Y gastric bypass is 100 cases. *Surg Endosc* 2003;17:212–5.

12 Schlachta C M, Mamazza J, Gregoire R, Burpee S E, Pace K T, Poulin E C. Predicting conversion in laparoscopic colorectal surgery. Fellowship training may be an advantage. *Surg Endosc* 2003;17:1288–91.

13 Ahlering T E, Skarecky D, Lee D, Clayman R V. Successful transfer of open surgical skills to a laparoscopic environment using a robotic interface: initial experience with laparoscopic radical prostatectomy. *J Urol* 2003;170:1738–41.

14 See W A, Cooper C S, Fisher R J. Predictors of laparoscopic complications after formal training in laparoscopic surgery. *JAMA* 1993;270:2689–92.

15 Menon M, Shrivastava A, Tewari A, Sarle R, Hemal A, Peabody J O, et al. Laparoscopic and robot assisted radical prostatectomy: establishment of a structured program and preliminary analysis of outcomes. *J Urol* 2002;168:945–9.

16 Mettler L, Semm K. Training and regulation for endoscopic surgery. *Baillieres Clin Obstet Gynaecol* 1994;8:881–94.

17 Mazur J E. *Learning and Behaviour.* 6th ed. Englewood Cliffs, NJ: Prentice Hall; 2005.

18 Bereiter C. Aspects of an educational learning theory. *Rev Educ Res* 1990;60:603–4.

19 Kolb D A. *Experiential Learning.* Englewood Cliffs, NJ: Prentice Hall; 1984.

20 Ramsden P. *Learning to Teach in Higher Education.* 2nd ed. London: Routledge; 2003.

21 Bruynzeel H, de Bruin A F, Bonjer H J, Lange J F, Hop W C, Ayodeji I D, et al. Desktop simulator: key to universal training? *Surg Endosc* 2007;21:1637–40.

22 Munz Y, Kumar B D, Moorthy K, Bann S, Darzi A. Laparoscopic virtual reality and box trainers: is one superior to the other? *Surg Endosc* 2004;18:485–94.

23 Youngblood P L, Srivastava S, Curet M, Heinrichs W L, Dev P, Wren S M. Comparison of training on two laparoscopic simulators and assessment of skills transfer to surgical performance. *J Am Coll Surg* 2005;200:546–51.

24 Scott D J, Young W N, Tesfay S T, Frawley W H, Rege R V, Jones D B. Laparoscopic skills training. *Am J Surg* 2001;182:137–42.

25 Grantcharov T P, Bardram L, Jensen P M, Rosenberg J. [Virtual reality-computer simulation as a tool for training and evaluating skills in laparoscopic surgery]. *Ugeskr Laeger* 2001;163:3651–3. Article in Danish.

26 Kanumuri P, Ganai S, Wohaibi E M, Bush R W, Grow D R, Seymour NE. Virtual reality and computer-enhanced training devices equally improve laparoscopic surgical skill in novices. *JSLS* 2008;12:219–26.

27 Kothari S N, Kaplan B J, DeMaria E J, Broderick T J, Merrell RC. Training in laparoscopic suturing skills using a new computer-based virtual reality simulator (MIST-VR) provides results comparable to those with an established pelvic trainer system. *J Laparoendosc Adv Surg Tech A* 2002;12:167–73.

28 Lehmann K S, Ritz J P, Maass H, Cakmak H K, Kuehnapfel U G, Germer C T, et al. A prospective randomized study to test the transfer of basic psychomotor skills from virtual reality to physical reality in a comparable training setting. *Ann Surg* 2005;241:442–9.

29 Jordan J A, Gallagher A G, McGuigan J, McClure N. Virtual reality training leads to faster adaptation to the novel psychomotor restrictions encountered by laparoscopic surgeons. *Surg Endosc* 2001;15:1080–4.

30 Seymour N E, Gallagher A G, Roman S A, O'Brien M K, Bansal V K, Andersen D K, et al. Virtual reality training improves operating room performance: results of a randomized, double-blinded study. *Ann Surg* 2002;236: 458–63.

31 Torkington J, Smith S G, Rees B I, Darzi A. Skill transfer from virtual reality to a real laparoscopic task. *Surg Endosc* 2001;15:1076–9.

32 Aggarwal R, Grantcharov T P, Eriksen, J R, Blirup D, Kristiansen V B, Funch-Jensen P, et al. An evidence-based virtual reality training program for novice laparoscopic surgeons. *Ann Surg* 2006;244:310–4.

33 Aggarwal R, Tully A, Grantcharov T, Larsen C R, Miskry T, Farthing A, et al. Virtual reality simulation training can improve technical skills during laparoscopic salpingectomy for ectopic pregnancy. *BJOG* 2006;113:1382–7.

34 Grantcharov T P, Rosenberg J. [Laparoscopic appendectomy]. *Ugeskr Laeger* 2005;167:2879–82. Article in Danish.

35 Stern D T, Mangrulkar R S, Gruppen L D, Lang A L, Grum C M, Judge R D. Using a multimedia tool to improve cardiac auscultation knowledge and skills. *J Gen Intern Med* 2001;16:763–9.

36 Rosser J C, Herman B, Risucci D A, Murayama M, Rosser L E, Merrell R C. Effectiveness of a CD-ROM multimedia tutorial in transferring cognitive knowledge essential for laparoscopic skill training. *Am J Surg* 2000;179:320–4.

37 Rogers D A, Regehr G, Howdieshell T R, Yeh K A, Palm E. The impact of external feedback on computer-assisted learning for surgical technical skill training. *Am J Surg* 2000;179:341–3.

38 Mahmood T, Darzi A. The learning curve for a colonoscopy simulator in the absence of any feedback: no feedback, no learning. *Surg Endosc* 2004;18:1224–30.

39 García Galisteo E, Del Rosal Samaniego J M, Baena González V, Santos García Baquero A. [Laparoscopic surgery training in pelvitrainer and virtual simulators]. *Actas Urol Esp* 2006;30:451–6. Article in Spanish.

40 Porte M C, Xeroulis G, Reznick R K, Dubrowski A. Verbal feedback from an expert is more effective than self-accessed feedback about motion efficiency in learning new surgical skills. *Am J Surg* 2007;193:105–10.

41 Obek C, Hubka M, Porter M, Chang L, Porter JR. Robotic versus conventional laparoscopic skill acquisition: implications for training. *J Endourol* 2005;19:1098–103.

42 Stefanidis D, Heniford B T. The formula for a successful laparoscopic skills curriculum. *Arch Surg* 2009;144:77–82.

43 Miskry T, Magos T, Magos A. If you're no good at computer games, don't operate endoscopically! *Gynecol Endosc* 2002;11:345–7.

44 De Cicco C, Corona R, Schonman R, Mailova K, Ussia A, Koninckx P. Bowel resection for deep endometriosis: a systematic review. *BJOG* 2011;118:285–91.

45 Sandadi S, Johannigman J, Wong V, Blebea J, Altoser M, Hurd D. Recognition and management of major vessel injury during laparoscopy. *J Minim Invasive Gynecol* 2010;17:692–702.

46 Stylopoulos N, Cotin S, Dawson S, Ottensmeyer M, Neumann P, Bardsley R, et al. CELTS: a clinically-based Computer Enhanced Laparoscopic Training System. *Stud Health Technol Inform* 2003;94:336–42.

47 Moorthy K, Munz Y, Sarker S K, Darzi A. Objective assessment of technical skills in surgery. *BMJ* 2003;327:1032.

7 Ovarian surgery

Valentine Akande and Sanjay Vyas

Introduction

Benign ovarian cysts are the most frequent abnormal anatomical gynaecological finding in women of reproductive age and are one of the top five reasons for hospitalisation in gynaecology.[1] The human ovary varies in function through a woman's lifetime. In the reproductive years, the ovary is dynamic in relation to reproductive and menstrual function. This predisposes the ovary to give rise to a variety of tumours or swellings, which could be cystic, solid or a combination of both. These tumours can be benign, malignant or borderline.

The gold standard approach to surgical treatment of ovarian cysts until recently was by laparotomy. The well-documented advantages of laparoscopy now make this the favoured approach. A Cochrane review concluded that in women undergoing surgery for benign ovarian tumours, laparoscopy is associated with a reduction in febrile morbidity, urinary tract infection, postoperative complications, postoperative pain, days in hospital and total cost.[2] However, we still face the crucial decision of the suitability of a woman with an adnexal mass for laparoscopic surgery.[3] Generally, laparoscopic surgery should be proposed only for benign lesions, so in the case of adnexal lesions the main difficulty lies in detecting the lesions that are malignant so that these women can be operated on by laparotomy.

The focus of this chapter is on benign conditions of the ovary and their surgical management. The management of ovarian malignancies or highly suspicious cysts of the ovary is beyond the scope of this book.

Anatomy

The ovaries are almond-shaped paired structures that lie either side of the uterus and measure up to 4 cm in length. Their anatomical location generally allows easy access for laparoscopic surgery. They lie in a shallow depression named the ovarian fossa, on the lateral wall of the pelvis; this fossa is bounded above by the external iliac vessels, in front by the obliterated umbilical artery and behind by the ureter. The lateral extremity is near the external iliac vein.

However, the ovary is quite variable in its position and can frequently be found in the pouch of Douglas or posterior to the uterus.[4] The blood supply is from the ovarian artery, which arises from the aorta at the level of the renal arteries. The ovarian vein drains on the right side to the inferior vena cava and on the left side to the left renal vein.[4] The ovary has no peritoneal covering; the serosa ends at the attachment of the mesovarium, which is connected to the uterus. The ovary consists mainly of stroma containing Graafian follicles at various stages of development, corpora lutea and corpora albicans. The fibrous capsule that covers the ovary is called the tunica albugenia.

Simple or functional ovarian cysts

The vast majority of ovarian cysts are benign and most can be described as physiological or functional. The wide availability and use of ultrasound scans has led to the frequent finding of such simple cysts. An accepted definition of an ovarian cyst is a fluid-containing structure of more than 30 mm in diameter within the ovary.[5] Functional cysts are rarely more than 6 cm in diameter. They result from disorders of the growing ovarian follicle that lead to either an estrogen-producing or a progesterone-producing cyst. They are best managed conservatively as most will resolve within 6 weeks and do not require surgery. Simple cysts of less than 30 mm in diameter are likely to be follicles and therefore do not usually require any follow-up. In a randomised study, women who had ovulation induction were observed for two cycles for resolution of the induced functional cysts.[6] All women who completed the trial showed complete resolution of their functional ovarian cysts after two cycles with or without treatment.

Previously, it was thought that suppressing pituitary hormone production, for example by using the oral contraceptive pill, would cause cysts to regress and this approach has been advocated for several years. Analysis of available evidence shows this not to be the case.[7] Placing women on the pill is no more effective than no treatment in producing resolution of simple cysts. Ovarian cysts that are noted to be persistent for over 3 months tend to be pathological and may warrant continued observation or surgery.

Aspiration of simple ovarian cysts seems to be no better than observation. A randomised controlled trial of 278 women revealed that after 6 months of follow-up, the rate of resolution was similar in those who had had their cysts aspirated and those who had had them observed.[8] Furthermore, the recurrence rates of simple cysts range from 53% to 84%.[8,9]

Diagnosis of ovarian cysts

Before laparoscopic surgery, it is essential to be as convinced as possible that the cyst is benign. If there is any doubt, referral should be made to an oncologist. Diagnostic preoperative assessment should include a thorough history, transvaginal or abdominal ultrasound and other imaging methods as appropriate. The ultrasound assessment should look for features suggestive of malignancy such as papillary nodules, septations, wall thickness, ascites and mobility. The history should establish whether the woman has a family history of ovarian or breast cancer, which is a risk factor for ovarian malignancy. The use of tumour makers such as serum CA125 may be helpful, but the results should be interpreted with caution and used in the context of the risk of malignancy index.[10,11]

Indications for ovarian surgery

Surgery for ovarian cysts is often indicated in the following situations:

- when significant pathology is noted
- when the woman is symptomatic
- when the cyst is persistent.

In women of reproductive age, the procedure is usually conservative, employing cystectomy or excision while preserving healthy ovarian tissue. However, if an ovary is significantly enlarged, it is usually appropriate to undertake a partial oophorectomy and cystectomy. Where disease is recurrent and the cyst is noted to be large, for example more than 15 cm, an oophorectomy is the preferred method.

Many adnexal masses that may have remained undetected before the era of liberal ultrasonography present problems to clinicians as unexpected incidental findings. The natural history of all incidentally detected cysts with a benign appearance on ultrasound is not known. Although surgery may be an option, expectant management with follow-up should also be considered.[12]

There is no consensus on the size above which surgical management should be considered. Some studies have used an arbitrary maximum diameter of 6 cm for their inclusion criteria to offer conservative management.[13] In a retrospective study of 2083 women with a preoperative diagnosis of benign adnexal mass who underwent laparoscopy, all women selected for surgical

TABLE 7.1 **Advantages and disadvantages of oophorectomy versus cystectomy**

Type of surgery	Advantages	Disadvantages
Oophorectomy	Whole ovary available for histological assessment	Earlier menopause and reduction in ovarian reserve for fertility
	Unlikely recurrence of cysts	Lower libido because source of testosterone production is removed
		May be surgically more challenging if the cyst or ovary is adherent to surrounding structures
Cystectomy	Less normal ovarian tissue removed	Risk of leaving disease and possible recurrence requiring further surgery
	Conservation of ovarian tissue for reproductive purposes	Risk of oophorectomy if significant haemorrhage is encountered

management had adnexal masses larger than 5 cm in diameter.[14] It would be reasonable to base the decision with regard to surgery on the woman's symptoms, past history, likely rate of cyst growth and possible risk of malignancy. Where the benefit of surgery is not clear in asymptomatic women, this should be clearly discussed, including the risks of surgery.

In postmenopausal women, an assessment of the risk of a cyst being malignant is made using the risk of malignancy index.[11] Where pathology is identified, the surgery employed is more radical and includes oophorectomy or salpingo-oophorectomy, which could be either unilateral or bilateral. There are advantages and disadvantages to undertaking oophorectomy as opposed to cystectomy, which are listed in Table 7.1.

Preoperative consent

Appropriate informed consent should be obtained for the intended procedure (ovarian cystectomy, oophorectomy or salpingo-oophorectomy, depending on the perceived nature of the cyst and the reproductive desires and age of the woman). The woman should also be informed of the risks and complications of surgery. These include bleeding, ureteric damage, scarring, oophorectomy, damage to adjacent organs such as bowel, thrombosis, pain and bruising. If complications are encountered, conversion to laparotomy may be required.

Equipment required for ovarian surgery

In uncomplicated ovarian surgery, not many instruments are required. The basic equipment that will suffice for most cases comprises the following:

- basic laparoscopy set to include telescope, gas and video screen

- two pairs of 5 mm grasping forceps

- some form of diathermy: unipolar or bipolar

- suction/irrigation

- disposable laparoscopic bag

- laparoscopic scissors.

Techniques for surgery

Your standard laparoscopic approach should be employed to gain intraperitoneal access. The woman should be placed in the Trendelenburg (head-down) position to allow good access to the pelvis. It is not usually necessary to prepare the bowel with laxatives before surgery as this offers no significant advantage; furthermore, there is evidence that this can increase perioperative discomfort.[15] The number and location of accessory ports depends on the complexity of the surgery with prior thought given to ergonomic comfort. For small and moderate-sized cysts of up to 8 cm in diameter, cyst removal via a 10–12 mm accessory port should be possible. Insertion of a uterine manipulator, while not essential, can be helpful in mobilising the uterus and placing it in a favourable position for surgery.

Where very large ovarian cysts are encountered, it may not be possible to undertake a total laparoscopic procedure. In such cases, minimal invasiveness can be maintained by undertaking a laparoscopically guided/assisted minilaparotomy.[16]

If a procedure is anticipated to be of long duration, it is good practice to insert a Foley catheter in the bladder to prevent its distension during the procedure.

Principles of ovarian surgery

Apart from giving the woman a prompt recovery, the key principles of ovarian surgery are:

- to remove diseased tissue

- to conserve fertility in women of reproductive age

- to avoid injury to adjacent organs.

Initial intraoperative assessment

A full abdominopelvic assessment is made as is routine during diagnostic laparoscopy. This includes detailed assessment for suspected or undiagnosed ovarian carcinoma. The ovary is examined for nodules, irregular vascularity and vegetations; if unsure, obtain frozen sections; if highly suspicious, seek a second opinion from an oncologist or remove the diseased ovary, preferably intact, by laparotomy. The omentum is examined and it is good practice to obtain free fluid for cytological assessment.

Approximately 25% of women with invasive epithelial ovarian carcinoma are first seen with disease confined to the ovary (International Federation of Gynecology and Obstetrics [FIGO] stage I). A large retrospective study of woman with FIGO stage I disease revealed that, after tumour differentiation, spillage of cyst contents was the most important unfavourable factor related to survival prognosis.[17] This suggests that if at the time of surgery the findings are suspicious, a laparotomy is the best course of action and an immediate staging laparotomy is warranted.

Approximately 10% of women suspected of having ovarian cysts will be found to have other adnexal pathology such as paratubal cysts, hydrosalpinges, pelvic cysts within adhesions or pelvic abscess.[18] Techniques similar to those applied during ovarian cystectomy and oophorectomy, including the use of adhesiolysis, can be employed to deal with these conditions.

Ovarian cystectomy for serous and mucinous tumours

The ovary is usually approached from the opposite side to the mesosalpinx. The ovarian cortex is incised and, depending on the nature of the cyst, it is either enucleated or drained to aid excision (Figure 7.1). If the cyst is com-

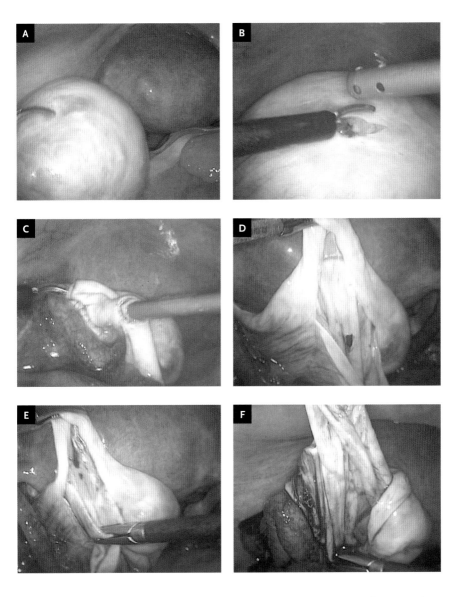

FIGURE 7.1 **Ovarian cystectomy for benign serous cyst**

(A) Left ovarian cyst
(B) Incision of ovarian capsule
(C) Aspiration of cyst contents
(D) Exposing cyst wall
(E) Beginning of stripping the cyst wall
(F) Cyst wall mostly stripped from ovary

pletely enucleated, it may be possible to drain the cyst in an endoscopic bag to prevent spillage.[16] Very often, if the correct plane is identified, it is relatively straightforward to peel away the cyst wall from the ovarian stroma and cortex. It is usual practice to employ a pair of grasping forceps to apply opposite traction to achieve a good stripping result. The forceps are carefully applied close to each other and careful traction is exerted to avoid tearing of the ovary.

The most vascular portion of the cyst wall is its attachment at the hilum of the ovary. Often, the ooze of blood clots quickly and no further action is required. Where bleeding is notable, options include diathermy or placing a figure-of-eight suture. In the absence of bleeding, there is no consensus as to whether it is better to suture the ovary once a cyst is excised. It is notable that routine practice during open surgery for cysts includes suturing the ovary. Accordingly, your approach to this would depend on your preference and experience with laparoscopic suturing. It is good practice to be able to suture should this be required for a complication or to secure haemostasis. In rare cases of intractable haemorrhage from a cyst, oophorectomy may be required.

Ideally, when removing cysts, only diseased tissue should be included and healthy ovarian tissue left behind. Studies reveal that you are more likely to remove ovarian tissue when removing endometriomas than when removing other cysts.[19] However, undertaking cystectomy by laparotomy rather than by laparoscopy does not seem to conserve more ovarian tissue.[20]

Excision of ovarian endometriomas

Women with ovarian endometriomas respond poorly to medical management,[21] leaving surgery as the most realistic option for treatment. Several laparoscopic techniques have been described for dealing with ovarian endometriomas: drainage, cyst wall ablation (laser/bipolar diathermy) and stripping. There is now convincing evidence that the best outcome for women in terms of recurrence, pain and fertility is achieved if the endometrioma is excised (stripped out).[22] However, a major concern following ovarian surgery – particularly in women with endometriosis and fertility issues – is the loss of follicles, which is quite significant regardless of whether excision or ablation of the cyst wall is undertaken.[23] One method to overcome this may be to use a combined method of stripping and coagulation.[24] This technique involves stripping the endometrioma in a conventional manner until the vascular hilum of the ovary is reached. The cyst is excised, leaving the hilar region to be ablated by bipolar coagulation.

One study[25] evaluated two different techniques of excising endometriomas by stripping: direct stripping of the cyst wall from the original adhesion site or circular excision around the original adhesion site. With both techniques, the remaining part of the cyst wall was stripped away in the conventional manner. The findings from this study indicated that the circular incision at the point of ovarian adhesions made the surgical stripping of the cyst wall easier.

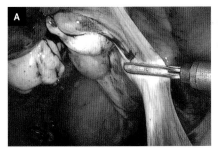
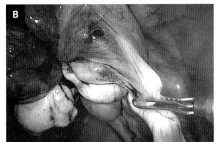
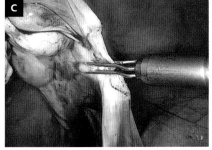
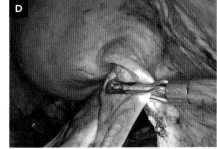
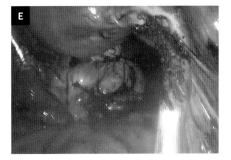

FIGURE 7.2 **Right salpingo-oophorectomy**

(A) Coagulation of the infundibulopelvic (IP) ligament with bipolar diathermy (B) Division of IP ligament (C) Coagulation extending into IP and broad ligament (D) Coagulation of fallopian tube (E) Salpingo-oophorectomy completed

Dermoid cysts (mature cystic teratomas)

Spillage of the contents of a dermoid cyst usually has no consequences.[26,27] However, in rare instances (fewer than 1% of women), chemical peritonitis can occur, which occasionally can be severe.[28] The spillage of contents is relatively common during ovarian surgery for large dermoid cysts and a thorough pelvic washout should be undertaken to reduce the risk of peritonitis.

Another technique to reduce the risk of spillage is to incise the ovarian capsule, avoiding puncture of the cyst wall.[29] While stabilising the ovary, the cyst wall is teased and dissected away from the ovarian stroma. The cyst is then placed in a bag and drained within the bag.

Oophorectomy and salpingo-oophorectomy

Oophorectomy tends to be undertaken in peri- and postmenopausal women to whom reproductive concerns no longer apply. This avoids recurrence and enables assessment of the whole ovary as the risk of malignancy is higher in this age group. Salpingo-oophorectomy is required when the ovary is much enlarged and the fallopian tube is stretched over the ovary and difficult to separate. The procedure includes first identifying the path of the ureter and, if necessary, undertaking adhesiolysis to free up the ovary. The ovary and tube are then grasped and traction is applied to position them medially with good vision of the infundibulopelvic pedicle (Figure 7.2). On occasions, it is necessary to dissect the sigmoid colon medially to obtain access to the left-sided pedicle.

Small ovaries can be removed following simple ligation of the ovary and tube with the infundibulopelvic ligament, using Endoloop® (Ethicon Endo-Surgery, Cincinnati, OH, USA) and then excision. Larger ovaries present larger pedicles and need haemostasis of the infundibulopelvic and ovarian ligaments separately with diathermy or ultrasonic energy followed by excision.

There is a body of evidence indicating that quality of life declines significantly in women who have both ovaries removed surgically compared with those undergoing natural menopause.[30] Studies also indicate changes in sexual function caused by a fall in androgen levels as well as increased cardiovascular risks, cognitive impairment and osteoporotic fractures. Thus, bilateral oophorectomy should not necessarily be routine practice in postmenopausal women unless otherwise clinically indicated. If undertaken, it is good practice to counsel women about these risks.

Oophorectomy after a hysterectomy

Some 4% of women who have a hysterectomy will have an ovarian lesion at a later date.[31] Removal of the residual ovary in these women presents a challenge because the incidence of pelvic and abdominal adhesions is much higher than in women who have not had previous surgery.[32] This requires greater skill from the surgeon.[33] For example, the left ovary may be more difficult to access because it is not uncommon for it to be adherent to the sigmoid colon, the left pelvic sidewall and even the bladder (Figure 7.3). These adhesions derive an additional blood supply from the peritoneum,[34] which can be difficult to dissect.

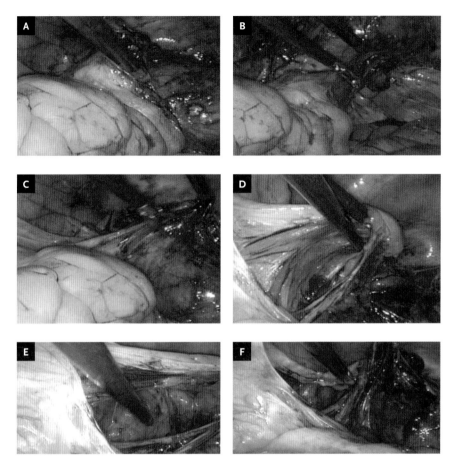

FIGURE 7.3 **Mobilising left ovary in hysterectomised pelvis**

(A) Left ovarian cyst identified adherent to sigmoid colon
(B) Division of adhesions
(C) Beginning to open the pelvic side wall
(D) Developing tissue planes in the pelvic side wall
(E) Identifying ureter
(F) Identifying ureter and blood vessels

The acute ovary and emergency surgical procedures

Ovarian torsion

An ovarian torsion is defined as a partial or complete rotation of the infundibulopelvic pedicle that causes obstruction to blood flow. In most instances, torsion affects the adnexa rather than the ovary alone.[35] It is notable that 15% of torsions occur in children.[36] Previous management of torsions was oophorectomy or partial oophorectomy if the ovary appeared engorged or ischaemic. It is now considered best practice to untwist the torted adnexa or ovary because this results in the preservation of ovarian function in 91–100% of women.[35]

Ovarian cyst rupture

Ovarian cyst rupture is usually physiological and most often occurs following ovulation. In most instances, ovarian cyst rupture can be managed expect-

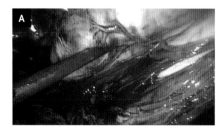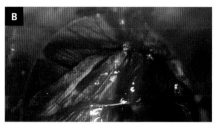

FIGURE 7.4 **Combined laparoscopic and minilaparotomy removal of very large ovarian cyst**

(A) Laparoscopic view of aspiration and mobilisation of ovary
(B) Laparoscopic view of ovary being removed via minilaparotomy incision

antly without surgery. If the woman is haemodynamically compromised or there is no relief of symptoms after 48 hours, laparoscopy should be considered. A cystectomy should be performed and haemostasis secured. In some women, this can prove challenging and suturing of the ovary or oophorectomy may be required.

Ovarian hyperstimulation syndrome

The ovaries often become significantly enlarged following assisted conception treatment requiring ovarian stimulation. This is usually self-limiting and resolves within days or a few weeks. In severe cases, the woman is uncomfortable, but surgery should be avoided at all costs unless a torsion is suspected, in which case management should be followed as described previously. It would be inappropriate to undertake a cystectomy as this is likely to result in severe haemorrhage from the multiple corpus luteum cysts, which could in turn lead to an unnecessary oophorectomy in an infertile woman wishing to conceive.

Very large ovarian cysts

Very large ovarian cysts present a different type of challenge to the laparoscopic surgeon. Removing such a cyst requires a combined approach of laparoscopy with open surgery such as minilaparotomy. Initially, the cyst can be drained either laparoscopically or by ultrasound-guided aspiration, following which an inspection of the cyst wall and peritoneal cavity is undertaken by laparoscopy to determine whether the cyst alone or the whole ovary should be excised (Figure 7.4). Once the cyst cavity is empty, the cystectomy or oophorectomy of the now flaccid ovary can be dealt with via a 2–3 cm minilaparotomy incision. In a study of 33 women with cysts measuring 10–30 cm, over 90% of procedures were successfully carried out laparoscopically.[37] The main reason for conversion to laparotomy was adhesions.

Ovarian surgery in pregnancy

The use of laparoscopy in the first trimester of pregnancy is relatively common. Although the enlarged uterus in the second and third trimesters requires a different approach, when undertaken by experienced surgeons a laparoscopic approach can be achieved.[38]

Insufflation requires different techniques from the usual blind Veress needle placement. Depending on the gestational age of the pregnancy and the size of the uterus, these include the open technique,[39] use of a blunt-tip optical trocar via the umbilicus or supraumbilically, subcostal entry or Palmer's point entry. Once a pneumoperitoneum has been achieved, it is advisable not to use a pressure of more than 12 mmHg or to place the woman in an extensive Trendelenburg position. The woman should also be placed in a left tilted position to prevent vena cava compression. Thereafter, standard laparoscopic techniques can be used to deal with the cyst.

Access to the cyst can be difficult if it is behind the uterus in the pouch of Douglas. Clearly, a uterine manipulator cannot be placed and the uterus should also not be touched by the laparoscopic instruments, for fear of provoking contractions or bleeding. It can be helpful to exert gentle traction on the cyst wall by use of blunt instruments, following suction aspiration if necessary.

There is a risk of uterine contractions and tocolytic agents should be considered. Depending on the duration of gestation, it may also be appropriate to consider preoperative administration of steroids to improve fetal lung maturity should premature delivery occur subsequently.

Postoperative care

Depending on the length and complexity of surgery, thromboprophylaxis should be considered and women can be discharged 6–24 hours after surgery. If significant haemorrhage was encountered intraoperatively, it would be good practice to check the haemoglobin level before discharge. Nonsteroidal analgesics and paracetamol are all that is normally required as analgesia postoperatively.

Summary and conclusions

Laparoscopic treatment of benign ovarian cysts by cystectomy or oophorectomy is now the optimal approach compared with laparotomy. This approach leads to a quicker recovery, fewer complications and greater patient satisfaction. It is now possible to remove virtually all cysts or ovaries either laparoscopically or, if very large, with minilaparotomy. As it is not feasible to guarantee removal of an ovary or cyst without rupture or spillage, it is paramount that the risk of malignancy is considered preoperatively.

References

1 Westhoff C, Clark C J. Benign ovarian cysts in England and Wales and in the United States. *Br J Obstet Gynaecol* 1992;99:329–32.

2 Medeiros L R, Fachel J M, Garry R, Stein A T, Furness S. Laparoscopy versus laparotomy for benign ovarian tumours. *Cochrane Database Syst Rev* 2005;(3):CD004751.

3 Chapron C, Dubuisson J B, Capella-Allouc S. Salpingo-oophorectomy for adnexal masses. Place and results for operative laparoscopy. *Eur J Obstet Gynecol Reprod Biol* 1997;73:43–8.

4 Ellis H. The ovary. In: Ellis H, editor. *Clinical Anatomy*. Oxford: Blackwell Scientific Publications, 1983. p. 173–4.

5 Ovarian and endometrial function during hormonal contraception. *Hum Reprod* 2001;16:1527–35.

6 MacKenna A, Fabres C, Alam V, Morales V. Clinical management of functional ovarian cysts: a prospective and randomized study. *Hum Reprod* 2000;15:2567–9.

7 Grimes D A, Jones L B, Lopez L M, Schulz K F. Oral contraceptives for functional ovarian cysts. *Cochrane Database Syst Rev* 2006;(4):CD006134.

8 Zanetta G, Lissoni A, Torri V, Dalla Valle C, Trio D, Rangoni G, et al. Role of puncture and aspiration in expectant management of simple ovarian cysts: a randomised study. *BMJ* 1996;313:1110–3.

9 Marana R, Caruana P, Muzii L, Catalano G F, Mancuso S. Operative laparoscopy for ovarian cysts. Excision vs. aspiration. *J Reprod Med* 1996;41:435–8.

10 Raza A, Mould T, Wilson M, Burnell M, Bernhardt L. Increasing the effectiveness of referral of ovarian masses from cancer unit to cancer center by using a higher referral value of the risk of malignancy index. *Int J Gynecol Cancer* 2010;20:552–4.

11 Royal College of Obstetricians and Gynaecologists. *Ovarian Cysts in Postmenopausal Women*. Green-top Guideline No. 34. London: RCOG; 2003 [www.rcog.org.uk/womens-health/clinical-guidance/ovarian-cysts-postmenopausal-women-green-top-34].

12 Valentin L. Use of morphology to characterize and manage common adnexal masses. *Best Pract Res Clin Obstet Gynecol* 2004;18:71–89.

13 Alcázar J L, Castillo G, Jurado M, García G L. Is expectant management of sonographically benign adnexal cysts an option in selected asymptomatic premenopausal women? *Hum Reprod* 2005;20:3231–4.

14 Leng J H, Lang J H, Zhang J J, Feng F Z, Liu Z F, Sun D W, et al. Role of laparoscopy in the diagnosis and treatment of adnexal masses. *Chin Med J (Engl)* 2006;119:202–6.

15 Muzii L, Bellati F, Zullo M A, Manci N, Angioli R, Panici P B. Mechanical bowel preparation before gynecologic laparoscopy: a randomized, single-blind, controlled trial. *Fertil Steril* 2006;85:689–93.

16 Panici P B, Palaia I, Bellati F, Pernice M, Angioli R, Muzii L. Laparoscopy compared with laparoscopically guided minilaparotomy for large adnexal masses: a randomized controlled trial. *Obstet Gynecol* 2007;110:241–8.

17 Vergote I, De Brabanter J, Fyles A, Bertelsen K, Einhorn N, Sevelda P, et al. Prognostic importance of degree of differentiation and cyst rupture in stage I invasive epithelial ovarian carcinoma. *Lancet* 2001;357:176–82.

18 Canis M, Botchorishvili R, Manhes H, Wattiez A, Mage G, Pouly JL, et al. Management of adnexal masses: role and risk of laparoscopy. *Semin Surg Oncol* 2000;19:28–35.

19 Muzii L, Bianchi A, Croce C, Manci N, Panici P B. Laparoscopic excision of ovarian cysts: is the stripping technique a tissue-sparing procedure? *Fertil Steril* 2002;77:609–14.

20 Alborzi S, Momtahan M, Parsanezhad M E, Dehbashi S, Zolghadri J, Alborzi S. A prospective, randomized study comparing laparoscopic ovarian cystectomy versus fenestration and coagulation in patients with endometriomas. *Fertil Steril* 2004;82:1633–7.

21 Muzii L. Medicated intrauterine systems for treatment of endometriosis-associated pain. *J Minim Invasive Gynecol* 2006;13:535–8.

22 Hart R J, Hickey M, Maouris P, Buckett W. Excisional surgery versus ablative surgery for ovarian endometriomata. *Cochrane Database Syst Rev* 2008;(2):CD004992.

23 Benaglia L, Somigliana E, Vighi V, Ragni G, Vercellini P, Fedele L. Rate of severe ovarian damage following surgery for endometriomas. *Hum Reprod* 2010;25:678–82.

24 Muzii L, Panici P B. Combined technique of excision and ablation for the surgical treatment of ovarian endometriomas: the way forward? *Reprod Biomed Online* 2010;20:300–2.

25 Muzii L, Bellati F, Palaia I, Plotti F, Manci N, Zullo M A, et al. Laparoscopic stripping of endometriomas: a randomized trial on different surgical techniques. Part I: clinical results. *Hum Reprod* 2005;20:1981–6.

26 Kocak M, Dilbaz B, Ozturk N, Dede S, Altay M, Dilbaz S, et al. Laparoscopic management of ovarian dermoid cysts: a review of 47 cases. *Ann Saudi Med* 2004;24:357–60.

27 Nezhat C R, Kalyoncu S, Nezhat C H, Johnson E, Berlanda N, Nezhat F. Laparoscopic management of ovarian dermoid cysts: ten years' experience. *JSLS* 1999;3:179–84.

28 Rubod C, Triboulet J P, Vinatier D. [Ovarian dermoid cyst complicated by chemical peritonitis. Case report]. *Gynecol Obstet Fertil* 2007;35:651–3. Article in French.

29 Mencaglia L, Wattiez A. *Management of Ovarian Cysts and Adnexal Masses*. Tuttlingen: Endo-Press; 2003.

30 Fenton A, Panay N. Out, damn ovary, out—the case for and against bilateral oophorectomy for benign disease. *Climacteric* 2008;11:441–2.

31 Plockinger B, Kolbl H. Development of ovarian pathology after hysterectomy without oophorectomy. *J Am Coll Surg* 1994;178:581–5.

32 Postoperative adhesion development after operative laparoscopy: evaluation at early second-look procedures. Operative Laparoscopy Study Group. *Fertil Steril* 1991;55:700–4.

33 Lee J H, Kyung M S, Jung U S, Choi J S. Laparoscopic management of adnexal tumours in post-hysterectomy women. *Aust N Z J Obstet Gynaecol* 2008;48:96–100.

34 Shemwell R E, Weed J C. Ovarian remnant syndrome. *Obstet Gynecol* 1970;36:299–303.

35 Bottomley C, Bourne T. Diagnosis and management of ovarian cyst accidents. *Best Pract Res Clin Obstet Gynaecol* 2009;23:711–24.

36 Adelman S, Benson C D, Hertzler J H. Surgical lesions of the ovary in infancy and childhood. *Surg Gynecol Obstet* 1975;141:219–26.

37 Eltabbakh G H, Charboneau A M, Eltabbakh N G. Laparoscopic surgery for large benign ovarian cysts. *Gynecol Oncol* 2008;108:72–6.

38 Mathevet P, Nessah K, Dargent D, Mellier G. Laparoscopic management of adnexal masses in pregnancy: a case series. *Eur J Obstet Gynecol Reprod Biol* 2003;108:217–22.

39 Hasson H M. Open laparoscopy: a report of 150 cases. *J Reprod Med* 1974;12:234–8.

8

Laparoscopic techniques for tubal pregnancy and tubal reconstructive surgery

Adrian M Lower and Geoffrey H Trew

Introduction

Disease of, or damage to, the fallopian tube accounts for 25–30% of the causes of infertility. The fallopian tubes can be damaged as a result of prior infection, previous pelvic surgery and endometriosis, but in some women a specific cause cannot be identified. Injury of the fimbrial ends of the fallopian tubes may interfere with the processes of ovum pick-up and transport. In addition, tubal transport abnormalities significantly increase the risk of an ectopic pregnancy. It is therefore appropriate to consider both tubal disease and tubal pregnancy in this chapter, although assessment and management are clearly quite different, one condition presenting as a surgical emergency, the other being an indication for an elective procedure that requires careful prior assessment.

Laparoscopic surgery embraces the principles of microsurgery, namely avoiding excessive tissue handling, preventing desiccation, enabling liberal irrigation of the operative field, facilitating haemostasis and magnifying the view of the operative field. Furthermore, all members of the theatre team can see the progress of the surgery and anticipate and assist with potential problems by virtue of the video screen.

In this chapter, we review the surgical techniques for treating tubal pregnancy. It is the aim of the Royal College of Obstetricians and Gynaecologists (RCOG) that all surgeons providing emergency gynaecological cover should be capable of performing a safe laparoscopy and safe laparoscopic management of the tubal pregnancy. We present an analysis of the surgical options for commonly presenting ectopic pregnancies and also talk briefly about the management of more complex conditions such as cornual pregnancy.

We also review the range of surgical procedures described for the management of tubal infertility and look at the evidence to be considered when selecting women for surgical management rather than assisted conception.

Finally, we consider the place of salpingectomy as a prelude to assisted conception and review the evidence supporting this management and the areas where caution is required.

Ectopic pregnancy

The incidence of ectopic pregnancy in the UK (11.1/1000 pregnancies) has remained static in recent years.[1] Nearly 32 000 ectopic pregnancies are diagnosed in the UK within a 3-year period.[1]

Guidelines[2,3] recommend that women with an ectopic pregnancy should be managed in dedicated early pregnancy units and clinicians should have received appropriate training in both open and laparoscopic management. This should include safe use of both monopolar and bipolar diathermy and attendance at an appropriate RCOG-approved course in basic or intermediate laparoscopic skills. The guidelines also state that clinicians should be supported by modern equipment to facilitate safe surgery.

For haemodynamically stable women, there is now Level Ia evidence supporting a laparoscopic approach to the surgical management of a tubal pregnancy in preference to an open approach.[2] Specifically, a meta-analysis of data from three randomised controlled trials comparing laparoscopic and open surgery revealed reductions in operation times, intraoperative blood loss, hospital stays and analgesic requirements if a laparoscopic procedure was used.[2] Overall tubal patency rates were similar with both approaches (relative risk [RR] 0.89, 95% CI 0.74–1.1). Subsequent intrauterine pregnancy rates among women who wished to conceive were also similar (RR 1.2, 95% CI 0.88–1.15) and laparoscopy tended to reduce the risk of a repeat ectopic pregnancy (RR 0.43, 95% CI 0.15–1.2). However, laparoscopic salpingotomy was less successful than open surgery in eliminating the tubal pregnancy (RR 0.90, 95% CI 0.83–0.97), a finding that was also reflected in a trend towards higher rates of persistent trophoblast (RR 3.6, 95% CI 0.63–21).

The surgical options for tubal pregnancy, whether performed by open surgery or laparoscopically, are salpingectomy and salpingotomy. The evidence comparing the two procedures is poor. There is low-grade evidence indicating that salpingotomy is associated with a higher rate of initial treatment failure. Therefore, in the presence of an apparently normal contralateral tube it may be preferable to perform a salpingectomy rather than attempting conservative management by salpingotomy.

Salpingotomy

By use of a needlepoint source of any energy modality such as diathermy or laser, the fallopian tube is incised longitudinally over the anti-mesosalpingeal border at the site of maximum distension of the affected fallopian tube. The trophoblast will usually begin to herniate out of the incision as soon as it is made (Figure 8.1). To avoid excessive bleeding and damage to the tubal mucosa, the temptation to grasp this tissue should be resisted. Irrigation using any irrigation fluid is the best method of removing the tissue. Usually, there will be no bleeding. On the odd occasion where bleeding is identified, it will usually respond to bipolar diathermy, but tubal function is more likely to be compromised and consideration should be given to performing a salpingectomy.

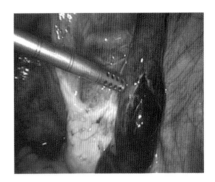

FIGURE 8.1 **Linear salpingotomy**

Salpingectomy

The fallopian tube is mobilised by dividing the mesosalpinx. Care should be taken to minimise damage to the vascular supply of the ovary. This can occur through the overuse of bipolar diathermy or through distortion of the vessels caused by inappropriate placement of Endoloop® (Ethicon Endo-Surgery, Cincinnati, OH, USA) ligatures.

One of the easiest instruments to use for haemostasis and division of the fallopian tube is the 'tripolar' forceps, a bipolar diathermy instrument with a central cutting blade (Figure 8.2, Video 8.1).

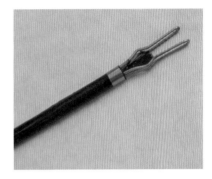

FIGURE 8.2 **Tripolar forceps**

Most haemostasis instruments assess the extent of haemostasis by measuring the impedance of the tissue, giving either an audible warning or shutting down power to the instrument when haemostasis is complete. The cutting blade is then advanced to divide the tissue. With this method, preferably starting at the cornual end of the tube, it is a fairly straightforward procedure to first divide the fallopian tube and then divide the mesosalpinx, staying close to the fallopian tube to minimise the risk of damage to the ovary (Figure 8.3). Any combination of haemostasis and cutting energy can be used. Commonly employed energy modalities include the ultrasonic scalpel, bipolar diathermy and scissors or laser. Some surgeons rely on Endoloop to achieve haemostasis (Figure 8.4). No useful data are available to support the use of one modality over another other than individual preference and the equipment available at the time.

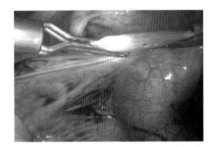

FIGURE 8.3 **Salpingectomy using tripolar forceps**

The divided fallopian tube should then be placed in a tissue retrieval bag to reduce the likelihood of losing trophoblastic tissue, which may implant elsewhere. The retrieval bag con-

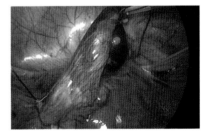

FIGURE 8.4 **Salpingectomy using Endoloop®** (Ethicon Endo-Surgery, Cincinnati, OH, USA)

taining the involved fallopian tube can be removed through the 10 mm umbilical port under the direct vision of a 5 mm laparoscope introduced in the left
iliac fossa trocar. If a second laparoscope is not available, the suprapubic trocar site can be slightly enlarged to facilitate tissue removal.

Tubal reconstructive surgery

Surgical modalities

When considering the options of corrective tubal surgery to improve a woman's fertility, it is always very important that all alternatives are discussed with
the woman to allow her to give informed consent to the best option for her
specific situation. This involves not only adequate investigation and work-up
of both partners of the couple wishing to conceive, but also consideration of
other factors that may help them make a decision as to whether to correct the
underlying tubal problem, such as a blockage or a sterilisation, or to bypass it
completely and go down the route of in vitro fertilisation (IVF).

Although success rates with IVF have continued to improve over the last
few years, this approach is still not always acceptable to all women for moral
or religious reasons. It is also important to take into account factors such as
the woman's age. The negative effect of maternal age may be more marked
on the outcome of assisted conception procedures than on that of corrective tubal surgery, particularly when one considers the cumulative conception
rates after attempts to conceive in multiple unstimulated cycles as opposed
to the conception rate after a single assisted conception cycle, where the
response to stimulation is probably poor so the benefit of multiple eggs collected during one cycle is likely to be absent.

Lastly, it should be remembered that correction of the underlying tubal
abnormality allows a woman to have more than one spontaneous pregnancy.
In addition, these pregnancies are generally singleton pregnancies and therefore do not have the increases in morbidity associated with multiple births,
which occur more frequently with IVF.

In recent years, the number of operative procedures for tubal reconstructive surgery has steadily declined, owing in part to the very high success rates
now obtained by assisted conception procedures. There are very few formally
trained reproductive surgeons currently practising in the UK. It is important
that surgeons performing reconstructive surgical procedures have completed
appropriate training in reproductive medicine so that they are aware of the
potential treatments and limitations offered by both assisted conception and
the surgical approach.

It is difficult to compare success rates achieved with IVF with those obtained at tubal surgery. This is because the success rates with IVF are expressed as pregnancies per cycle initiated or per embryo transfer. By contrast, the pregnancy rates after surgery are usually expressed as cumulative pregnancy rates per unit of time after a variable period of follow-up.

Maternal age

The fecundability of women declines with advancing age. The primary mechanism is age-related changes in the oocyte. Pregnancy rates decrease for both IVF and tubal surgery with advancing maternal age. Funding issues may mean that assisted conception is not available for older women and tubal surgery is the only treatment open to them. This may negatively affect the year audited results of tubal surgery in comparison with IVF. Conversely, IVF may not be acceptable to some women for ethical, religious or financial reasons.

Preoperative assessment

Hysterosalpingography remains the primary diagnostic test in the identification of tubal damage. In addition to providing information about the patency of the fallopian tubes, hysterosalpingography can help to diagnose other abnormalities such as intrauterine adhesions and polyps. The diagnostic accuracy of the hysterosalpingography is good when tubal patency is demonstrated, but only moderate confidence can be placed on a diagnosis of tubal blockage. This is because spasm of the fallopian tubes can lead to an incorrect assessment of proximal tubal obstruction.

Is important that a full evaluation is completed on couples where tubal problems are anticipated. In particular, it is important to rule out male factor problems and ovulatory disorders.

Where tubal abnormalities are identified or anticipated, a laparoscopy and hysteroscopy may be required to confirm the diagnosis. Full informed consent should be obtained before the laparoscopy to enable the surgeon to treat any abnormality encountered that may be amenable to surgery.

The traditional process of a diagnostic laparoscopy to establish the extent of pathology is rapidly becoming a thing of the past. Most centres are adopting a 'see and treat' policy, where a laparoscopy is performed with full consent from the woman to proceed to definitive management of any pathology identified. The extra time required to perform an adhesiolysis is small in comparison with the administrative time required to get the woman to theatre and anaesthetised in order for the laparoscopy to be performed, and of course the see and treat policy avoids a further operative procedure and general anaesthetic for the woman. Therefore, the see and treat approach is better for the woman and potentially saves costs for the provider.

Proximal tubal disease

Proximal tubal occlusion can be diagnosed both by hysterosalpingography and by hysterosonography. These diagnostic tests show the proximal tubal pathology but do not give any information about the distal portion of the tube. If there is significant distal disease and bilateral hydrosalpinges are visible by ultrasound, it can reasonably be assumed that the woman has bilateral bipolar disease that is not amenable to corrective tubal surgery. Generally, however, the distal portion is more fully examined at a subsequent laparoscopy and the cause of the proximal tubal disease can also be further elucidated.

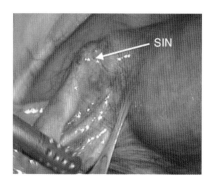

FIGURE 8.5 **Laparoscopic view of cornual portion of the fallopian tube enlarged by salpingitis isthmica nodosa**

The most common cause of true proximal disease (as opposed to tubal spasm or an incorrectly performed test) is salpingitis isthmica nodosa, a progressive inflammatory disease of unknown aetiology. It is most commonly found in women with secondary infertility and affects the intramural portion of the tube extending down to the isthmic portion. It can be obstructive or nonobstructive; both result in infertility (Figure 8.5).

Other causes of proximal tubal occlusion are large polyps, which can completely occlude the fallopian tube, and adenomyosis. Adenomyosis can occlude the intramural portion by the resultant thickening of the myometrium from the adenomyotic tissue. It can be important to clarify the underlying cause of proximal tubal occlusion because adenomyosis is not treated surgically. If deemed necessary, it can be treated medically with prolonged suppression through gonadotrophin-releasing hormone agonist therapy. Salpingitis isthmica nodosa and significant cornual polyps, on the other hand, can be treated surgically with excellent results.

Cornual polyps are treated by a linear salpingostomy performed over the proximal isthmic portion by use of a very fine monopolar diathermy needle. The cut is made through the full thickness of the uterine cornu over the fallopian tube down to the tubal lumen and the polyp often extrudes immediately on opening. The polyp is then gently grasped and cut at its base with fine laparoscopic scissors, without the application of diathermy. Diathermy is unnecessary and can damage the delicate tubal mucosa. The resulting linear incision is then closed in one layer with fine (5-0 or 6-0) interrupted sutures.

Proximal tubal occlusion from salpingitis isthmica nodosa is generally treated by a minilaparotomy with an operating microscope. The operation can also be performed laparoscopically, but this is one of the most complex laparoscopic microsurgical procedures. Laparoscopic tubocornual resection and subsequent anastomosis was pioneered by Charles Koh in Milwaukee, WI, USA. Indeed, he is one of the few people still performing this complex procedure and is getting excellent pregnancy results of over 60%.[4] He has developed laparoscopic microsurgical instruments and often takes 5–6 hours to perform a bilateral procedure. The diseased area is identified and resected back until a healthy proximal portion and a healthy distal portion are seen. This can often be the case after two-thirds of the intramural tube have been resected. The healthy tubes are splinted and a two-layer closure performed. The first layer is with interrupted 8-0 sutures and the serosal layer with either continuous or interrupted 6-0 sutures. The splint is then removed and patency checked transcervically. Dilute Pitressin® (Goldshield Pharmaceuticals, Croydon, UK) is often injected into the cornual portion of the tubes before the resection to reduce bleeding.

Reversal of sterilisation

Reversal of sterilisation can be one of the most successful operations on the fallopian tube because the surgeon is dealing with an otherwise healthy tube that has been iatrogenically occluded. Generally, there is no other disease process present and hence the results are significantly better than those for any other form of tubal surgery. The usual work-up investigations have to be performed. There is no point in reversing a sterilisation only to find there is a severe male factor present and the woman still does not become pregnant. Reversal of sterilisation is an excellent surgical option as long as there are no other significant factors contributing to the overall fertility situation.

Over the last 15 years, the vast majority of sterilisations in the UK have been performed by placement of a single Filshie® (Femcare; Romsey, UK) clip over the isthmic portion of each fallopian tube. Other forms of sterilisation, however, are still seen and these can range from the use of the Falope-Ring® (Gyrus ACMI; Southborough, MS, USA) to segmental diathermy. Generally, all of these forms of sterilisation can be reversed as long as there is a considerable portion of the fallopian tube left and, in particular, the fimbrial end of the fallopian tube has not been damaged in any way. The success rates of the reversal procedure are directly proportional to the amount of tube that has been damaged. Therefore, the higher success rates are generally seen from the reversal of sterilisations where a single clip, such as a Filshie or Hulka–Clemens clip, has been used and hence the amount of tube that has been damaged is minimal.

A diagnostic laparoscopy is performed first in the usual way to confirm that reversal of either one or both sides is possible. Most surgeons would use a three-port technique. As with any laparoscopic procedure, the exact location of the ports is left to the surgeon's own personal preference.

The surgeon must be adept at gentle manipulation of the tubes and skilled in laparoscopic suturing. The most commonly performed reversal technique is one that is taken from Dubuisson and Chapron [5] and is a single-stitch approach. This involves removal of the clip if it has not already fallen off, and then the occluded or damaged side of the tube is prepared in the usual microsurgical fashion. The tube is mobilised and circumcised both proximally and distally, normally either with fine monopolar scissors or with needlepoint diathermy to coagulate the serosal surface. Under tension, the damaged end of the tube is then excised with laparoscopic scissors and the tubal lumen revealed. If possible, both sides of the tube are then stented with a fine nylon splint, which is either passed down the distal portion of the fallopian tube to be removed from the fimbrial end later or it is removed before the anastomosis is complete. Any deficit in the broad ligament from this mobilisation is then repaired with a single interrupted suture. A further single interrupted suture is placed through the opposing parts of the fallopian tube, which are then sutured together. The placement of this suture is critical not only to match up the correct parts of the fallopian tube, but also to make sure that the suture is not passed into the lumen of the tube, hence damaging it as the suture is reabsorbed.

This is the procedure in its most simple fashion. It has been modified by several surgeons to include the further placement of one or two other interrupted sutures to further approximate the tubal lumen. These sutures are generally placed in an interrupted fashion by use of a fine material such as a 5-0 or 6-0 absorbable suture. The pelvis is then thoroughly washed out, preferably with an anti-adhesion agent such as 4% icodextrin solution (Adept®; Baxter Healthcare Corporation, Deerfield, IL, USA), and further icodextrin solution is left in at the end of the procedure. Finally, routine closure is made.

Distal tubal disease

Unfortunately, there is a distinct lack of good data on which to base decisions regarding tubal surgery. However, as discussed, it is reasonable to expect that tubal adhesions may interfere with ovum pick-up and tubal transport even if the fallopian tubes are patent. Where fine adhesions exist that tether the fimbrial end of the fallopian tube to the ovary, it can be a relatively simple matter to divide them. The extra time taken to perform this procedure by a skilled and appropriately trained surgeon may at least offer the woman a chance of conception and thus avoidance of assisted conception procedures. If she does not conceive, the outcome of assisted conception procedures will not be adversely affected by having had surgery, so there seems to be no disadvantage in this approach.

No difference has been demonstrated in the success rates of any surgical modality over another. Equivalent pregnancy rates have been quoted after the use of carbon dioxide or fibre laser technology, needlepoint diathermy or fine surgical scissors. The important practice point is to ensure gentle handling of the tissues and to recognise the normal physiological adhesions between the fallopian tube and the ovary and the pathological adhesions.

The best data available indicate that if the fallopian tubes are patent but tethered, a pregnancy rate of up to 60% may be expected, depending on the duration of follow-up (usually 1 year or more).

If the fallopian tubes are blocked distally (hydrosalpinx), the chance of conception declines to only 30%. However, this still represents an advantage if assisted conception is avoided. The problem with hydrosalpinges is that they often reocclude, in which case the chance of success with assisted conception is reduced by 50%. Some surgeons would therefore prefer to perform a neosalpingostomy at the time of diagnostic laparoscopy, rather than performing a salpingectomy, as this allows a chance of conception. If the hydrosalpinx re-forms, salpingectomy may be offered as definitive management if the woman has not already conceived either spontaneously or with assisted conception procedures.

Neosalpingostomy

Again, there is no clear advantage of one surgical modality over another. Essentially, management is by forming a cruciate incision in the distal end of the fallopian tube at the site of the thin eschar formed over the lumen. The correct site at which to commence the incision can be identified by injecting methylene blue dye into the fallopian tube via the cervix. Once the incision has been made, some effort must be made to reduce the chance of the tube resealing. This can be achieved by causing mild cicatrisation of the external surface of the tube using a source of heat energy such as laser or diathermy. Alternatively, if the surgeon is skilled at laparoscopic suturing, a more perma-

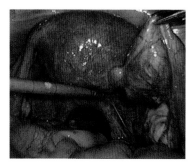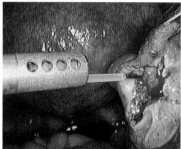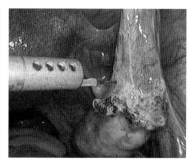

FIGURE 8.6
Hydrosalpinx (A)
opened with a cruciate
incision (B); the outside
of the tube is then
moulded back by heat
shrinkage caused by the
application of the laser
fibre (C)

nent solution would be to use 5-0 or 6-0 monofilament sutures to create a cuff salpingostomy (Figure 8.6, Video 8.2).

Laparoscopic tubal surgery to improve in vitro fertilisation success rates

It has been known since Strandell's innovative work published back in 1994 that hydrosalpinges detectable by ultrasound can have a significant effect on implantation rates.[6] This work has since been repeated by others.[7-9] This is practical, evidence-based medicine at its best. Of equal importance is the fact that removal of the tubes was subsequently shown to significantly improve the implantation rates.[10] This has been confirmed by a meta-analysis[11] and a Cochrane review.[12]

The exact mechanism of this is debatable. It is generally thought that the hydrosalpingeal fluid leaks back into the uterine cavity and is toxic to the embryos trying to implant in the cavity. The fluid may also have a direct physical action by 'washing' the embryos out of the implantation site.[13] It has also been thought that the tube itself might have some adverse effect on the embryos, but more recent work[14,15] has shown that blocking the tube in the isthmic to cornual portion – but not removing it – significantly improves pregnancy rates. This operation can be performed by bipolar coagulation or clipping.[14,15] The fluid within the hydrosalpinx itself is in a low-pressure environment and the tube does not necessarily have to be drained at the time of clipping or coagulation. Pressures are equivalent to approximately 18–20 mmHg and a woman's worries that the tube will carry on increasing in size and eventually rupture can be allayed as it seems to be a self-limiting situation.

Possible problems with salpingectomy

Given that salpingectomy may have a deleterious effect on future ovarian function,[16,17] it is possible that this procedure, when performed for ectopic pregnancy, can compromise the ovarian response to controlled hyperstimulation in the ipsilateral ovary. This probably results from surgery-related compromise to the ovarian blood supply. This may therefore decrease the ovarian response to gonadotrophins in subsequent IVF cycles, although this has been contradicted by findings from other studies.[18] In particular, if there is severe adnexal disease that makes the tube not suitable for corrective surgery, it is more likely that surgery to remove the tube will also be difficult, however carefully the dissection is performed.

The work described in the preceding paragraph was further corroborated in an excellent paper by Gelbaya et al.[19] These authors compared women with hydrosalpinges who had salpingectomy with those who underwent proximal division of the fallopian tubes and showed that the number of oocytes obtained in the salpingectomy group was significantly lower than that in the proximal division group.

It is also recognised that some of the aetiological causes of tubal disease can also damage the ovaries. An infection that caused the distal disease in the first place can produce an oophoritis, which can subsequently result in a poorer than expected result to ovarian stimulation. Recurrent endometriotic cysts can, in some women, also result in a poor response. If the initial ovarian damage is then compounded by subsequent compromise to the ovarian vasculature from a salpingectomy, the net result in some women can be very few eggs, or no eggs at all, from an IVF cycle.

What techniques should be used on an irreparable tube?

Both salpingectomy and coagulation or clipping of the tube can be performed laparoscopically. Indeed, these days there would be very few occasions when the laparoscopic approach would not be the option of choice. Given that blocking of the proximal portion of the tube laparoscopically is a simpler, and therefore probably safer, operation than salpingectomy and given that it is less likely to affect the ovarian response, it could be argued that blocking the proximal portion of the tube should be the treatment of choice. There are, however, some circumstances where a salpingectomy might be beneficial. The two occasions when this is likely to be the case would be:

- the woman who suffered from recurring episodes of salpingitis

- the woman with chronic pelvic pain in whom the hydrosalpinges are thought to be a significant contributing factor.

These women would have the additional benefit of improved implantation rates, in addition to removal of the cause of their recurring pain. Salpingectomy in such women should be performed laparoscopically by a suitably qualified laparoscopic surgeon paying particular care to the dissection of the tube.

Unilateral hydrosalpinx

Some women have unilateral disease that has been caused by localised aetiology but the contralateral tube is still healthy. Sagoskin et al.[20] showed that salpingectomy of the affected side significantly improved spontaneous pregnancy rates after the diseased side was removed. The explanation for this improvement could be similar to that of the effect seen in IVF. In this case, the woman could well be forming a healthy embryo, which is transported down the healthy tube but has a lower chance of successfully implanting because of the hydrosalpingeal fluid entering the uterine cavity from the diseased side. Sagoskin's work elegantly showed that these carefully chosen women do not have to go straight to IVF but have an excellent spontaneous pregnancy rate after surgery. Indeed, 88% of women achieved a spontaneous pregnancy after an average of 5.6 months.[20]

References

1 Department of Health, Scottish Executive Health Department, and Department of Health, Social Services and Public Safety, Northern Ireland. *Why Mothers Die. Fifth Report on Confidential Enquiries into Maternal Deaths in the United Kingdom, 1997–1999*. London: RCOG Press; 2001.

2 Royal College of Obstetricians and Gynaecologists. *The Management of Tubal Pregnancy*. Green-top Guideline No. 21. London: RCOG; 2004 [www.rcog.org.uk/womens-health/clinical-guidance/management-tubal-pregnancy-21-may-2004].

3 Centre for Maternal and Clinical Enquiries. Saving Mothers' Lives. Reviewing maternal deaths to make motherhood safer: 2006–2008. The Eighth Report on Confidential Enquiries into Maternal Deaths in the United Kingdom. *BJOG* 2011;118 Suppl 1:1–203.

4 Koh C, personal communication.

5 Dubuisson J B, Chapron C. Single suture laparoscopic tubal re-anastomosis. *Curr Opin Obstet Gynecol* 1998;10:307–13.

6 Strandell A, Lindhard A, Waldenström U, Thorburn J, Janson PO, Hamberger L. Hydrosalpinx and IVF outcome: a prospective, randomised, multicentre trial in Scandinavia on salpingectomy prior to IVF. *Hum Reprod* 1994;9:2762–9.

7 Vandromme J, Chasse E, Lejeune B, Van Rysselberge M, Delvigne A, Leroy F. Hydrosalpinges in in vitro fertilization: an unfavourable prognostic feature. *Hum Reprod* 1995;10:576–9.

8 Akman MA, Garcia JE, Damewood MD, Watts LD, Katz E. Hydrosalpinx affects the implantation of previously cryopreserved embryos. *Hum Reprod* 1996;11:1013–4.

9 Blazar AS, Hogan JW, Seifer DB, Frishman GN, Wheeler CA, Haning RV. The impact of hydrosalpinx on successful pregnancy in tubal factor infertility treated by in vitro fertilization. *Fertil Steril* 1997;67:517–20.

10 Strandell A, Lindhard A. Hydrosalpinx and ART. Salpingectomy prior to IVF can be recommended to a well-defined subgroup of patients. *Hum Reprod* 2000;15:2072–4.

11 Camus E, Poncelet C, Goffinet F, Wainer B, Merlet F, Nisand I, et al. Pregnancy rates after IVF in cases of tubal infertility with and without hydrosalpinx: A meta-analysis of published comparative studies. *Hum Reprod* 1999;14:1243–9.

12 Johnson N, van Voorst S, Sowter MC, Strandell A, Mol BW. Surgical treatment for tubal disease in women due to undergo in vitro fertilisation. *Cochrane Database Syst Rev* 2010;(1):CD002125.

13 Eytan O, Azem F, Gull I, Wolman I, Elad D, Jaffa AJ. The mechanism of hydrosalpinx in embryo implantation. *Hum Reprod* 2001;16:2662–7.

14 Stadtmauer LA, Riehl RM, Toma SK, Talbert LM. Cauterization of hydrosalpinges before in vitro fertilization is an effective surgical treatment associated with improved pregnancy rates. *Am J Obstet Gynecol* 2000;183:367–1.

15 Surrey ES, Schoolcraft WB. Laparoscopic management of hydrosalpinges before in vitro fertilization–embryo transfer: salpingectomy versus proximal tubal occlusion. *Fertil Steril* 2001;75:612–7.

16 Lass A, Ellenbogen A, Croucher C, Trew G, Margara R, Becattini C, et al. Effect of salpingectomy on ovarian response to superovulation in an in vitro fertilization–embryo transfer programme. *Fertil Steril* 1998;70:1035–8.

17 Chan CCW, Ng EHY, Li CF, Ho PC. Impaired ovarian blood flow and reduced antral follicle count following laparoscopic salpingectomy for ectopic pregnancy. *Hum Reprod* 2003;18:2175–80.

18 Strandell A, Lindhard A, Waldenstrom U, Thorburn J. Prophylactic salpingectomy does not impair the ovarian response in IVF treatment. *Hum Reprod* 2001;16:1135–9.

19 Gelbaya TA, Nardo LG, Fitzgerald CT, Horne G, Brison DR, Lieberman BA. Ovarian response to gonadotropins after laparoscopic salpingectomy or the division of fallopian tubes for hydrosalpinges. *Fertil Steril* 2006;85:1464–8.

20 Sagoskin AW, Lessey BA, Mottla GL, Richter KS, Chetkowski RJ, Chang AS, et al. Salpingectomy or proximal tubal occlusion of unilateral hydrosalpinx increases the potential for spontaneous pregnancy. *Hum Reprod* 2003;18:2634–7.

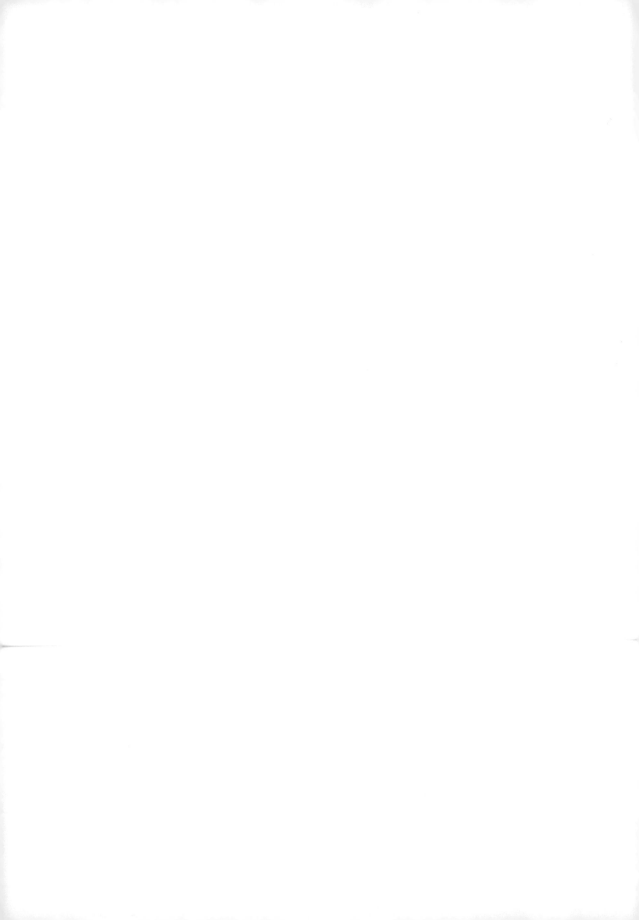

9 Laparoscopic myomectomy

Hayden Homer and Ertan Saridogan

Introduction

Uterine fibroids or leiomyomas are abnormal growths of uterine smooth-muscle cells and are the most common benign tumours in women. Indeed, fibroids can be identified by ultrasound in about 80% of African American women and in almost 70% of white American women by the time of the menopause.[1] At least 50% of fibroids are asymptomatic, however, and are usually discovered incidentally during ultrasonography for other indications or during pelvic surgery.

Myomectomy remains the best treatment option for women with symptomatic fibroids who wish to retain their uterus for fertility purposes. Although laparotomy is the traditional route for performing myomectomy, in recent years laparoscopic myomectomy (LM) has undergone extensive evaluation and benefited from technological improvements. In addition, at least seven randomised controlled trials (RCTs), six of which have recently been subjected to meta-analysis,[2] have now compared LM with open myomectomy and provide compelling conclusions regarding the benefits of LM. Although LM is still a technically challenging procedure that requires advanced laparoscopic surgical skills and has a long learning curve, electrical morcellators have greatly aided the retrieval of tissue from the abdominal cavity and improvements in laparoscopic suturing techniques have enabled better repair of the uterine wall defect. Thus, although LM was initially met with scepticism because of prolonged operating times, excessive blood loss, high conversion rates to laparotomy and suboptimal postsurgical uterine integrity, many such concerns have dissipated. Indeed, some authors now contend that LM is a wholly acceptable and perhaps even preferable option to open myomectomy for treating fibroids.[3,4]

In this chapter, we focus on the technique of LM and explore some of the recent evidence related to this minimally invasive surgical modality. We conclude with a brief overview of some alternative laparoscopic approaches for fibroid treatment.

Fibroid-related symptoms and impact of fibroids on reproductive outcome: rationale for myomectomy

The most common symptoms ascribable to fibroids are excessive uterine bleeding (30%) and pelvic pain and pressure effects (20–50%), for which various modalities of fibroid treatment have been evaluated. Myomectomy results in an overall 81% resolution of menorrhagia, with similar efficacy for alleviating pressure symptoms.[5]

Fibroids may also be associated with reduced fertility and adverse pregnancy sequelae such as miscarriage during the early stages and fetal malpresentation during more advanced gestation.[6] Whereas myomectomy clearly has a role in the treatment of bleeding and pressure symptoms, the role of fibroid treatment in improving reproductive parameters is far less certain. Fibroids are present in 5–10% of women treated for infertility and may be the sole factor identified in 2–3% of such women. Myomas could quite plausibly affect fertility through anatomical distortion of the endometrial cavity, dysfunctional uterine contractility, obstruction of the tubal ostia, altered uterine vasculature and chronic endometrial inflammation.

Two systematic reviews[6,7] have focused on the issue of fibroids and fertility and have pooled data from several series in an attempt to furnish meaningful guidance. Importantly, conclusions from both papers are remarkably consistent and provide convincing evidence supporting submucosal and intramural fibroids as harbingers of an adverse pregnancy outcome. Thus, Pritts et al.[7] found that submucosal fibroids were associated with lower rates of clinical pregnancies (odds ratio [OR] 0.36, 95% CI 0.18–0.74), implantations (OR 0.28, 95% CI 0.12–0.65) and ongoing pregnancies and live births (OR 0.32, 95% CI 0.12–0.85) and with higher rates of spontaneous miscarriages (OR 1.68, 95% CI 1.37–2.05). Similarly, Klatsky et al.[6] found a reduction in the rates of implantations (OR 0.39, 95% CI 0.24–0.65) and clinical pregnancies (OR 0.44, 95% CI 0.28–0.70) and an increased rate of miscarriages (OR 3.85, 95% CI 1.12–13.27) in women with submucosal myomas. Like submucosal fibroids, intramural fibroids were found to be associated with lower clinical pregnancy rates (OR 0.81, CI 0.70–0.94), reduced implantation rates (OR 0.68, CI 0.59–0.80), lower ongoing pregnancy and live birth rates (OR 0.70, CI 0.58–0.85) and higher miscarriage rates (OR 1.75, CI 1.23–2.49).[7] Unlike the other two fibroid variants, subserosal fibroids do not seem to exert a deleterious effect on fertility or pregnancy outcome.[6,7]

The evidence related to the influence of myomectomy on reproductive parameters is comparatively sparse and less clear. Myomectomy for submucous fibroids virtually doubles clinical pregnancy rates compared with no treatment (relative risk [RR] 2.034, 95% CI 1.08–3.83).[7] Somewhat surprisingly, however, although showing a trend towards reduction, the spontaneous miscarriage rate remained statistically unchanged following myomectomy (RR 0.77, 95% CI 0.36–1.66).[7] In contrast to submucosal fibroids, myomectomy for intramural fibroids did not impart any significant benefit to either pregnancy rate or outcome.[7]

In summary, therefore, submucosal fibroids are counterproductive to fertility and the available evidence supports improved reproductive outcome following treatment. For intramural fibroids, there is an undeniable association with adverse pregnancy outcome. However, further prospective studies are required to determine the role of myomectomy for intramural fibroids in improving reproductive performance.[6,7] According to these two reviews, subserosal fibroids do not seem to consistently exert adverse effects on pregnancy and do not routinely require consideration within a fertility context.

Preoperative evaluation

Preoperative evaluation seeks to determine the appropriateness of myomectomy, the feasibility of the laparoscopic approach, the health status of the affected woman and the need for preoperative treatment.

Indications for myomectomy

Myomectomy is appropriate when symptoms can reasonably be ascribed to the presence of fibroids and there is a desire to preserve the uterus. Surgery is most commonly considered when conservative management has failed to control intolerable bleeding problems, especially if the bleeding induces iron deficiency anaemia or compromises quality of life in other ways.[8] Surgery may also be warranted for pain or pressure effects on contiguous structures leading to constipation, dyspareunia, urinary incontinence or frequency or more serious urinary compression effects such as urinary outflow obstruction or hydronephrosis.

As discussed, the role of myomectomy in otherwise asymptomatic women purely for purposes of fertility enhancement is controversial. On the basis of current evidence, however, a lower threshold for treating certain fibroids, such as submucosal fibroids and intramural fibroids, which distort the endometrial cavity, seems justifiable. At the other extreme, subserosal fibroids do not generally warrant treatment unless they are associated with symptoms such as menorrhagia or pain.[3,6,7] Whether treatment is required for intramural fibroids that do not distort the cavity is less clear, but such fibroids should probably be a minimum of about 4 cm before being considered of clinical significance.[3]

Feasibility of laparoscopic myomectomy

Before considering LM, the number, size and location of fibroids must be carefully mapped. This not only helps determine the feasibility of LM versus an open approach but also identifies submucosal fibroids that, as a group, are generally better treated hysteroscopically.[9] Notably, however, because of the potential for heavy bleeding and incomplete resection, some larger type I (intracavitary component more than 50%) and type II (intracavitary component less than 50%) submucosal fibroids may be more effectively treated by the laparoscopic route. There is also concern that hysteroscopic resection of deeply infiltrating type II fibroids, which leaves only a thin residual myometrial layer, may increase the risk of uterine rupture in a subsequent pregnancy, so that women with such fibroids would be better served by an abdominal approach.

There is no absolute restriction to the number and size of fibroids that can be removed laparoscopically,[10] this being determined by the surgeon's experience and expertise. However, the risks of conversion to laparotomy, blood loss and surgical duration increase with fibroid size and number, with an anterior location and with accompanying adenomyosis.[4,10,11] Some authors consider LM to be appropriate for a maximum of three or four myomas whose sizes should not exceed 8 cm,[3,12] whereas others believe in individual choice based on surgical skill.[13]

Using high-quality machines and in experienced hands, transvaginal ultrasound examination is usually adequate for evaluating fibroids preoperatively. Important parameters to be derived from ultrasound include fibroid dimensions, fibroid subtype (submucosal, intramural or subserosal) and fibroid location (for example anterior wall, posterior wall). Saline infusion sonohysterography may also assist in identifying submucosal fibroids and may be particularly useful when there is significant uterine distortion from several other fibroids.[14] Submucosal fibroids may also be identified incidentally on hysterosalpingography as a filling defect or a distorted uterine cavity. When ultrasound findings are atypical, magnetic resonance imaging, which has a high degree of accuracy in characterising fibroids, or computed tomography scanning may help to confirm the diagnosis and to differentiate fibroids from adenomyosis.[8] This is an important distinction to be made because adenomyosis presents an added challenge during laparoscopy owing to the lack of a clearly defined dissection plane. Hysteroscopy and three-dimensional ultrasound are additional modalities that may be useful in delineating fibroids (Figure 9.1, Video 9.1).

In spite of meticulous preoperative evaluation, the final decision as to whether LM is feasible may only be possible at the time of surgery. A decision to convert to an open approach on the basis of the initial laparoscopic findings should be considered a sign of wisdom, not evidence of defeat.[3] It is therefore imperative that the woman be made aware of the possibility of an open approach and that this is reflected in the preoperative consultation and consent.

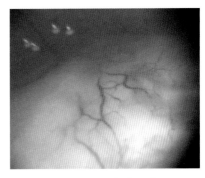

FIGURE 9.1 **Hysteroscopic view of a 7 cm posterior wall type II submucosal fibroid with a significant intramural component**

Pretreatment with gonadotrophin-releasing hormone agonists

There are pros and cons to the use of gonadotrophin-releasing hormone (GnRH) agonists before LM. The main advantages include correction of anaemia presurgery, attenuation of blood loss, reduction of the uterine and fibroid size and reduction of adhesion formation.[15,16] The downsides include added cost and menopausal adverse effects. In addition, GnRH agonists may increase the difficulty in identifying surgical dissection planes, increase the duration of the procedure and increase the risk of conversion to laparotomy.[11] Preoperative GnRH agonists have also been reported as a risk factor for fibroid recurrence,[17] presumably because smaller fibroids shrink and are overlooked at surgery only to regrow when the analogue's effects wear off.

Overall, given that GnRH analogues may increase the risk of recurrence, and given the complexity of surgery and hence its duration and risk of laparotomic conversion, the routine use of these agents is not justified. This is especially so since other agents such as intraoperative vasopressin do not increase surgical intricacy and are of proven efficacy in reducing intraoperative bleeding.[18] A potential benefit to be derived from GnRH agonist use might be reduced fibroid and uterine size, an effect that enables a larger number of hysterectomies to be performed vaginally rather than abdominally.[16] If GnRH agonist use makes the laparoscopic approach similarly more feasible for larger fibroids, it may be considered worthwhile in these circumstances, albeit at the expense of rendering surgical planes less distinct. Some authors do not consider such a trade-off to be surgically advantageous and restrict GnRH agonist usage to women with serious anaemia preoperatively.[13]

Additional preoperative issues

Because many LM operations will be performed for intractable menorrhagia, many women will be anaemic and require preoperative intervention to resurrect the haemoglobin concentration to anaesthetically safe levels. As already mentioned, GnRH analogues constitute one effective means for achieving this by temporarily reducing heavy periods in the run-up to surgery. Some authors advocate recombinant erythropoietin,[8] with an Italian prospective study[19] showing a significant increase in haemoglobin concentrations before and after gynaecological surgery (which included hysterectomy for large symptomatic fibroids) after using recombinant human erythropoietin for 8–16 days. Women with borderline haemoglobin levels should also be advised on the use of oral ferrous sulphate.

Regardless of the preoperative haemoglobin level, it should be ensured that cross-matched blood is readily accessible at the time of surgery. It is important that the woman undergoing surgery be made aware of the possibility of conversion to laparotomy and of the less frequent need for hysterectomy in addition to other standard complications associated with laparoscopic surgery. Bowel preparation using a mild laxative may provide better exposure of the operative field, especially for posterior wall fibroids or when there is coexisting disease requiring simultaneous treatment such as endometriosis.

Surgical technique

Preparation of the woman

Under general endotracheal anaesthesia, the woman is placed in the lithotomy position with the thighs slightly flexed and with the arms at the sides. The cervix is grasped with a vulsellum forceps and a uterine manipulator is placed in the cervical canal. This is useful for exerting countertraction during fibroid enucleation, for manipulating the uterus during suturing and for methylene blue dye instillation if tubal patency testing is required. If there is any uncertainty from preoperative imaging regarding the presence and/or type of submucous fibroids and whether hysteroscopic resection is preferable to LM, a diagnostic hysteroscopy is undertaken.

Trocar placement

Trocar placement is at the surgeon's discretion and should be such that it allows for fibroid dissection and countertraction during enucleation and facilitates intracorporeal suturing. The laparoscope is most often inserted through a 10 mm umbilical trocar, although a Palmer's point entry with a 5 mm scope may be preferable for larger fibroids or where periumbilical adhesions are anticipated as a result of prior surgery.[20] The authors' preference is to use three further ports: two 5 mm high paraumbilical ports placed lateral to the epigastric vessels and a 10 mm suprapubic port placed slightly off-centre and approximately 4 cm superior to the symphysis pubis. The suprapubic port provides suture access, facilitates mechanical enucleation by allowing the use of either a heavy self-locking claw grasper or myomectomy screw and will later be enlarged to 15 mm and replaced by the morcellator. Other port arrangements have been described, such as two contra- and ipsilateral ports, which are suggested to be more ergonomic for suturing.[21]

As an initial step, it is important to carefully survey the pelvis and reassess whether the laparoscopic approach remains feasible. For deeper-sited fibroids that may not be readily evident on inspection, an intraoperative ultrasound evaluation to identify and map fibroid dimensions is invaluable to compensate for the lack of a tactile element in LM.[22]

Having decided that LM is the optimal procedure and that target fibroids are clearly delineated, there are three main steps involved in LM. These include uterine incision and fibroid enucleation, establishment of haemostasis and repair of the uterine wall, and removal of the specimen.

Minimising intraoperative bleeding

Before incising the serosa, a dilute solution of Pitressin® (20 U/ml; Goldshield Pharmaceuticals, Croydon, UK), a synthetic vasopressin, is injected. We dilute 20 U of Pitressin in 20 ml of saline and administer it using an 18-gauge spinal needle placed directly through the abdominal wall. Pitressin is instilled bilaterally into the broad ligament just inferior to the round ligaments and subserosally over the fibroid in the plane that allows the solution to 'spread' over the fibroid, accompanied by blanching (Figure 9.2, Video 9.2).

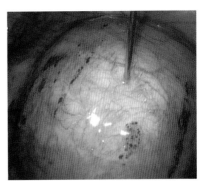

FIGURE 9.2 **Subserosal Pitressin® injection with accompanying blanching**

Vasopressin causes constriction of vascular smooth muscle and may cause untoward cardiovascular complications, making it important to forewarn the anaesthetist prior to its instillation. Pitressin use in myomectomy is an off-label use of the drug. A recent meta-analysis affirmed the efficacy of vasopressin in reducing intraoperative bleeding during myomectomies, alternatives being vaginal misoprostol or a combination of 0.25% bupivacaine and epinephrine.[18]

Uterine incision

An incision is made in the uterine serosa overlying the fibroid using a monopolar hook or scissors with unmodulated high-wattage current (50 W or more) together with a smoke extractor to maintain a clear operative field (Video 9.3). Alternatively, an ultrasonic scalpel (Harmonic Scalpel®; Johnson & Johnson, New Brunswick, NJ, USA) may be used, which has the advantages of avoiding thermal damage, reducing the need for smoke evacuation and inducing less blood loss,[23] the trade-off being increased cost. Recent RCT data cite additional benefits for the Harmonic Scalpel over electrosurgical approaches including reduced postoperative pain and reduced operating times.[24]

The direction of the incision depends on the location of the fibroid and must take into account avoidance of tubal injury and ease of suturing. Some feel that horizontal incisions cause less bleeding than vertical ones by virtue of avoiding cutting across the transversely running arcuate vessels.[21] In practice, however, when highly effective haemostatic adjuvants such as Pitressin are employed, the overwhelming factor influencing the choice of incisional direction is the extent to which it facilitates suturing. The repair of horizontal incisions is easier with ipsilaterally placed ports,[21] whereas when ports are sited contralaterally, vertical incisions are more amenable to suturing. Horizontal incisions may risk inadvertent extension into the cornua and interstitial portions of the tubes. In a recent report of 2050 LMs, all incisions were made vertically.[4] Some advocate the use of elliptical as opposed to linear incisions to enable resection of some of the overlying myometrium and to reduce redundant tissue, thereby facilitating closure.

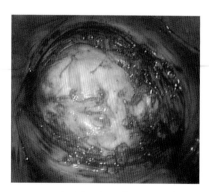

FIGURE 9.3 **Incision through serosa and myometrium into the myoma**

Fibroid dissection and enucleation

Identification of the correct plane helps fibroid extraction. The incision is carried through the serosa, the myometrium, the pseudocapsule and into the myoma itself (Figure 9.3, Video 9.3). So-called onion-skinning allows the myometrium to retract and the fibroid to progressively become extruded, thereby allowing the correct plane to declare itself. This plane, which is avascular, is often deeper than is commonly recognised.

Primary traction on the exposed fibroid is applied with a self-locking claw grasper or fibroid screw placed through the 10–12 mm suprapubic port (Figure 9.4, Video 9.3). A blunt probe together with a grasper such as a Manhes forceps to hold the myometrial/serosal edge via the paraumbilical ports is used to push the myometrial edge off the fibroid. This enables the space along the pseudocapsule to be gradually extended circumferentially. Tension on the fibroid by use of the suprapubic 10 mm claw forceps with simultaneous countertraction from the blunt probe and/or Manhes forceps and the uterine manipulator, aided by division of more stubborn bands using the monopolar hook, progressively coaxes the fibroid from its uterine bed (Figure 9.5, Video 9.3). Once removed, the fibroid can be placed in the pouch of Douglas. Larger fibroids may be placed in the upper abdomen, but it would be better to keep smaller fibroids in the pelvis to avoid difficulty in locating them later in the upper abdomen among the loops of bowel and the omentum.

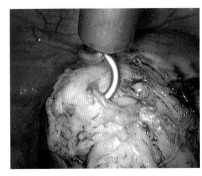

FIGURE 9.4 **Myomectomy screw is inserted into the fibroid through the 11 mm suprapubic port**

Haemostasis and repair of the myometrial defect

It is often felt that a distinct primary vascular pedicle will be found at the fibroid base. However, this is not supported by vascular corrosion casting with electron microscopic examination, which demonstrates that the vascular supply completely surrounds the fibroid as a dense vascular capsule.[25] The appearance of a vascular pedicle may actually represent myometrium under tension.[21]

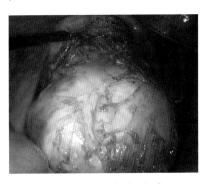

FIGURE 9.5 **Myoma enucleation is almost complete**

Instead of indiscriminate use of electrocautery, individual bleeding vessels should be isolated and cauterised between the jaws of a bipolar forceps, thereby limiting thermal spread and tissue charring. Use of a vasoconstrictor such as vasopressin is effective in maintaining a relatively bloodless field so that prompt suturing is often all that is required to control the majority of bleeding. As far as possible, electrocoagulation should be avoided as it has been implicated in an increased risk of uterine rupture in subsequent pregnancy,[12,26,27] possibly through tissue damage and compromised wound healing. Consistent with this theory, two studies[28,29] have reported on pregnancies following LM during which electrocoagulation was avoided and haemostasis secured by suturing; no uterine ruptures were observed in 111 deliveries[28] and 106 deliveries.[29]

Repair of the uterine wall is the most technically demanding component of the procedure. In one series,[11] difficulties encountered with suturing were a major cause of conversion to laparotomy, accounting for 30/48 (63%) conversions. The uterine defect can be closed using conventional laparoscopic needle drivers and delayed absorbable sutures (Figures 9.6 and 9.7). Knot tying may be either intra- or extracorporeal. If the endometrial cavity is breached, the endome-

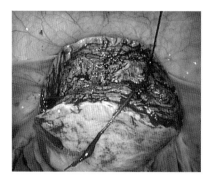

FIGURE 9.6 **Beginning of first layer of repair after myoma enucleation**

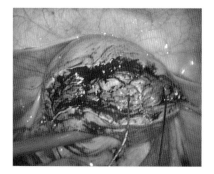

FIGURE 9.7 **First layer of uterine repair is complete**

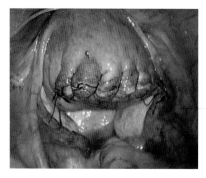

FIGURE 9.8 **Completion of uterine serosa repair**

trium is closed with interrupted 3-0 monofilament polyglactin. The myometrium is closed using large curved needles swaged to 1-0 or 0 polyglactin in one or two continuous running layers depending on the depth of fibroid invasion and the thickness of the myometrium to be approximated (Figure 9.7, Video 9.4). Although continuous running sutures may not necessarily be more expedient, they are associated with a significantly smaller drop in haemoglobin levels.[13] Suturing is made more convenient with an anchoring suture placed on the proximal end of the defect, on which the assistant exerts traction so as to bring the target into a favourable position for placing the running suture, which commences at the distal end. A separate layer of 0 monofilament polyglactin is used to close the serosa (Figure 9.8).

Because of the two-dimensional view and lack of tactile sensation during laparoscopy, simply loading a curved needle properly on to a needle driver can be frustrating. Technological innovations such as self-righting needle drivers that snap the needle into place with the correct orientation and ready-made clips that obviate the need for knot tying may therefore simplify suturing,[3] especially at the beginning of the learning curve.

A significant advance with the potential for greatly simplifying LM is the barbed suture, which has tiny barbs cut into the length of the thread. These barbs face either in one direction with a needle swaged to one end (V-Loc™ device; Covidien, Mansfield, MA, USA) or in opposite directions from the midpoint with needles at either end (Quill™ SRS; Angiotech Pharmaceuticals, Vancouver, BC, Canada). The barbed suture distributes tension more uniformly along the length of the uterine incision and self-anchors, thereby obviating the need for knot tying. Evaluations of this suture design indicate that it can be safely and effectively applied to LM.[30] Moreover, in keeping with the elimination of a technically challenging step during LM, retrospective comparisons indicate a significant shortening of the operating time with the barbed suture as opposed to conventional smooth sutures.[31]

Fibroid removal and anti-adhesion agents

The fibroid is usually removed using a single-use or reusable electromechanical morcellator. The 10 mm suprapubic trocar is removed and the skin incision extended to accommodate the 15 mm morcellator trocar. The fibroid is drawn into the morcellator via a heavy grasper and the morcellator is activated, taking extreme care that its tip is free of the abdominal wall and in a pocket of pneumoperitoneum having proper 360° clearance from bowel and adjacent structures (Video 9.5). The morcellator blade is kept retracted except when actively morcellating the fibroid (Figure 9.9).

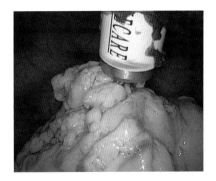

FIGURE 9.9 **Morcellation using a single-use morcellator inserted suprapubically**

After removing the main bulk of the fibroid, meticulous inspection of the abdominopelvic cavity and removal of fibroid fragments is imperative as morcellated fragments of fibroid have been implicated in the development of disseminated peritoneal leiomyomatosis. Miyake et al.[32] reported the case of a woman who developed 17 fibroids in the pelvic cavity after LM. Molecular genetic analysis revealed that all fibroids, 14 of which were resected 6 years after the initial myomectomy, were identical to the fibroid removed during the primary surgery.

Another option for fibroid removal is via a colpotomy incision, which may be faster than morcellation.[23] However, colpotomy leaves the woman with a vaginal incision, may increase the risk of infection and cannot be used for very large fibroids.

Once the fibroid has been removed, the uterus is irrigated and haemostasis confirmed.

Barriers to adhesion may be used upon completion of suturing. A Cochrane review[33] found that oxidised regenerated cellulose (Interceed®; Johnson & Johnson, New Brunswick, NJ, USA) reduces adhesions following laparoscopy (Figure 9.10, Video 9.6) and that expanded polytetrafluoroethylene (Gore-Tex®; WL Gore and Associates, Newark, DE, USA) may be superior to Interceed, although its usefulness is limited by the need for suturing and later removal. There was no evidence of effectiveness for the hyaluronic-acid-based membrane Sepra-film® (Genzyme, Cambridge, MA, USA) and the sheet-type fibrin sealant TachoComb® (Nycomed Austria, Linz, Austria) in preventing adhesion formation.[33] As yet, however, there is no substantial evidence that any of these agents improve fertility, reduce pain or decrease the incidence of postoperative bowel obstruction.[34]

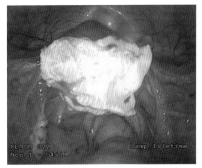

FIGURE 9.10 **Interceed® laid over the sutured incision**

Finally, when closing the abdominal wall incisions, it is important to repair the rectus sheath defect within the 15 mm suprapubic incision used for grasper, suture and morcellator access to avoid subsequent herniation. Closure can be effected with either a J-shaped needle or a suture passer needle.

Complications

Anxiety has been expressed that the rate of complications following LM may be unacceptably high. However, these fears may have been fuelled by earlier sensational case reports that focused attention on adverse effects; in these reports, suboptimal technique such as complete failure to undertake suturing[35,36] or use of too fine a suture calibre (e.g. 4-0)[37] could well have consigned these women to disaster. In light of results from larger series in which LM was undertaken using rigorous techniques, earlier apprehension now seems exaggerated.

A study[4] in 2007 reported on 2050 LM procedures undertaken in four Italian referral centres. This is the single largest prospective study to look at complications of LM and is instructive regarding rates and types of adverse effects associated with LM. The overall complication rate was 11.1%, of which 9.1% were considered minor and 2% (38 of 2050) major.

With regard to major complications, intraoperative bleeding occurred in 0.68% (14/2050) of women, of whom only one woman required a blood transfusion.[4] There were two (0.10%) women with serious secondary haemorrhage, both requiring a transfusion; one woman required laparoscopic hysterectomy because of bleeding from the left uterine artery and the other required ultrasound-guided drainage of a broad ligament haematoma. Failure to complete planned surgery occurred in seven (0.34%) instances; one of these procedures was converted to laparoscopic hysterectomy because of a large intraligamentous fibroid. Conversion to laparotomy occurred in the other six women (0.29%) – in three women because of anaesthetic problems, in one woman because of a suspected sarcoma and in only two women because of insufficient space limiting mobilisation for very large myomas. This relatively low conversion rate was not related to the selection of women with a low risk because fibroids of up to 20 cm were removed in this study and up to 15 fibroids per woman were considered feasible.

In this series,[4] only one (0.05%) woman suffered a bowel injury, this woman having had a prior myomectomy before presenting with leiomyomatosis peritonealis disseminata. This woman presented with late bowel perforation on day 13 after surgery and was treated laparoscopically and avoided a colostomy. One (0.05%) woman had an unrecognised episode of prolonged hypotension resulting in acute kidney failure, which resolved after 2 days of dialysis, and two (0.10%) women had an unexpected sarcoma. Among 386 women who became pregnant, one (0.26%) woman had a uterine rupture at 33 weeks of gestation; this woman had had an 8 cm adenomyoma.

The most common complications were minor and included unexplained transient pyrexia (105/2050 women; 5.12%) and urinary tract infections

(70/2050 women; 3.41%).[4] There were 12 (0.60%) episodes of uterine manipulator injury. Overall, the mean drop in haemoglobin levels was 1.6 g/dl and mean hospital stay was about 2 days.

Therefore, in the hands of expert laparoscopic surgeons, exclusion criteria for LM in terms of numbers and sizes of fibroids are very few indeed.[4] Moreover, it is extremely reassuring that very low rates of major haemorrhage requiring transfusion (0.14%), conversion to laparotomy (0.34%), bowel injury (0.05%) and uterine rupture in a subsequent pregnancy (0.26%) are attainable. Although their rate is low, complications do correlate positively with fibroid number and size,[4] as also noted previously.[11] Thus, although these figures may not accurately reflect problems encountered by less experienced laparoscopic surgeons, they reinforce the importance of ensuring that the selection of women for surgery is proportionate to surgical skill.

It should be remembered that, compared with open myomectomy, LM is a relatively new procedure that is still evolving. Furthermore, some of the skills needed for LM are not readily transferable from more routinely performed procedures, as might be the case for open myomectomy. As such, many operators are still on their learning curve and as their repertoire of laparoscopic skills continues to be honed, complication rates will undoubtedly fall. Added to this, improvements and new innovations in laparoscopic equipment to aid suturing and fibroid removal have (and will continue to have) an impact on LM. In this regard, it is noteworthy that some of the surgeons involved in the Italian multicentre study that reported the impressively low complication rates discussed previously (such as a 0.05% rate of intraoperative transfusions[4]) reported considerably higher rates (such as a 2.6% rate of intraoperative transfusions) in a study published 6 years earlier.[38] Furthermore, in a very insightful study, some of these authors appraised their own practice over a 13-year period.[13] They found that as their dexterity improved and they supplemented their practice with electromechanical morcellation and vasoconstrictive agents, they could cope with considerably larger fibroids while at the same time decreasing their operating times and blood loss.[13]

Laparoscopic myomectomy versus open myomectomy

LM has been performed since the late 1970s and is a much more recently described technique than its abdominal counterpart, which was described as far back as 1840.[9] Abdominal myomectomy has been considered the gold standard in conservative surgical treatment for uterine fibroids. As such, before embracing the minimal access approach, this approach must be

TABLE 9.1 **Randomised controlled trials comparing laparoscopic myomectomy with open myomectomy**

Study	Laparoscopic myomectomy (n)	Laparotomy (n)	Advantages of laparoscopic myomectomy	Disadvantages of laparoscopic myomectomy	Notes
Mais et al., 1996[42]	20	20	Less pain Shorter hospitalisation Faster recovery	None	No difference in fibroid recurrence Similar operative times
Serrachioli et al., 2000[39]	66	65	Less fever Less blood loss Shorter hospitalisation	None	No difference in fibroid recurrence Similar operative times
Rossetti et al., 2001[17]	41	40	None	None	No difference in fibroid recurrence Data available for recurrence rates only
Alessandri et al., 2006[41]	74	74	Less pain Less blood loss Less ileus Shorter hospitalisation Faster recovery	Longer operative time Two complications (one conversion to laparotomy for bleeding and one ileal perforation)	No difference in fibroid recurrence
Holzer et al., 2006[66]	19	21	Less pain	None	Data available for pain only
Palomba et al., 2007[43,44]	68	68	Less pain Less blood loss Shorter hospitalisation	None	Similar operative tines Fibroid location was the most significant determinant of surgical difficulty
Sesti et al., 2008[40]	50	50	Shorter operative times Less pain Less blood loss Less fever Less ileus Faster recovery	None	Used isobaric gasless laparoscopy

shown to be at least as safe as open surgery. What head-to-head comparisons have been made and what do they tell us about the two procedures?

Since the last review[3] of LM when three RCTs comparing LM and open myomectomy were identified, there have been at least four further RCTs (Table 9.1) and one meta-analysis. Reduced pain and bleeding are consistent features after laparoscopy, identified in five and four studies, respectively (Table 9.1). Randomised controlled data also support reduced febrile morbidity following laparoscopy[39,40] and a shorter duration of postoperative ileus[40,41] (Table 9.1). Although the lack of a tactile component during laparoscopy could plausibly allow smaller fibroids to be missed, this does not seem to be of any clinical consequence because four RCTs[17,39–41] reveal no difference between the two approaches in terms of fibroid recurrence (Table 9.1). Notably, none of the RCTs demonstrated a higher rate of complications for any of these variables following LM. The meta-analysis by Jin et al.[2] reaffirms the benefits of LM and led the authors to propose that the laparoscopic approach is a better choice than the open approach in appropriately selected women. Thus, we can conclude that LM is associated with reduced rates of postoperative pain, bleeding, febrile morbidity and postoperative ileus, all culminating in faster recovery and shorter hospital stay.

Owing to the technical challenges of laparoscopic suturing and the time taken for removal of fibroids from the abdominal cavity, LM would be expected to be a longer procedure than open myomectomy. Interestingly, however, major differences in operating times are not consistently apparent from RCTs. One study[41] did report significantly shorter times for minilaparotomy compared with laparoscopy, although the times were relatively short for both arms (85 minutes versus 98 minutes). However, three studies[39,42,43] reported no difference in operating times between the two modalities and in one study[40] in which gasless laparoscopy was used, operating times were significantly shorter for LM (Table 9.1). Increasingly acceptable operating times for LM probably reflect a refinement of laparoscopic skills along with access to better surgical equipment. In support of this hypothesis, an Italian group recently analysed their LM operating times over a 13-year period, during which time they operated on 332 women. As their learning curve evolved and they introduced electromechanical morcellation and vasoconstrictive agents, they found that operating times declined significantly from 142.2 minutes to 118.7 minutes.[13] Similar to this, the large Italian multicentre study reported a mean operating time of 107.7 minutes for 2050 LM procedures.[4] Overall, therefore, there does not seem to be a huge gulf in surgical duration between the two modalities. Instead, the most consistent conclusion from recent studies is that the two approaches are of comparable duration (Table 9.1).

One of the major criticisms levelled against LM has been that the integrity of uterine repair is inferior to that attainable following open myomectomy. Indeed, many of the sensational reports that attracted unwanted attention to LM were based on uterine rupture in pregnancies following LM.[26,35–37] As discussed previously, however, in many instances suboptimal operative technique may have contributed to poor outcome. It is hard to establish how the risk of uterine rupture following LM compares with that following open surgery. Nevertheless, technical inadequacies that may predispose to rupture after LM have been exposed.[29] It is also clear from recent series[4] that when good surgical discipline is maintained, dehiscence rates well below 1% can be expected.

Fertility and reproductive outcomes after LM and open myomectomy have been addressed in two RCTs.[39,44] The first RCT involved 131 infertile women and found no difference in the rates of pregnancy, miscarriage or preterm delivery between the two approaches.[39] The more recent paper included 136 women, 74 of whom had symptomatic fibroids and no fertility issues and 62 of whom had unexplained infertility.[44] Consistent with the findings by Seracchioli et al.,[39] the outcomes in terms of cumulative pregnancy, live birth and miscarriage rates among the women with unexplained infertility were similar regardless of the surgical approach used.[44] Interestingly, however, reproductive parameters were significantly better following LM among women with symptomatic fibroids. As a group, women having LM had significantly higher rates of pregnancies and live births per cycle and a shorter time to first conception.[44] Thus, there is a suggestion that fertility prospects might improve with the laparoscopic approach.

One mechanism by which LM could be advantageous to fertility is through reduced adhesion formation. One recent prospective study compared adhesion rates after LM with those after open myomectomy and found a nonsignificant trend towards reduced adhesion formation with the laparoscopic approach. Added to this, two case–control studies[45,46] indicate that LM induces less adhesion formation than laparotomy. Nevertheless, such links, if they do exist, remain tenuous because they imply that reduced adhesions correlate with improved fertility, an association that is not borne out by studies on anti-adhesion agents.[34]

Laparoscopic alternatives to laparoscopic myomectomy for fibroid management

Laparoscopically assisted myomectomy

Laparoscopically assisted myomectomy (LAM) has been proposed as an alternative to LM that may incorporate some of the benefits of the laparoscopic approach, such as reduced hospital stay, while at the same time being less technically demanding than LM and thus more widely applicable.[47] The technique usually incorporates a minilaparotomy incision up to 7 cm long. The uterine incision can be made either laparoscopically prior to laparotomy or via the laparotomy incision.[48,49] An alternative to classic LAM has also been described in which fibroid removal and uterine repair are conducted through a posterior colpotomy instead of a minilaparotomy.[50]

Although initially described in 1994,[51] to date LAM has been evaluated in only two RCTs [48,49] (both involving minilaparotomy) and only one of these has compared LAM with LM.[49] In their study of 52 women, Tan et al.[49] found that LAM was superior to LM in terms of operating time and intraoperative blood loss. Similar to these data, a recent nonrandomised prospective study [52] of 116 women that compared LAM with LM found shorter operating times for LAM but less blood loss for LM.

Although LAM is almost two decades older than LM, it has been far less extensively evaluated. Furthermore, LAM can involve a skin incision of considerable length, which goes against the ethos of laparoscopic surgery and must therefore be cosmetically inferior to LM. Consequently, LAM should not be considered a laparoscopic approach per se and is perhaps more appropriately regarded as a minilaparotomy myomectomy that has the benefit of laparoscopy for pre- and postmyomectomy pelviuterine evaluation and treatment of associated pathology such as endometriosis.

Laparoscopic uterine artery occlusion and ligation

Driven by the benefit of improved fibroid-related symptoms associated with fibroid devascularisation by uterine artery embolisation (UAE), uterine artery ligation undertaken by the laparoscopic route has been pursued. The advantage of laparoscopic uterine artery occlusion (LUAO) is that it avoids off-target embolisation of other organs, most notably the ovaries, which may result in ovarian failure in up to 5% of women following UAE.[53] However, given that myomectomy with uterine preservation is often performed for women wishing to retain (or indeed improve) their fertility, the impact of LUAO on subsequent reproductive performance is paramount. This is especially so since pregnancies following UAE seem to be at increased risk of miscarriage[54] and pregnancy outcome following LM is superior to that following UAE.[55,56] It is reassuring, however, that LUAO seems to have less of a negative impact on miscarriage rates than UAE, as indicated by a prospective study.[57] Given that LUAO requires a general anaesthetic and carries many of the risks of LM, and that temporary uterine artery occlusion using a transvaginal Doppler-guided clamp offers a potential noninvasive alternative,[53] further evaluation of LUAO will be required. Thus far, no head-to-head comparisons between LUAO as an isolated treatment modality and LM have been reported.

Laparoscopic uterine artery ligation (LUAL) performed at the time of LM has been pursued with the intention of reducing bleeding and thereby simplifying the procedure. One prospective nonrandomised study[58] compared LM alone with LM in combination with LUAL and found significantly reduced blood loss and reduced myoma recurrence rates but longer operating times when LUAL was incorporated. Another prospective comparison[59] returned similar outcomes with regard to myoma recurrence but found no differences with regard to blood loss or operating times. Thus, one consistent finding is reduced myoma recurrence when LUAL is incorporated into the LM procedure, perhaps because the resulting ischaemia prevents de novo fibroid formation or the growth of small residual fibroids. As alluded to above, there are concerns that such ischaemia could plausibly be detrimental to fertility prospects. Reassuringly, however, one study[58] found no difference in live birth rates between infertile women who underwent LM only and those in whom LUAL was included.

In recognition of the potential risks to fertility incurred by LUAL-induced ischaemia, one study[60] explored the use of transient occlusion of the uterine artery at the time of LM. When compared with women undergoing LM alone, those undergoing transient LUAO had significantly less blood loss. Notably, there was no difference in pregnancy rates between the two groups. Interestingly, however, unlike LUAL, transient LUAO did not reduce the recurrence rate of myomas, indicating that this benefit is derived only when more severe ischaemia is induced.

Laparoscopic myolysis

A reduction in fibroid volume of 50% or more can be achieved using energy delivered directly to the fibroid via electrocautery or laser (thermomyolysis) or by inserting a super-cooled cryoprobe to reduce the core fibroid temperature to −90°C (cryomyolysis).[61] However, myolysis has been associated with high rates of dense adhesions and is yet to be evaluated against more established treatment modalities.[3] Furthermore, other experimental means of delivering energy to fibroids, such as focused ultrasound energy guided and monitored by magnetic resonance imaging, may prove more attractive because of their noninvasiveness.

Robot-assisted laparoscopic myomectomy

Although most extensively used so far for laparoscopic hysterectomies, computer-assisted or robotic technology is increasingly being applied to LM.[62] Robot-assisted LM (RALM) is still in its infancy with no prospective trials yet available that compare RALM and LM. One recent retrospective matched-control study[63] found similar blood loss, postoperative complication rates and hospital stay for RALM and LM but significantly longer operating times for RALM. Another retrospective analysis[64] did not find that RALM significantly increased surgical time and advocated robotic technology as a means for enabling a laparoscopic approach in women who would otherwise require open surgery because of a larger fibroid size or a difficult location. It remains to be seen how the benefits offered by RALM such as three-dimensional images, superior instrument articulation, absence of tremor, downscaling of movements and increased comfort for the surgeon compare with its downsides such as bulkiness, cost of equipment and lack of haptic feedback.

Conclusions

Modern LM represents the results of years of refinement, often in response to weaknesses highlighted by adverse effects, combined with key advances such as the development of intraoperative vasoconstrictors and electromechanical morcellation. The end result is a technique with impressive efficacy and safety profiles. Regrettably, in the UK the uptake of LM seems low, with a recent survey[65] reporting that only 16% of 735 consultants performed LM compared with 75% undertaking open myomectomy.

Although there are no preset restrictions, surgeons must be pragmatic in matching their skill to fibroid burden, opting for a laparotomy approach when fibroids are too many or too large. In such circumstances, LAM may be of value. Compared with conventional myomectomy, LM is – apart from its obvious aesthetic superiority – consistently associated with reduced rates of pain, bleeding, febrile morbidity and ileus, shorter hospital stay and faster recovery. Importantly, recent evidence indicates that with careful attention to surgical detail, the rate of uterine ruptures in pregnancies following LM is low and operating times are not dissimilar to open surgery. Moreover, LM is superior to UAE in terms of reproductive outcomes in subsequent pregnancies and may offer advantages over the open approach. Further research is required regarding the potential reproductive benefits of LM and the role of alternative modalities such as LAM, LUAO and RALM.

References

1 Day Baird D, Dunson D B, Hill M C, Cousins D, Schectman J M. High cumulative incidence of uterine leiomyoma in black and white women: ultrasound evidence. *Am J Obstet Gynecol* 2003;188:100–7.

2 Jin C, Hu Y, Chen X C, Zheng F Y, Lin F, Zhou K, et al. Laparoscopic versus open myomectomy – a meta-analysis of randomized controlled trials. *Eur J Obstet Gynecol Reprod Biol* 2009;145:14–21.

3 Hurst B S, Matthews M L, Marshburn P B. Laparoscopic myomectomy for symptomatic uterine myomas. *Fertil Steril* 2005;83:1–23.

4 Sizzi O, Rossetti A, Malzoni M, Minelli L, La Grotta F, Soranna L, et al. Italian multicenter study on complications of laparoscopic myomectomy. *J Minim Invasive Gynecol* 2007;14:453–62.

5 Buttram V C, Reiter R C. Uterine leiomyomata: etiology, symptomatology, and management. *Fertil Steril* 1981;36: 433–45.

6 Klatsky P C, Tran N D, Caughey A B, Fujimoto V Y. Fibroids and reproductive outcomes: a systematic literature review from conception to delivery. *Am J Obstet Gynecol* 2008;198:357–66.

7 Pritts E A, Parker W H, Olive D L. Fibroids and infertility: an updated systematic review of the evidence. *Fertil Steril* 2008;91:1215–23.

8 Parker W H. Uterine myomas: management. *Fertil Steril* 2007;88:255–71.

9 Saridogan E, Cutner A. Endoscopic management of uterine fibroids. *Hum Fertil (Camb)* 2006;9:201–8.

10 Sinha R, Hegde A, Mahajan C, Dubey N, Sundaram M. Laparoscopic myomectomy: do size, number, and location of the myomas form limiting factors for laparoscopic myomectomy? *J Minim Invasive Gynecol* 2008;15:292–300.

11 Dubuisson J B, Fauconnier A, Fourchotte V, Babaki-Fard K, Coste J, Chapron C. Laparoscopic myomectomy: predicting the risk of conversion to an open procedure. *Hum Reprod* 2001;16:1726–31.

12 Dubuisson J B, Fauconnier A, Deffarges J V, Norgaard C, Kreiker G, Chapron C. Pregnancy outcome and deliveries following laparoscopic myomectomy. *Hum Reprod* 2000;15:869–73.

13 Rossetti A, Sizzi O, Chiarotti F, Florio G. Developments in techniques for laparoscopic myomectomy. *JSLS* 2007;11: 34–40.

14 Lindheim S R, Adsuar N, Kushner D M, Pritts E A, Olive D L. Sonohysterography: a valuable tool in evaluating the female pelvis. *Obstet Gynecol Surv* 2003;58:770–84.

15 Imai A, Sugiyama M, Furui T, Takahashi S, Tamaya T. Gonadotrophin-releasing hormones agonist therapy increases peritoneal fibrinolytic activity and prevents adhesion formation after myomectomy. *J Obstet Gynaecol* 2003;23:660–3.

16 Lethaby A, Vollenhoven B, Sowter M. Pre-operative GnRH analogue therapy before hysterectomy or myomectomy for uterine fibroids. *Cochrane Database Syst Rev* 2001;(2):CD000547.

17 Rossetti A, Sizzi O, Soranna L, Cucinelli F, Mancuso S, Lanzone A. Long-term results of laparoscopic myomectomy: recurrence rate in comparison with abdominal myomectomy. *Hum Reprod* 2001;16:770–4.

18 Kongnyuy E J, van den Broek N, Wiysonge C S. A systematic review of randomized controlled trials to reduce hemorrhage during myomectomy for uterine fibroids. *Int J Gynaecol Obstet* 2008;100:4–9.

19 Sesti F, Ticconi C, Bonifacio S, Piccione E. Preoperative administration of recombinant human erythropoietin in patients undergoing gynecologic surgery. *Gynecol Obstet Invest* 2002;54:1–5.

20 Vilos G A, Ternamian A, Dempster J, Laberge P Y, The Society of Obstetricians and Gynaecologists of Canada. Laparoscopic entry: a review of techniques, technologies, and complications. *J Obstet Gynaecol Can* 2007;29:433–65.

21 Koh C, Janik G. Laparoscopic myomectomy: the current status. *Curr Opin Obstet Gynecol* 2003;15:295–301.

22 Lin P C, Thyer A, Soules M R. Intraoperative ultrasound during a laparoscopic myomectomy. *Fertil Steril* 2004;81: 1671–4.

23 Ou C S, Harper A, Liu Y H, Rowbotham R. Laparoscopic myomectomy technique. Use of colpotomy and the harmonic scalpel. *J Reprod Med* 2002;47:849–53.

24 Litta P, Fantinato S, Calonaci F, Cosmi E, Filippeschi M, Zerbetto I, et al. A randomized controlled study comparing harmonic versus electrosurgery in laparoscopic myomectomy. *Fertil Steril* 2010;94:1882–6.

25 Walocha J A, Litwin J A, Miodonski A J. Vascular system of intramural leiomyomata revealed by corrosion casting and scanning electron microscopy. *Hum Reprod* 2003;18: 1088–93.

26 Hasbargen U, Summerer-Moustaki M, Hillemanns P, Scheidler J, Kimmig R, Hepp H. Uterine dehiscence in a nullipara, diagnosed by MRI, following use of unipolar electrocautery during laparoscopic myomectomy: Case report. *Hum Reprod* 2002;17:2180–2.

27 Nezhat F, Seidman D S, Nezhat C, Nezhat C H. Laparoscopic myomectomy today. Why, when and for whom? *Hum Reprod* 1996;11:933–4.

28 Kumakiri J, Takeuchi H, Itoh S, Kitade M, Kikuchi I, Shimanuki H, et al. Prospective evaluation for the feasibility and safety of vaginal birth after laparoscopic myomectomy. *J Minim Invasive Gynecol* 2008;15:420–4.

29 Seracchioli R, Manuzzi L, Vianello F, Gualerzi B, Savelli L, Paradisi R, et al. Obstetric and delivery outcome of pregnancies achieved after laparoscopic myomectomy. *Fertil Steril* 2006;86:159–65.

30 Einarsson J I, Vellinga T T, Twijnstra A R, Chavan N R, Suzuki Y, Greenberg J A. Bidirectional barbed suture: an evaluation of safety and clinical outcomes. *JSLS* 2010;14: 381–5.

31 Einarsson J I, Chavan N R, Suzuki Y, Jonsdottir G, Vellinga T T, Greenberg J A. Use of bidirectional barbed suture in laparoscopic myomectomy: evaluation of perioperative outcomes, safety, and efficacy. *J Minim Invasive Gynecol* 2011;18:92–5.

32 Miyake T, Enomoto T, Ueda Y, Ikuma K, Morii E, Matsuzaki S, et al. A case of disseminated peritoneal leiomyomatosis developing after laparoscope-assisted myomectomy. *Gynecol Obstet Invest* 2008;67:96–102.

33 Ahmad G, Duffy J M, Farquhar C, Vail A, Vandekerckhove P, Watson A, et al. Barrier agents for adhesion prevention after gynaecological surgery. *Cochrane Database Syst Rev* 2008;(2):CD000475.

34 Practice Committee of the American Society for Reproductive Medicine, Society of Reproductive Surgeons. Pathogenesis, consequences, and control of peritoneal adhesions in gynecologic surgery. *Fertil Steril* 2007;88:21–6.

35 Oktem O, Gökaslan H, Durmusoglu F. Spontaneous uterine rupture in pregnancy 8 years after laparoscopic myomectomy. *J Am Assoc Gynecol Laparosc* 2001;8:618–21.

36 Pelosi M A, Pelosi M A. Spontaneous uterine rupture at thirty-three weeks subsequent to previous superficial laparoscopic myomectomy. *Am J Obstet Gynecol* 1997;177:1547–9.

37 Harris W J. Uterine dehiscence following laparoscopic myomectomy. *Obstet Gynecol* 1992;80:545–6.

38 Landi S, Zaccoletti R, Ferrari L, Minelli L. Laparoscopic myomectomy: technique, complications, and ultrasound scan evaluations. *J Am Assoc Gynecol Laparosc* 2001;8: 231–40.

39 Seracchioli R, Rossi S, Govoni F, Rossi E, Venturoli S, Bulletti C, et al. Fertility and obstetric outcome after laparoscopic myomectomy of large myomata: a randomized comparison with abdominal myomectomy. *Hum Reprod* 2000;15:2663–8.

40 Sesti F, Capobianco F, Capozzolo T, Pietropolli A, Piccione E. Isobaric gasless laparoscopy versus minilaparotomy in uterine myomectomy: a randomized trial. *Surg Endosc* 2008;22:917–23.

41 Alessandri F, Lijoi D, Mistrangelo E, Ferrero S, Ragni N. Randomized study of laparoscopic versus minilaparotomic myomectomy for uterine myomas. *J Minim Invasive Gynecol* 2006;13:92–7.

42 Mais V, Ajossa S, Guerriero S, Mascia M, Solla E, Melis G B. Laparoscopic versus abdominal myomectomy: a prospective, randomized trial to evaluate benefits in early outcome. *Am J Obstet Gynecol* 1996;174:654–8.

43 Palomba S, Zupi E, Russo T, Falbo A, Marconi D, Tolino A, et al. A multicenter randomized, controlled study comparing laparoscopic versus minilaparotomic myomectomy: short-term outcomes. *Fertil Steril* 2007;88:942–51.

44 Palomba S, Zupi E, Falbo A, Russo T, Marconi D, Tolino A, et al. A multicenter randomized, controlled study comparing laparoscopic versus minilaparotomic myomectomy: reproductive outcomes. *Fertil Steril* 2007;88:933–41.

45 Bulletti C, Polli V, Negrini V, Giacomucci E, Flamigni C. Adhesion formation after laparoscopic myomectomy. *J Am Assoc Gynecol Laparosc* 1996;3:533–6.

46 Stringer N H, Walker J C, Meyer P M. Comparison of 49 laparoscopic myomectomies with 49 open myomectomies. *J Am Assoc Gynecol Laparosc* 1997;4:457–64.

47 Seidman D S, Nezhat C H, Nezhat F, Nezhat C. The role of laparoscopic-assisted myomectomy (I AM). *JSLS* 2001;5:299–303.

48 Cagnacci A, Pirillo D, Malmusi S, Arangino S, Alessandrini C, Volpe A. Early outcome of myomectomy by laparotomy, minilaparotomy and laparoscopically assisted minilaparotomy. A randomized prospective study. *Hum Reprod* 2003;18:2590–4.

49 Tan J, Sun Y, Dai H, Zhong B, Wang D. A randomized trial of laparoscopic versus laparoscopic-assisted minilaparotomy myomectomy for removal of large uterine myoma: short-term outcomes. *J Minim Invasive Gynecol* 2008;15:402–9.

50 Pelosi M A, Pelosi M A. Laparoscopic-assisted transvaginal myomectomy. *J Am Assoc Gynecol Laparosc* 1997;4:241–6.

51 Nezhat C, Nezhat F, Bess O, Nezhat C H, Mashiach R. Laparoscopically assisted myomectomy: a report of a new technique in 57 cases. *Int J Fertil Menopausal Stud* 1994;39:39–44.

52 Prapas Y, Kalogiannidis I, Prapas N. Laparoscopy vs laparoscopically assisted myomectomy in the management of uterine myomas: a prospective study. *Am J Obstet Gynecol* 2009;200:144–6.

53 Tropeano G, Amoroso S, Scambia G. Non-surgical management of uterine fibroids. *Hum Reprod Update* 2008;14:259–74.

54 Homer H, Saridogan E. Uterine artery embolization for fibroids is associated with an increased risk of miscarriage. *Fertil Steril* 2010;94:324–30.

55 Goldberg J, Pereira L. Pregnancy outcomes following treatment for fibroids: uterine fibroid embolization versus laparoscopic myomectomy. *Curr Opin Obstet Gynecol* 2006;18:402–6.

56 Mara M, Maskova J, Fucikova Z, Kuzel D, Belsan T, Sosna O. Midterm clinical and first reproductive results of a randomized controlled trial comparing uterine fibroid embolization and myomectomy. *Cardiovasc Intervent Radiol* 2008;31:73–85.

57 Holub Z, Mara M, Kuzel D, Jabor A, Maskova J, Eim J. Pregnancy outcomes after uterine artery occlusion: prospective multicentric study. *Fertil Steril* 2008;90:1886–91.

58 Alborzi S, Ghannadan E, Alborzi S, Alborzi M. A comparison of combined laparoscopic uterine artery ligation and myomectomy versus laparoscopic myomectomy in treatment of symptomatic myoma. *Fertil Steril* 2009;92: 742–7.

59 Bae J H, Chong G O, Seong W J, Hong D G, Lee Y S. Benefit of uterine artery ligation in laparoscopic myomectomy. *Fertil Steril* 2011;95:775–8.

60 Liu L, Li Y, Xu H, Chen Y, Zhang G, Liang Z. Laparoscopic transient uterine artery occlusion and myomectomy for symptomatic uterine myoma. *Fertil Steril* 2011;95:254–8.

61 Zupi E, Sbracia M, Marconi D, Munro M G. Myolysis of uterine fibroids: is there a role? *Clin Obstet Gynecol* 2006;49:821–33.

62 Quaas A M, Einarsson J I, Srouji S, Gargiulo A R. Robotic myomectomy: a review of indications and techniques. *Rev Obstet Gynecol* 2010;3:185–91.

63 Nezhat C, Lavie O, Hsu S, Watson J, Barnett O, Lemyre M. Robotic-assisted laparoscopic myomectomy compared with standard laparoscopic myomectomy – a retrospective matched control study. *Fertil Steril* 2009;91:556–9.

64 Barakat E E, Bedaiwy M A, Zimberg S, Nutter B, Nosseir M, Falcone T. Robotic-assisted, laparoscopic, and abdominal myomectomy: a comparison of surgical outcomes. *Obstet Gynecol* 2011;117:256–65.

65 Chapman L, Magos A. Surgical and radiological management of uterine fibroids in the UK. *Curr Opin Obstet Gynecol* 2006;18:394–401.

66 Holzer A, Jirecek S T, Illievich U M, Huber J, Wenzl R J. Laparoscopic versus open myomectomy: a double-blind study to evaluate postoperative pain. *Anesth Analg* 2006; 102:1480–4.

10 Laparoscopically assisted vaginal hysterectomy

Kevin G Cooper

Introduction

Despite overwhelming evidence supporting the vaginal over the abdominal route for benign hysterectomy, there remains a preference for the abdominal approach in the UK and many other countries. The reasons for this remain unclear and are undoubtedly multifactorial, but a change in the mindset of gynaecologists is required. Perceived difficulty of the vaginal approach to hysterectomy in combination with familiarity with the abdominal route, particularly for teaching, are reasons frequently cited. The reduction in exposure to surgeries and to a mix of surgical problems, enforced by shortened training programmes and the European Working Time Directive, will make it even more difficult for trainees to attain the requisite levels of skills. Unfortunately, the situation until recently was more difficult for UK trainees because abdominal and vaginal hysterectomy were in separate Advanced Training Specialist Modules, with laparoscopic hysterectomy in yet another.

If there is a perceived or real difficulty with learning and undertaking vaginal hysterectomy, then any technique that helps make it easier should be considered. The laparoscopic approach simplifies the most difficult components of the vaginal hysterectomy, the adnexal pedicles, facilitating conversion from an abdominal to a vaginal procedure.

Laparoscopy has been used by gynaecologists for many years, initially as a diagnostic tool, but over the last 30 years it has been used for a diverse number of operative procedures across an ever increasing number of surgical specialties. Most procedures traditionally undertaken by an open technique have been successfully performed endoscopically, although this does not prove the efficiency, efficacy or safety of the approach. What is undeniably proven to be advantageous is laparoscopic adnexal surgery. It is currently a requirement for all gynaecology trainees to become proficient in undertaking laparoscopic surgery for ectopic pregnancy. With a few additional skills, which are easily learnt, most gynaecologists could therefore reduce their abdominal hysterectomy rate through releasing the upper pedicles of a hysterectomy laparoscopically.

TABLE 10.1 **Recommended staging of laparoscopic hysterectomy**

Stage	Procedure	Content
Level 0	Vaginal hysterectomy with laparoscopic assessment/haemostasis	Laparoscopy at start of procedure to exclude disease that would preclude vaginal hysterectomy; laparoscopy at end of procedure to ensure haemostasis and washout
Level 1	Laparoscopically assisted vaginal hysterectomy	Release of upper pedicles to level of uterine arteries, which are secured vaginally
Level 2	Laparoscopic hysterectomy	The uterine arteries are divided laparoscopically, the uterosacral ± cardinal ligaments are secured vaginally; the vaginal vault is closed vaginally
Level 3	Total laparoscopic hysterectomy	Whole procedure completed laparoscopically with no vaginal component

Laparoscopically assisted vaginal hysterectomy (LAVH) was first undertaken and described by Harry Reich in 1989.[1] The procedure took some time, not least because this was a completely new technique. The specialist laparoscopic equipment that we take for granted nowadays did not exist, including simple methods of achieving haemostasis, such as laparoscopic bipolar diathermy. There is little doubt that the procedure described by Reich would otherwise have been performed using an abdominal approach.

It is widely believed that if a hysterectomy can be safely undertaken vaginally, this is the route of choice. When a totally vaginal approach is not appropriate, consideration should be given to undertaking an LAVH, thus reducing the abdominal hysterectomy rate. Cynics would argue that 3 months after the surgery there is no difference in outcome among the different routes, and this is correct. In those first 3 months, however, there are significant and important differences for the woman, healthcare provider and purchaser in favour of the less invasive procedure. Furthermore, contrary to widespread belief, there is evidence from randomised trials to suggest that LAVH is quicker than abdominal hysterectomy.[2]

Classification of hysterectomy

In this chapter, laparoscopic hysterectomy beyond securing the uterine arteries is not discussed and chapter 12 should be consulted. LAVH specifies that the procedure stops before division of the uterine arteries. The generally agreed classification is described in Table 10.1.

TABLE 10.2 **Staging of laparoscopic hysterectomy**[3]

Stage	Laparoscopic content
0	Laparoscopy done but no laparoscopic procedure before vaginal hysterectomy
1	Procedure includes laparoscopic adhesiolysis and/or excision of endometriosis
2	Either or both adnexa freed laparoscopically
3	Bladder dissected from the uterus laparoscopically
4	Uterine artery transected laparoscopically
5	Anterior and/or posterior colpotomy or entire uterus freed laparoscopically

Many other more extensive classifications have been published, but the one described in Table 10.1 is useful as it has clearly understood definitions. It is a modification of the description by Richardson et al.[3] in 1995 (Table 10.2). From this we see that LAVH incorporates stages 1–3, stage 4 becomes laparoscopic hysterectomy and stage 5 becomes total laparoscopic hysterectomy. A standardised classification is particularly helpful when auditing operative and clinical outcomes and, importantly, morbidity. Widespread use and acceptance of this classification ensures clarity when reporting on laparoscopic hysterectomy. This has been recommended by a Cochrane review[2] to minimise the confusion that has prevailed in the literature to date.

Indications

It was originally thought that LAVH might replace vaginal hysterectomy altogether. It was assumed that there would be more accurate haemostasis leading to a lower incidence of vault haematoma, transfusion, infection and hence quicker recovery. This has not been borne out in randomised trials, with the laparoscopic approach being slower and more costly than a vaginal hysterectomy.[2] In addition, there are the specific risks related to trocar insertion, which are outlined in chapter 2.

The ability to undertake a vaginal hysterectomy varies greatly between surgeons. The personal level of training and experience will determine whether an individual chooses a vaginal hysterectomy or an abdominal approach. Although using the laparoscope can undoubtedly make a vaginal hysterectomy easier, it cannot replace it altogether and should certainly not be seen as a way of being able to reduce training in vaginal surgery.

There are widely accepted reasons other than surgeon experience for not undertaking a vaginal hysterectomy. These include known or suspected pelvic disease, pelvic pain, fibroids, enlarged uterus and adnexal mass. Endometrial and cervical carcinoma would also fall into this category. No previous vaginal delivery with resulting poorer vaginal access and perhaps caesarean scarring will also be included by many surgeons. In these situations, a laparoscopic approach may convert the planned abdominal hysterectomy into a vaginal hysterectomy or an LAVH.

A diagnostic laparoscopy will demonstrate whether any disease processes are present. If this determines that a vaginal hysterectomy is suitable, then this is what should be done. Adhesiolysis or excision/treatment of endometriosis can be performed in conjunction. The laparoscope can also facilitate the opening of the posterior fornix vaginally if the light from the laparoscope is placed in the pouch of Douglas. This along with the pneumoperitoneum makes opening the posterior fornix a simple task. This should result in less stripping of pelvic peritoneum from the vaginal submucosa and hence less troublesome bleeding. Once the vaginal hysterectomy is completed, haemostasis can be checked for and secured laparoscopically. If necessary, a peritoneal washout can be performed.

Should laparoscopy determine that a vaginal hysterectomy would not normally be performed, proceeding to LAVH may be appropriate. This is particularly the case when one or both ovaries are to be removed, or in the presence of adnexal masses, an enlarged or fibroid uterus (where access is deemed adequate) and early endometrial carcinoma. More advanced grades of endometrial cancer and cervical cancer where more radical dissection and lymph node sampling is expected should be undertaken only by advanced laparoscopic surgeons who are preferably also gynaecological oncologists or are supervised by one. For women with poor vaginal access or a fixed uterus, a total laparoscopic hysterectomy may be required, but again this should be undertaken only by laparoscopic surgeons with advanced skills.

Risks

If an LAVH is being considered, it is imperative that the woman is counselled with regard to the risks and benefits involved. This should be based on best evidence but influenced by the surgeon's own figures, making self-audit mandatory. Written information sheets and relevant websites should be given to the woman well in advance of the procedure so that when consent is sought a meaningful discussion can be had and consent is truly informed. It should be made clear why the operation is being performed, that alternative options have been discussed and what the expected outcomes should be. When consent is sought, the woman should be specifically asked whether she has read and understood the information sheet and whether she has any further questions. The woman should also be directed to the National Institute for Health and Clinical Excellence (NICE) website,[4] where an excellent document entitled *Keyhole Hysterectomy*, written for the layperson, is available. The statistics quoted in the subsequent paragraphs in this section are those quoted by NICE.[5]

The specific risks associated with LAVH are modifications of the risks of vaginal and abdominal hysterectomy and those of laparoscopic surgery. Obviously, trocar injuries do not occur in nonlaparoscopic procedures and contribute to a significant proportion of complications from laparoscopic surgery. The risks of injury to the urinary tract also seem to be higher. The ureter is up to five times more likely to be injured during laparoscopic hysterectomy (in approximately 1% of women undergoing this surgery). Ureteric injury is more likely when the anatomy is distorted, in particular with endometriosis. It is also more common if one or both ovaries are to be removed as the ureter at the pelvic brim is potentially vulnerable. Most ureteric injuries are low and occur as a result of securing haemostasis of the uterine artery.

Bladder injury occurs in 1.3% of procedures – almost three times the incidence at open hysterectomy. This is more common where the bladder is adherent, as can be the case after a caesarean section. The risk of major haemorrhage is twice as great as with a nonlaparoscopic approach, although less than 1% of women will require a transfusion. The risk of a fistula is approximately 0.2%, slightly higher than with open surgery, but there seems to be no difference in the incidence of bowel injury. As with all inadvertent injuries, immediate detection and repair will often result in little or no sequelae in the medium or long term.

Approximately 3% of laparoscopic hysterectomies will require laparotomy. This should not be seen as a complication but as prudence on behalf of the surgeon. Conversion to laparotomy was classified as a major complication in the eVALuate study (evaluating the relative roles of Vaginal, Abdominal, and Laparoscopic hysterectomy) and if it had not, then major complication rates would have been comparable for abdominal and laparoscopic hysterectomy.[6] A laparoscopic procedure should only be planned and continued in that mode if it is safe and appropriate. If a complication arises, this will often necessitate a laparotomy. As these are women who would otherwise have undergone abdominal hysterectomies, the vast majority will still avoid a significant abdominal incision.

The Vaginal, Abdominal or Laparoscopic Uterine Excision (VALUE) study[7] demonstrated almost twice as many operative complications for those undergoing a laparoscopic approach (6% compared with 3.6%). It must be remembered that this was in 1995 when formal training programmes were not available and camera equipment, monitors and other laparoscopic equipment were not of today's standards. In experienced centres, there is little difference in risks between laparoscopic, open and vaginal hysterectomy.[8] Care must be taken when quoting these data as they are retrospectively collected. Although generalisability of results obtained from a single specialist centre is limited, these results do show what might be achieved. There is no doubt that a surgeon on the learning curve has higher rates of complications and the learning curve for laparoscopic surgery is certainly greater than that for open or vaginal hysterectomy.

There is an increased risk of thromboembolic phenomena with prolonged procedures with the woman in the head-down Trendelenburg position, the legs in the low lithotomy or modified Lloyd–Davies position and a pneumoperitoneum. Thromboprophylaxis using surgical stockings or pneumatic boots should be used in conjunction with an injection of low-molecular-weight heparin. If the legs have been positioned thus for 2 hours, they should be brought to a neutral position for a period of at least 10 minutes before returning them to the modified Lloyd–Davies position. This exercise is undertaken for three reasons: firstly, to reduce the risk of lower limb compartment syndrome; secondly, to allow a rest for the operating team; and lastly, to re-evaluate the operation, its progress and whether it is prudent to continue laparoscopically. The time of legs up should be formally noted on the theatre whiteboard.

Equipment

The set-up for undertaking LAVH is similar to that in other operative gynaecological laparoscopic procedures and the chapter describing this should be read.

A safe and effective means of securing haemostasis is mandatory. There are numerous energy sources available that can speed up and often simplify haemostasis and dissection. The Ligasure™ (Valleylab, Boulder, CO, USA) tissue sealing system and linear (Harmonic Scalpel®; Johnson & Johnson, New Brunswick, NJ, USA) and torsional (Lotus™; SRA Developments, Bremridge, UK) ultrasonic coagulating shears are three such devices. While convenient when undertaking LAVH or adnexal surgery, they are costly compared with bipolar electrocautery and monopolar scissors or hook. Stapling devices require a 12 mm port, are expensive and cannot be justified for LAVH. These operations can be undertaken effectively using an umbilical 5–10 mm trocar, two or three 5 mm trocars, a laparoscope, a light source and camera unit, bipolar forceps, scissors, a monopolar and bipolar energy source, grasping forceps, a suction/irrigation system and, occasionally, a needle holder.

There are reusable versions of all this equipment, although disposable scissors will be required if monopolar diathermy is to be used through them because monopolar energy will blunt scissor blades quickly.

Before using electrical energy for surgery, open or laparoscopic, it is essential that its characteristics and applications are fully understood (see chapter 5). Both bipolar and monopolar electrosurgery should be available for operative laparoscopic surgery.

A good-quality uterine manipulator will markedly improve presentation of the uterus and can be more useful than having another port. Reusable instruments such as the Valtchev® (Conkin Surgical Instruments, Toronto, Canada) or Pelosi (Apple Medical Corporation, Marlboro, MA, USA) manipulators allow the uterus to be presented at an angle of retroversion of up to 20° through to an angle of anteversion of over 90°, while lateral movement to each pelvic sidewall is possible. Although not essential when only taking the upper pedicles of a hysterectomy, manipulators facilitate access when there is associated pathology and aid presentation of the uterine pedicles and vagina in more difficult procedures. For most LAVH procedures, polyp forceps opened into the cornuae of the uterine cavity or a Spackman cannula will be adequate.

Although an ability to stitch is not absolutely necessary for performing an LAVH, it gives the operator another option for repair or haemostasis without having to resort to laparotomy. It should be a skill practised and attained by all who aspire to undertake operative laparoscopy and can prove an invaluable asset in many situations.

The laparoscopic approach is significantly more costly than the purely vaginal route. When expensive disposables are not used, costs are similar to abdominal hysterectomy.[9] Additional savings are made in the reduced inpatient stay. Increasing operative costs through the use of disposable equipment can be justified only if it results in a meaningful reduction in operating times or reduced morbidity.

The procedure

The simplest version of LAVH is division of the infundibulopelvic ligament if undertaking oophorectomy, or of the ovarian ligament and fallopian tube if retaining the ovary. This is essentially little more than is technically undertaken for laparoscopic ectopic surgery, but in this case it is performed bilaterally. Division of the round ligament and dissection of the broad ligament – exposing the uterine artery and releasing the bladder – are additional procedures that can be undertaken. The remainder of the hysterectomy would then be completed vaginally, but the laparoscope would be reintroduced at the end of the procedure to ensure full haemostasis and washout. The different steps in undertaking the procedure are outlined below.

All operative laparoscopic procedures should be performed under general anaesthesia with muscle relaxation to allow safe maintenance of an adequate pneumoperitoneum. The woman should be intubated with a cuffed tube to reduce the risk of introducing gas into the stomach. If there is concern regarding gastric gas, a nasogastric tube can be passed. A surgical safety checklist[10] (surgical pause) should be applied to establish that all theatre staff and surgeons involved are fully aware of each other, the woman present and the procedure planned. Antibiotic prophylaxis is administered.

Initial preparation

The woman is positioned as described for myomectomy (page 142). The abdomen and perineal region are cleaned, taking particular care to ensure that all debris is removed from the umbilicus. The bladder should be catheterised and careful vaginal examination should take place before inserting the trocars to assess size, mobility and descent of the uterus. This can help determine what type of hysterectomy is to be undertaken. A uterine manipulator or alternatively a Spackman cannula or polyp forceps opened in the uterine cavity will allow mobilisation of the uterus.

The umbilical trocar can be inserted directly into the peritoneal cavity following a cut-down (Hasson technique)[11] or following the creation of a pneumoperitoneum using a Veress needle with the woman in a level, untilted position.

The laparoscope is then introduced and the size of the uterus is checked as this might influence the number and placement of the lateral trocars. The anterior abdominal wall is inspected and the inferior epigastric artery with its attending venae comitantes on either side is identified (Figure 10.1). The accessory 5 mm ports should be placed lateral to this and the rectus abdominis muscle under direct vision. A third 5 mm trocar, if required, can be placed in the midline suprapubically. If this position is chosen, it must be more than 8 cm from the umbilical port, otherwise it will

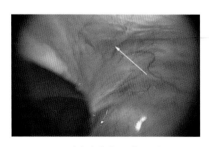

FIGURE 10.1 **Right inferior epigastric artery (arrow)**

interfere with the laparoscope. The woman should then be positioned in the head-down Trendelenburg position at 15–30° to optimise visualisation of the pelvic organs. The small bowel is displaced out of the pelvis using atraumatic graspers.

Careful inspection of the pelvis and its organs can then be undertaken and any pathology documented, videoed or photographed. Mobility of the uterus and ovaries should be noted.

The ureters

The next structures that need to be identified are the ureters. The ureters enter the pelvis over the pelvic brim, crossing the external iliac artery on the right. As the ureter is more medial on the left, it crosses over the common iliac artery. On the left at this point, the ureter is hidden by the sigmoid colon. The ureters continue distally, retroperitoneally, along the pelvic sidewall. Both ureters are initially crossed by the infundibulopelvic ligament containing the ovarian vessels. If the overlying peritoneum is not diseased, the ureters should be easily visible through the peritoneum along the pelvic sidewall until reaching the ureteric canal, where the uterine artery crosses above it. Retroperitoneal structures become more difficult to see as operating time increases because the carbon dioxide pneumoperitoneum causes mild inflammation of the peritoneum, reducing visibility through it. Vermiculation (a slow wriggling movement) as opposed to pulsation is peculiar to the ureter, although this reduces with increasing operation time.

If there is distortion of the anatomy, endometriosis involving the sidewall or an inability to identify a ureter clearly, the ureter should be formally displayed. It is usually easiest to open the pelvic peritoneum at the pelvic brim, where the ureter can be clearly found on the right, the peritoneum is opened just lateral to it and the incision extended distally using a blunt instrument (Video 10.1). On the left side, the physiological adhesions tethering the sigmoid to the pelvic brim may need to be released if the ureter cannot be easily identified. The sigmoid, once released, is moved medially to reveal the iliac vessels and ureter. The peritoneum can then be opened at the pelvic brim (Video 10.2). Sharp dissection may be required if there is overlying disease, but usually blunt extension of the pelvic peritoneum caudally will reduce the risk of injury to the ureter. The left ureter is thus displayed and can be released and exposed in the same way as the right (Video 10.3). The pneumoperitoneum itself and aquadissection with the irrigator aid ureteric dissection markedly. Adhesions should be divided and treatment of endometriosis performed if required and within the capability of the surgeon.

Concomitant salpingo-oophorectomy

The uterus is deviated to the contralateral side and pushed cephalad. The peritoneum filling the triangle bounded by the round ligament, infundibulopelvic ligament/fallopian tube and external iliac artery is opened by lifting the central peritoneum with grasping forceps and dividing the peritoneum with cutting diathermy (Video 10.4). This 'triangle' is easily viewed from above or, by anteverting the uterus and elevating the tube, from below. A window is thus created through the triangle, which is extended so that the infundibulopelvic ligament is skeletonised, making haemostasis of the ovarian vessels and division of this pedicle easier. The distance between pedicle and ureter is also increased, reducing the risk of ureteric injury.

The ovarian pedicle can be secured effectively using bipolar diathermy, Ligasure™, a linear or torsional ultrasonic device or suture. If using bipolar diathermy (30–40 W), pulsed bursts of energy are used so that the bipolar paddles do not 'weld' to the tissue. Energy should be applied until tissue bubbling just stops. Continuing to apply energy can result in charring and then fracturing with loss of haemostasis and unwanted, increased lateral thermal spread. A grasper in the other port can ensure optimal presentation of the infundibulopelvic ligament. The bipolar or ultrasonic forceps should be placed away from the pelvic sidewall (Video 10.5) to remove the risk of injury to sidewall structures. If diathermy is applied too laterally and the pedicle is cut but bleeds, achieving haemostasis can be difficult with increased risk of thermal injury to pelvic wall structures. The cut vessels can retract into the sidewall and retroperitoneal bleeding makes identification and isolation of the bleeding vessel difficult. The application of pressure is often a safer option than applying diathermy in this circumstance.

No concomitant salpingo-oophorectomy

There is no need to formally open the 'triangle' of pelvic peritoneum described in the previous section if the ovaries are to be retained. Whereas there is only one pedicle to secure when taking the ovary, there are two to secure when conserving it. Once more the uterus is deviated to the contralateral side and pushed cephalad. An atraumatic grasper holding the ovary laterally helps presentation of the ovarian ligament, which can then be secured using the energy mode of choice as previously described (Video 10.6). The fallopian tube is dealt with in the same manner and the blades of the energy source advanced onto untreated tissue until bubbling ceases. It is important not to divide the tissue too close to the body of the uterus because bleeding from the organ is difficult to stop and becomes a nuisance. The ovarian ligament, fallopian tube and the interposing adventitial tissue of the mesosalpinx are divided, either by use of the energy modality (Ligasure, linear or torsional ultrasonic shears) or with scissors and monopolar energy if necessary.

The ovary should be checked for haemostasis and, if necessary, bipolar energy applied to any bleeding points.

Exposing the uterine artery

The round ligaments are desiccated and divided (Video 10.7). The posterior leaf of the broad ligament is then divided to the uterine insertion of the utero-sacral ligament with scissors and monopolar diathermy if necessary. There is often a significant artery just below the round ligament; this is sometimes referred to as Samson's vessel and may require formal coagulation before dividing. The pneumoperitoneum should separate the loose areolar tissue within the broad ligament, greatly facilitating dissection and identification of structures. Traction of the obliterated hypogastric artery will aid identification of the uterine artery. Once the uterine vessels are clearly identifiable and skeletonised (Video 10.8), the hysterectomy can be completed vaginally. One simple step can further simplify the procedure. A posterior culdotomy is easily performed laparoscopically (Video 10.9). If a uterine manipulator with a vaginal barrel is being used, the uterus should be anteverted maximally. The barrel of the manipulator will be easily seen and felt in the posterior fornix, delineating the junction between cervix and vagina. Using a cutting or blended current and a monopolar hook, making a transverse cut onto the barrel of the manipulator, the vagina is entered and the incision can be extended if desired (Video 10.10). Cutting onto the barrel of an all-metal manipulator will not cause a vaginal burn away from the incision site because the energy is dissipated over the large surface area of the whole manipulator. If there are concerns, a nonmetal manipulator can be used instead. Alternatively, culdotomy is easily achieved by inserting sponge forceps into the posterior fornix, opening them slightly and cutting between the blades with monopolar scissors or hook. The sponge forceps are then pushed through and opened, stretching the hole or holding it open for extension using monopolar scissors. This is also a useful technique for removing larger specimens at other laparoscopic procedures such as myomectomy and the removal of ovarian masses.

The bladder

Although the intra-abdominal portion of an LAVH can directly mimic that of an abdominal hysterectomy, there are some steps that can help the operator. If the bladder is mobilised first, further deflection occurs throughout the operation from the pressure created by the pneumoperitoneum. The uterus is pushed cephalad and posterior using the uterine manipulator. The bladder edge is usually easily identified, but this can be aided by pushing the catheter upwards and seeing the balloon at the upper bladder margin or instilling 30 ml of saline with methylene blue into the bladder.

The uterovesical peritoneum is easily lifted with atraumatic grasping forceps and the peritoneum opened with scissors and a cutting monopolar current at 50–80 W. The peritoneum is elevated with the lower scissor blade and the incision extended horizontally and then cephalad on each side, opening the anterior leaf of the broad ligament towards the round ligament (Figure 10.2, Video 10.11). Blunt dissection and, if necessary, aquadissection will deflect the bladder further caudally, whereas the pneumoperitoneum will open the broad ligament further. If there is scarring from a caesarean section, the bladder is released further by scissors and monopolar diathermy to maintain haemostasis, with care being taken not to extend laterally off the uterine isthmus/cervix, which will increase the risk of bleeding. Division of the condensations of connective tissue that represent the bladder pillars on each side releases the bladder from the cervix. The bladder pillars are vascular and will require division using scissors with monopolar diathermy. This allows the bladder to be deflected further caudally and with this the ureters are displaced laterally away from the cervix.

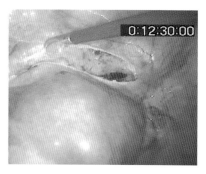

FIGURE 10.2 **Opening the uterovesical fold**

Generalised ooze can be safely stopped by holding the slightly opened blades of bipolar forceps sideways on, just over the area that is bleeding. As the current is travelling between the two blades without tissue interposed, there is some lateral thermal spread over a short distance, which can be very effective at securing haemostasis. This is particularly useful when close to organs where monopolar energy is best avoided. The slightly open blades are kept moving over the area and irrigation with glycine allows visualisation while using electrical energy and reduces thermal spread further.

Vaginal component

The woman is levelled and the legs will need to be repositioned into lithotomy, ensuring that they are well supported. There are a variety of techniques for completing the procedure vaginally and the surgeon should use a technique that they are comfortable with, that is safe and that works. Adapting the technique for each woman will certainly be necessary. A simple and proven method of completing the procedure is described.

If a posterior culdotomy has not been performed laparoscopically, this is undertaken next. With the tenaculum on the posterior cervical lip and upward traction, the reflection of the posterior fornix onto the cervix should be visible. Moving the cervix in and out will demonstrate the reflection of the posterior fornix and anterior bladder. Alternatively, reinflating the abdomen with gas will help delineate the posterior fornix, while placing the laparoscope with the light on into the cul-de-sac further demonstrates the correct point for vaginal incision. Incising the posterior cervix first is sensible so that bleeding is not a problem. Incising anteriorly first can lead to blood dripping into the operating field, which is an avoidable nuisance. The cervix is incised circumferentially and the skin reflected slightly. The peritoneum of the posterior fornix is then opened and extended laterally while trying to minimise stripping of the pelvic peritoneum from the vaginal skin.

The anterior cervical skin is freed by scissors cutting onto the body of the cervix, developing the plane between bladder and uterus. Once the abdomen is entered anteriorly, the bladder is elevated by placing a retractor between the bladder and the uterus. Heavy curved clamps can then secure the uterosacral/cardinal ligaments on each side. These are then divided and transfixed with a number 1 suture, keeping a long end on each side so that the uterosacral ligaments can be plicated to the vault at the end of the procedure. The second and final pedicle on each side should be the uterine vessels. Care should be taken not to put undue traction on the uterus at this stage because it is attached only by its arteries on each side. Further curved clamps are placed over the uterine pedicles and the uterus is removed. The pedicles are transfixed with number 1 polyglycolic sutures or equivalent. Clamps are then placed on the angles of the vault, the posterior vaginal wall and peritoneum, and the anterior vaginal wall. The vault is then closed with figure-of-eight haemostatic sutures, ensuring that the long ends from the uterosacral pedicles exit into the vagina through the vault centrally. These are tied together vaginally once laparoscopic inspection and washout have taken place.

Final inspection

The woman is returned to the position for laparoscopic surgery. The abdomen is reinflated and inspection of the pelvis commences. Each pedicle should have residual blood clots removed to ensure full haemostasis. Any bleeding points should be identified and haemostasis obtained by use of bipolar or, on occasion, monopolar diathermy or suture. Irrigation should be copious over the whole operative field and continue until complete haemostasis is achieved and the fluid is clear. The ureters should be inspected carefully and a urologist should be called if injury is suspected. The sigmoid colon and rectum should also be examined. If there is concern regarding wall integrity, the pelvis should be filled with irrigation fluid, the sigmoid at the pelvic brim should be occluded with an atraumatic instrument and air should be injected per rectum using a 50 ml catheter-tipped syringe to distend the rectosigmoid. Air bubbles visualised laparoscopically indicate a perforation. If there is serosal damage to bowel, it should be inspected by a surgeon, although it can usually be sutured laparoscopically.

Finally, the woman should be flattened out or go slightly head-up to allow blood and fluid that will have collected in the upper abdomen to return to the pelvis and be removed. Failure to do this can lead to avoidable pelvic collections occurring postoperatively. Alternatively, a drain can be placed in the pouch of Douglas for removal 6–12 hours postoperatively.

Postoperative care

Care postoperatively is essentially as for vaginal hysterectomy. As there has been little or no handling of the bowel, ileus is extremely unusual. Oral intake can commence as soon as the woman wishes in uncomplicated cases. There has, however, been considerable bladder mobilisation and a urinary catheter should remain in position for 12–24 hours. Early mobilisation should be encouraged and adequate analgesia prescribed. Intravenous fluid support can be discontinued once oral intake is adequate. Routine nursing observations are undertaken and daily thromboprophylaxis continued while the woman is in hospital. In uncomplicated cases, the woman can be discharged the following day if she feels ready, has support at home and observations are normal. Ideally, all women discharged following operative laparoscopic surgery should receive an information sheet. This should outline what to expect in the recovery phase and mention any developments that would be of concern and require medical review. Contact numbers should be included on this sheet.

Conclusion

The fact that over two-thirds of benign hysterectomies are still performed abdominally in the UK is inexcusable. With pressure on inpatient beds and the increasing costs of hospitalisation, in addition to the advantages to the woman from avoiding an abdominal incision, we should be striving to reduce these rates. It is obviously not possible for all procedures to be performed vaginally, but many women could avoid an abdominal hysterectomy if an operative laparoscopic approach were adopted.

For this to happen, there will have to be a dramatic change in the mindset of many gynaecologists and improvements in training to attain the requisite skills. The trainees themselves should be asking the question: why are we doing this procedure abdominally? The ability to undertake a laparoscopic salpingectomy and attendance at a laparoscopic training course are requirements of specialist registrar training for gynaecology in the UK, so the basic underlying laparoscopic skills are there. Gaining the training for the vaginal component of the procedure may be the harder goal for many. The development of a combined benign gynaecology Advanced Training Specialist Module that brings the different routes for hysterectomy together, as opposed to the present situation where the different routes are dealt with in separate modules, will help greatly.

Finally, surgeons should familiarise themselves with the varied equipment and energy options available for undertaking laparoscopic procedures. The manufacturers can be very helpful in arranging training and support for their products. Surgeons should choose the equipment that enables them to undertake procedures comfortably, effectively and safely. Ultimately, costs will influence what the gynaecologist is able to use. It should be remembered that diathermy and suturing are cheap and effective options that should ideally be understood and mastered.

References

1 Reich H, Decaprio J, McGlynn F. Laparoscopic hysterectomy. *J Gynecol Surg* 1989;5:213–6.

2 Nieboer T E, Johnson N, Barlow D, Lethaby A, Tavender E, Curr E, et al. Surgical approach to hysterectomy for benign gynaecological disease. *Cochrane Database Syst Rev* 2009;(3):CD003677.

3 Richardson R E, Bournas N, Magos AL. Is laparoscopic hysterectomy a waste of time? *Lancet* 1995;345:36–41.

4 National Institute for Health and Clinical Excellence. *Keyhole Hysterectomy*. Interventional Procedure Guidance 239. London: NICE; 2007 [www.guidance.nice.org.uk/IPG239/publicinfo/pdf/English].

5 National Institute for Health and Clinical Excellence. *Laparoscopic Techniques for Hysterectomy*. Interventional Procedure Guidance 239. London: NICE; 2007 [www.egap.evidence.nhs.uk/IPG239].

6 Garry R, Fountain J, Mason S, Napp V, Brown J, Hawe J, et al. The eVALuate study: two parallel randomised trials, one comparing laparoscopic with abdominal hysterectomy, the other comparing laparoscopic with vaginal hysterectomy. *BMJ* 2004;328:129–33.

7 McPherson K, Metcalfe M A, Herbert A, Maresh M, Casbard A, Hargreaves J, et al. Severe complications of hysterectomy: the VALUE study. *BJOG* 2004; 111:688–94.

8 Donnez O, Jadoul P, Squifflet J, Donnez J. A series of 3190 laparoscopic hysterectomies for benign disease from 1990 to 2006: evaluation of complications compared with vaginal and abdominal procedures. *BJOG* 2009;116:492–500.

9 Sculpher M, Manca A, Abbott J, Fountain J, Mason S, Garry R. Cost effectiveness analysis of laparoscopic hysterectomy compared with standard hysterectomy: results from a randomised trial. *BMJ* 2004;328:134.

10 Haynes A B, Weiser T G, Berry W R, Lipsitz S R, Breizat A H, Dellinger E P, et al. A surgical safety checklist to reduce morbidity and mortality in a global population. *N Engl J Med* 2009;360:491–9.

11 Hasson H M. Open laparoscopy: a report of 150 cases. *J Reprod Med* 1974;12:234–8.

11   Laparoscopic subtotal hysterectomy

John Erian and Anastasios Pachydakis

Introduction

Hysterectomy was mentioned in Greek manuscripts 2000 years ago.[1] Soranus of Ephesus described a vaginal hysterectomy for a prolapsed gangrenous uterus in the 2nd century AD. The first abdominal hysterectomy was performed by Charles Clay in Manchester in 1844. During the 19th century, the postoperative mortality of the procedure was over 70%,[2] mainly as a result of haemorrhage and sepsis. The first abdominal total hysterectomy was performed by Edward H Richardson in Baltimore in 1929.[3] He also advocated the removal of the cervix for the prevention of cancer of the cervical stump, which at the time had a reported incidence of 0.4%.[4] However, subtotal abdominal hysterectomy remained the operation of choice for benign uterine disease until 1940,[3] when antibiotics were introduced, because not opening the vaginal vault reduced the risk of infection and thus death.

Following an intense debate after the introduction of antibiotics and transfusion in the 1950s, total abdominal hysterectomy prevailed as it offered protection against cervical cancer. The incidence of cervical cancer dropped to 0.14–0.16% in the 1970s, with a further drop to 0.084% attributed to the uptake of cervical screening.[5]

In 1989, the first total laparoscopic hysterectomy was described by Harry Reich in Pensylvania,[6] and 2 years later the first laparoscopic subtotal hysterectomy was described by Kurt Semm.[7] This was performed via 'pelviscopy' (gynaecological laparoscopy); the word 'laparoscopy' was forbidden because it was associated with great intraoperative morbidity. The procedure carrying the unfortunate acronym CASH (classic abdominal serrated-edge macromorcellator hysterectomy) involved complete excision of the endocervix with the aid of a transcervical guide wire and removal of the uterine corpus. The procedure was long and expensive, had relatively high morbidity and required advanced laparoscopic surgical skills. Preservation of the ectocervix also contradicted the belief of gynaecologists, built over three decades, that the cervix is 'better removed'.

During recent years, the interest in subtotal hysterectomy through the laparoscopic approach has been revived. Indeed, the USA has seen a four-fold increase in the number of subtotal hysterectomies performed.[8] However, grade A evidence is lacking. As different women have different pathologies and are treated by surgeons with different skills, any attempt at randomisation is likely to be impossible. We describe our own experience with laparoscopic subtotal hysterectomy with reference to the literature when available.

Preoperative preparation

Laparoscopic subtotal hysterectomy includes morcellation of the myometrium and of the endometrium; therefore, it is very important to exclude endometrial hyperplasia and malignancy. Preoperative endometrial assessment with transvaginal ultrasound scanning and, where appropriate, outpatient hysteroscopy and endometrial sampling is of paramount importance for all women undergoing the procedure.

Women are advised that there is a small chance of developing cyclical bleeding despite diathermy of the endocervix and it is impossible to predict which women will develop this symptom. This cyclical bleeding invariably lasts for 1 day only in a periodic pattern and will never evolve into a heavy period. We believe that women who are informed of the possibility of cyclical bleeding are much less likely to be disturbed by its occurrence and much less likely to request a trachelectomy following a laparoscopic subtotal hysterectomy. The importance of continued cervical screening is also reinforced.

Contraindications to laparoscopic subtotal hysterectomy include the following:

- uterus of a bigger size than a uterus at 20 weeks of gestation

- stoma

- adhesions

- unfitness for anaesthesia

- poor compliance with cervical screening

- dyskariosis/cervical intraepithelial neoplasia

- suspected malignancy.

We consider it good practice to offer the results of our own continuous audit to the women attending our clinic.

Surgical technique

This is a comprehensive account of our standardised technique. In other units, alternative forms of thermal energy and different types of morcellating devices and uterine manipulators are used with equally good results.

The procedure is performed under general anaesthesia by two surgeons, with the woman in the Lloyd–Davies position. Preparation of the woman includes indwelling bladder catheterisation and placement of a Pelosi Uterine Manipulator (Apple Medical Corporation, Marlborough, MA, USA) in the cervix. This is an articulated manipulator that allows extreme anteversion and retroversion as well as lateral manipulation of the uterus even in the absence of an assistant. The use of an indwelling catheter is essential as it will keep the bladder empty as the suprapubic port is placed later during the procedure and the collecting bag will immediately fill with carbon dioxide if the bladder is injured. If Palmer's point entry is indicated, a nasogastric tube is inserted to decompress the upper gastrointestinal tract after the induction of anaesthesia.

The procedure is performed through a four-port operative laparoscopy: a 10 mm infraumbilical port for the laparoscope, two 5 mm lateral ports and a suprapubic 12 mm port for morcellation. The lateral ports are placed high in the abdomen, at the same level as the umbilicus. This allows more space for handling pedicles in large uteruses and also facilitates the angle of coagulation as the line of the instrument is parallel to the lateral margin of the uterus and away from the pelvic sidewall.

Laparoscopic subtotal hysterectomy is a two-surgeon procedure, with both surgeons predominantly operating with their right hand. The surgeon on the left uses the right hand to handle instruments through the left port and the left hand to manipulate the Pelosi Uterine Manipulator and maximise exposure of the operating field. The surgeon on the right of the woman under surgery uses the right hand to handle instruments through the right port and the left hand to handle the laparoscope.

The laparoscopic steps include coagulation and transection of the infundibulopelvic ligament in the case of bilateral salpingo-oophorectomy or the ovarian ligament in the case of conservation of the ovaries. The round ligament is coagulated and transected (Figure 11.1). The broad ligament is incised and the uterovesical fold is deflected to allow more space for the Lap Loop (Roberts Surgical Healthcare, Kidderminster, UK) monopolar diathermy device at the level of the cervical isthmus. The broad ligament is incised lateral to the uterus so that the uterine plexus in not inadvertently injured.

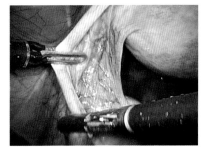

FIGURE 11.1 **Plasma Kinetic® (Gyrus Medical, Cardiff, UK) division of tube and ovarian ligament**

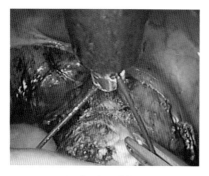

FIGURE 11.2 **Application of the Lap Loop system and amputated cervix**

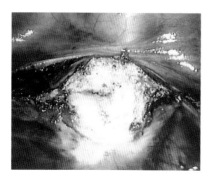

FIGURE 11.3 **Conisation effect of the Lap Loop device**

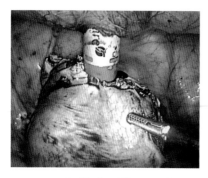

FIGURE 11.4 **Positioning of the morcellator at the midline: maximum distance from adjacent viscera**

Transection of the uterine vessels is performed at the same time as the detachment of the uterine corpus using the Lap Loop monopolar wire after removal of the uterine manipulator (Figure 11.2). The Lap Loop device is inserted through the suprapubic port to the left of the uterus and the wire is grasped by the surgeon on the right, advanced behind the cervix and attached to the Lap Loop applicator. The pouch of Douglas is checked with the wire under tension to avoid bowel entrapment inside the monopolar wire. The diathermy is set at 100 W coagulation and the surgeon on the left keeps the uterus retroflexed. With this technique, the angle of cutting is vertical and the Lap Loop device provides a conisation effect (Figure 11.3) removing a wedge off the endocervix.

When the uterine vessels are cut with the wire, they remain attached on the sides of the cervical stump instead of retracting to the pelvic sidewall. All pedicles are cross-coagulated (coagulated from the left and the right side trocars at right angles) by the surgeon and the assistant. Any complementary coagulation to the uterine vessels is easy, does not require any additional dissection and, most importantly, does not jeopardise the integrity of the ureters and the major vessels of the pelvic sidewall.

The uterus is then morcellated by drawing the specimen into the morcellator using a single-tooth or a gallbladder forceps while the surgeon on the right is lifting and stabilising the specimen (Figure 11.4). The tip of the rotating electromechanical morcellator is always kept within 2 cm of the lower abdominal wall[9] and the single-tooth forceps is only advanced 3–4 cm beyond the edge of the trocar to avoid inadvertent grasping of bowel or omentum during the morcellation. We routinely use the suprapubic port for the morcellator as we feel this provides more space inferiorly and laterally from the blade of the morcellator to the abdominal viscera and the pelvic sidewall, therefore minimising the risk of accidental damage to vital structures (Figure 11.4).

After morcellation is completed, the peritoneal cavity is cleared of any collected blood and fragments of myometrium by collection and irrigation with normal saline solution followed by suction. The bowel is not displaced before all the visible fragments are removed to minimise missing uterine corpus fragments in between bowel loops. The clearance of the pelvis, paracolic gutters and upper abdomen (as the woman is in deep head-down position) is of paramount importance as there have been reports of pelvic seeding of morcellated uterine tissue and subsequent development of adenomyotic masses (morcelloma)[10,11] in the peritoneal cavity or the cervical stump. Meticulous clearance of the peritoneal cavity has been advocated[12] because several complications may be attributed to incomplete collection of uterine fragments. The endocervix is cauterised with bipolar diathermy.

Haemostasis is checked after decompressing the peritoneal cavity. Then the abdominal cavity is reinflated and a 16-gauge drain is passed through the lateral port to the pouch of Douglas. The drain is connected with a decompressed collection container as suction drainage may draw small or large bowel into the drain and cause ischaemia and subsequent perforation.[13] Finally, the laparoscopic instruments and trocars are removed under direct vision and the port sites are closed with a J-shaped needle and number 1 Vicryl® (polyglactin 910; Ethicon Endo-Surgery, Cincinnati, OH, USA) under laparoscopic control before decompression of the pneumoperitoneum.

See Video 11.1 for an example of subtotal laparoscopic hysterectomy for adenomyosis.

Learning curve

As with all new procedures, mentoring and preceptorship are essential to minimise the risk of complications.[14] Once introduced as routine practice, the complication rate of minimal access hysterectomy seems to fall by 11–13% per year, reaching a plateau after about 5–7 years of practice.[15,16] The fall in complication rates may be associated with the early identification of potential visceral injury and laparoscopic repair of the injured viscera.

The operating time seems to be longer in the first operations but stabilises after the first 30 procedures.[17] The effect of surgical volume was seen in a double-parallel randomised trial in the UK,[18] in which laparoscopic hysterectomy was performed in a limited number of centres, with participating surgeons performing on average only 13 procedures over 4 years. In this study, the complication rate (including preoperative conversion to laparotomy) for the laparoscopic hysterectomy group remained as high as 11%.[18] Similarly, cyclical bleeding after the procedure has been demonstrated to be more common with the most inexperienced surgeons.[19] This may be related to the correct level of detachment of the uterine corpus or smoothness of the incision line in the cervical stump. In our experience, the Lap Loop system offers a fairly standard level of a smooth uterine incision even in the hands of less

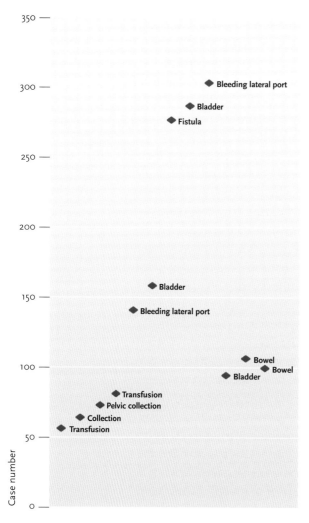

FIGURE 11.5 **Timing of major complications**

experienced surgeons, which may offer an advantage over the monopolar hook or spatula, the ultrasonic hook or the Plasma Kinetic® (Gyrus Medical, Cardiff, UK) hook techniques. However, this advantage has not been assessed in comparative studies.

In our series, the major complication rate was 1.2%,[20] which is in agreement with results found by Wattiez et al.[16] All complications associated with haemostasis (haematoma, pelvic collection and transfusion) occurred during the first 81 operations[20] (Figure 11.5) and this reflects the duration of the learning curve. Visceral injuries occurred later, after the first 100 operations[21] or 2 years of practice, probably reflecting the confidence to undertake more difficult procedures in women with a complex previous surgical history. These findings are in accordance with those from Wattiez et al.[16] It is notable that none of the visceral injuries that occurred in our series was related to thermal energy or morcellation.

In our technique, reflection of the bladder is essential prior to placement of the Lap Loop wire, but we understand that in other units this step is not considered to be essential, with equally good but unpublished results. We have changed the technique of bladder dissection and now each surgeon dissects their side of the bladder. Following this change, we have not had any bladder damage. All bladder injuries in our series (0.75%) occurred in women with three or four previous caesarean sections.[20]

Laparoscopic subtotal hysterectomy as same-day surgery

The Foley indwelling catheter and the drain are removed 4 hours after the procedure. Women are reviewed by the medical team 6 hours postoperatively and discharged. They are advised to call the 24-hour helpline service if they are experiencing any symptoms. If there has been bladder damage during surgery, the home care team will allocate a nurse who will remove the catheter at the appropriate time (5 days postoperatively) and ensure there is an acceptable postvoiding residual of urine. In our series of over 400 women, we have not had to intervene surgically or transfuse any women intra- or postoperatively. Two women required transfusion preoperatively because of menorrhagia-induced anaemia. The readmission rates seem very low (4/400, or 1%, in our series)[22] and the duration of surgery is short (mean duration 46.4 minutes),[20] even with large uteruses approaching 1 kg in weight. The postoperative management protocol is simple but requires a team effort and multiprofessional education to organise a setting where laparoscopic subtotal hysterectomy can be performed safely as a 6-hour discharge procedure.

Urinary tract injuries: diagnosis, surgical and postoperative management

In our series, there were no ureteric injuries in the first 500 women (unpublished results). This was probably the case because there is no need to dissect the paracervical tissues. The distance between the cervix and the ureter is less than 5 mm in over 10% of women;[23] the lateral thermal spread of coagulating devices varies from 2 mm to 4 mm,[24] and they are usually 2–5 mm wide. It is easy to understand how ureteric thermal injury occurs in these conditions. The possibility of avoiding this area altogether gives laparoscopic subtotal hysterectomy a distinct advantage over total laparoscopic hysterectomy.

In a series published in 2008,[25] the incidence of ureteric injury was 0.34%. It is noteworthy, however, that all ureteric injuries in this series occurred when a colpotomy was used to remove the uterus from the peritoneal cavity. When colpotomy was replaced by morcellation, there was no ureteric injury for over 10 years. We can safely say that ureteric injury during laparoscopic subtotal hysterectomy is very rare when morcellation is used to remove the uterine corpus.

Bladder injury is not so uncommon. If a suprapubic trocar is used, catheterisation is absolutely essential. In our experience, bladder injury only occurs in the presence of multiple (more than two) previous caesarean sections and this is a counselling point that needs to be stressed. The results from Donnez et al.[26] are in agreement with this point because all their bladder injuries happened in women with previous caesarean sections as well. The incidence reported was 0.25%, which is lower than that in our series (0.75%). Bladder injuries are easy to detect intraoperatively as the catheter bag is inflated with carbon dioxide that escapes through the bladder incision. Bladder injury is repaired by laparoscopic suturing using a single-layer closure. Antibiotic prophylaxis is administered and the bladder is catheterised for 5 days on free flow (the catheter is draining freely in a urine collector and no tap is used, ensuring continuous decompression of the bladder) on an outpatient basis. The catheter is then removed at home and the postvoiding residual urine is measured.

Patient satisfaction

In our series, 98% of the women were satisfied with the operation and the same number would recommend the procedure to a friend. In previous studies, there was clear evidence that the laparoscopic approach resulted in a shorter convalescence time, less postoperative pain and rapid improvement in quality of life indicators.[18,27] This percentage is higher than that in a report by Lieng et al.,[19] who presented a satisfaction rate of 90%. However, in that study about 50% of the women did not expect to have any bleeding postoperatively. In our opinion, the procedure is offered to treat menorrhagia and not to induce complete amenorrhoea. When this is clearly conveyed to the women preoperatively, they are less likely to be disappointed because of cyclical bleeding. The incidence of cyclical bleeding in our series was 2% and some surgeons would argue that this is the reason why our satisfaction rate is 98%.[20] This is incorrect as there are women who are dissatisfied because of other problems such as residual pain, postoperative infection, communication with medical and nursing staff and waiting time.

Laparoscopic subtotal hysterectomy and cervical cancer

One of the main arguments of those supporting total hysterectomy is the potential for the cervical stump to develop cervical intraepithelial neoplasia or cancer. We do not offer a laparoscopic subtotal hysterectomy to women with smear abnormalities. A study of 1.87 million women has shown that the risk of cervical cancer after a normal smear history is 1 : 5546 (0.018%).[28] The incidence of cervical cancer in women who have undergone subtotal hysterectomy is 0.1–0.2%.[29] To put this into context, the risk of cervical cancer in women who undergo laparoscopic subtotal hysterectomy is smaller than the risk of uterine rupture in labour in women with a previous caesarean section (0.3%) – and vaginal birth after a caesarean section is considered routine practice.

In the rare case when cervical cancer does occur in the cervical stump, the prognosis is no different from that in women who have not had a hysterectomy.[30] However, the treatment of cervical intraepithelial neoplasia with large loop excision of the transformation zone (LLETZ) is more hazardous as the uncontrolled spread of thermal energy towards the bladder in the absence of a uterine corpus may result in fistulae. In these circumstances, laparoscopic dissection of the anterior peritoneum with a relatively full bladder, acting as a heat sink, should be considered.

Cervical stump symptoms

The rate of persistent vaginal bleeding in other series can be as high as 24%,[19] but 90% of the women are satisfied with the procedure. This reinforces the need for appropriate preoperative counselling regarding this potential symptom. In our series, 2% of the women complained of chronic vaginal bleeding and this low rate may be attributed to the low amputation of the cervical stump with the Lap Loop device and the meticulous destruction of the cervical canal with high-frequency pulsatile bipolar diathermy.

Disturbing symptoms, namely pain and bleeding from the cervical stump, have been reported to be more common in women who have endometriosis.[31] However, later studies have contradicted this notion.[32] The degree of treatment of peritoneal disease, the presence of ovaries and the pre- and post-operative medical treatment of the disease would affect these results.

The effect of trachelectomy on the resolution of the symptoms attributed to the retained cervix has not been assessed in a clinical study. Therefore, the suggestion of a trachelectomy to a woman who is symptomatic following a supracervical hysterectomy should be made with caution as the resolution of symptoms after the trachelectomy cannot be guaranteed.

In a large retrospective Scandinavian study,[33] at least one-third of the women undergoing hysterectomy had chronic pain 1 year later and the main risk factors appeared to be pelvic pain, pain in another part of their body and, of course, endometriosis. In women who have persistent pain, therefore, other causes of pain must also be considered, in addition to the retained cervical stump.

Conclusion

Laparoscopic subtotal hysterectomy is an effective procedure that can be performed safely in a day-care setting. It is not proven to be superior or inferior to total laparoscopic hysterectomy, but it seems to carry less febrile morbidity and a lower risk of hospital admission, making it more suitable for same-day surgery. The procedure offers an early return to normal activities and an early resumption of sexual function.

Advances in coagulation and morcellation technology have reduced the operating time and have dramatically changed the safety profile of the procedure compared with the 1990s. The long-term risks are small and mostly theoretical, whereas the benefits in the immediate and late postoperative period are documented and substantial.

References

1 Baskett T F. Hysterectomy: evolution and trends. *Best Pract Res Clin Obstet Gynaecol* 2005;19:295–305.

2 Sutton C. Hysterectomy: A historical perspective. *Baillieres Clin Obstet Gynaecol* 1997;11:1–22.

3 Sutton C. Subtotal hysterectomy revisited. *Endosc Surg Allied Technol* 1995;3:105–8.

4 Johns A. Supracervical versus total hysterectomy. *Clin Obstet Gynecol* 1997;40:903–13.

5 Quinn M, Babb P, Jones J, Allen E. Effect of screening on incidence of and mortality from cancer of cervix in England: evaluation based on routinely collected statistics. *BMJ* 1999;318:904–8.

6 Reich H, DeCaprio J, McGlynn E. Laparoscopic hysterectomy. *J Gynecol Surg* 1989;5:213–6.

7 Semm K. [Hysterectomy via laparotomy or pelviscopy. A new CASH method without colpotomy]. *Geburtshilfe Frauenheilkd* 1991;51:996–1003. Article in German.

8 Merrill R M. Hysterectomy surveillance in the United States, 1997 through 2005. *Med Sci Monit* 2008;14:CR24–31.

9 Erian J, Hassan M, Hill N. Electromechanical morcellation in laparoscopic subtotal hysterectomy. *Int J Gynaecol Obstet* 2007;99:67–8.

10 Donnez O, Squifflet J, Leconte I, Jadoul P, Donnez J. Posthysterectomy pelvic adenomyotic masses observed in 8 cases out of a series of 1405 laparoscopic subtotal hysterectomies. *J Minim Invasive Gynecol* 2007;14:156–60.

11 Hilger W S, Magrina J F. Removal of pelvic leiomyomata and endometriosis five years after supracervical hysterectomy. *Obstet Gynecol* 2006;108:772–4.

12 Lieng M, Istre O, Busund B, Qvigstad E. Severe complications caused by retained tissue in laparoscopic supracervical hysterectomy. *J Minim Invasive Gynecol* 2006;13:231–3.

13 Reed M W R, Wyman A, Thomas W E, Zeiderman M R. Perforation of the bowel by suction drains. *Br J Surg* 1992;79:679.

14 Cutner A, Erian J. Training in minimal access surgery. *Br J Hosp Med* 1995;53:226–8.

15 Brummer T H, Seppälä T T, Härkki P S. National learning curve for laparoscopic hysterectomy and trends in hysterectomy in Finland 2000–2005. *Hum Reprod* 2008;23:840–5.

16 Wattiez A, Soriano D, Cohen S B, Nervo P, Canis M, Botchorishvili R, et al. The learning curve of total laparoscopic hysterectomy: comparative analysis of 1647 cases. *J Am Assoc Gynecol Laparosc* 2002;9:339–45.

17 Ghomi A, Littman P, Prasad A, Einarsson J I. Assessing the learning curve for laparoscopic supracervical hysterectomy. *JSLS* 2007;11:190–4.

18 Garry R, Fountain J, Mason S, Napp V, Brown J, Hawe J, et al. The eVALuate study: two parallel randomised trials, one comparing laparoscopic with abdominal hysterectomy, the other comparing laparoscopic with vaginal hysterectomy. *Br Med J* 2004;328:129–36.

19 Lieng M, Qvigstad E, Istre O, Langebrekke A, Ballard K. Long-term outcomes following laparoscopic supracervical hysterectomy. *BJOG* 2008;115:1605–10.

20 Erian J, Hassan M, Pachydakis A, Chandakas S, Wissa I, Hill N. Efficacy of laparoscopic subtotal hysterectomy in the management of menorrhagia: 400 consecutive cases. *BJOG* 2008;115:742–8.

21 Erian J, El-Toukhy T, Chandakas S, Theodoridis T, Hill N. One hundred cases of laparoscopic subtotal hysterectomy using the PK and Lap Loop systems. *J Minim Invasive Gynecol* 2005;12:365–9.

22 Erian J, Lee C, Chandakas S, Watkinson S, Hill N. Feasibility of 6 hour discharge following laparoscopic subtotal hysterectomy; analysis of 492 consecutive cases. *J Minim Invasive Gynecol* 2008;15:5S.

23 Simon N V, Laveran R L, Cavanaugh S, Gerlach D H, Jackson J R. Laparoscopic supracervical hysterectomy vs. abdominal hysterectomy in a community hospital. A cost comparison. *J Reprod Med* 1999;44:339–45.

24 Carbonell A M, Joels C S, Kercher K W, Matthews B D, Sing R F, Heniford B T. A comparison of laparoscopic bipolar vessel sealing devices in the hemostasis of small-, medium-, and large-sized arteries. *J Laparoendosc Adv Surg Tech A* 2003;13:377–80.

25 Jung S K, Huh C Y. Ureteral injuries during classic intrafascial supracervical hysterectomy: an 11-year experience in 1163 patients. *J Minim Invasive Gynecol* 2008;15:440–5.

26 Donnez, P Jadoul, J Squifflet, J Donnez. A series of 3190 laparoscopic hysterectomies for benign disease from 1990 to 2006: evaluation of complications compared with vaginal and abdominal procedures. *BJOG* 2009;116:492–500.

27 Garry R. The place of subtotal/supracervical hysterectomy in current practice. *BJOG* 2008;115:1597–1600.

28 Morrell S, Taylor R, Wain G. A study of Pap test history and histologically determined cervical cancer in NSW women, 1997–2003. *J Med Screen* 2005;12:190–6.

29 Thakar R, Ayers S, Clarkson P, Stanton S, Manyonda I. Outcomes after total versus subtotal abdominal hysterectomy. *N Engl J Med* 2002;347:1318–25.

30 Hellström A C, Sigurjonson T, Pettersson F. Carcinoma of the cervical stump. The radiumhemmet series 1959–1987. Treatment and prognosis. *Acta Obstet Gynecol Scand* 2001;80:152–7.

31 Okaro E O, Jones K D, Sutton C. Long term outcome following laparoscopic supracervical hysterectomy. *BJOG* 2001;108:1017–20.

32 Ghomi A, Hantes J, Lotze EC. Incidence of cyclical bleeding after laparoscopic supracervical hysterectomy. *J Minim Invasive Gynecol* 2005;12:201–5.

33 Brandsborg B, Nikolajsen L, Hansen C T, Kehlet H, Jensen T S. Risk factors for chronic pain after hysterectomy: a nationwide questionnaire and database study. *Anesthesiology* 2007;106:1003–12.

12 Total laparoscopic hysterectomy

Alan Farthing

Introduction

Laparoscopic hysterectomy was first performed over 20 years ago with a view to decreasing the morbidity associated with total abdominal hysterectomy (TAH). The advantages of laparoscopic surgery in general have been discussed elsewhere in this book and they all apply to using minimal access techniques to perform hysterectomies. Unlike oophorectomy or excision of endometriosis, a hysterectomy could already be performed through minimal access techniques before the advent of laparoscopy, through the vagina. However, for the majority of surgeons vaginal hysterectomy was an awkward operation that was difficult to teach and arguably required greater surgical skill to perform well. Perhaps for these reasons, it tended to be confined to women with prolapse and, despite the advantages, in the 1980s nearly 90% of hysterectomies in the UK were being performed abdominally.[1]

Initially, there was an enthusiasm to use some aspects of laparoscopic surgery to make a vaginal hysterectomy possible. These techniques became known as the laparoscopically assisted vaginal hysterectomy (LAVH). This allowed the surgeon to inspect the peritoneal cavity, divide adhesions, mobilise the adnexae for removal and ensure there was no unrecognised pathology when the vaginal part of the procedure was commenced.

The enthusiasm of the early pioneers of LAVH ensured that many studies were performed to demonstrate the superiority of the new techniques over the old techniques. Not surprisingly, the results of many of these studies were open to interpretation and undoubtedly influenced by the relative lack of experience of those using the laparoscopic techniques. It seemed acceptable to consider a surgeon who had performed only 20 laparoscopic hysterectomies as someone sufficiently skilled to enter women into trials. Of course, these surgeons would be comparing their laparoscopic skills with their TAH techniques, which they would have practised hundreds of times previously; however, excluding these surgeons would have prevented the trials from taking place at all. A Cochrane database review[2] indicated that laparoscopic techniques were not superior and were probably inferior to vaginal hysterectomy, while both approaches allowed for quicker recovery than TAH. However, much of this evidence is based on those flawed studies from inexperienced surgeons.

Although we did not necessarily think it at the time, most of us who performed laparoscopic surgery would admit, in retrospect, that it takes many more than 20 operations to be able to gain the laparoscopic skills required to take on those difficult procedures where complications are more likely. It is perhaps only now that we have a group of surgeons who have performed as many laparoscopic hysterectomies as they have TAHs. In the last few years, studies have been published detailing the experience of complications in very large series involving over 3000 women from a single centre[3] and nearly 14 000 from multiple centres.[4] These studies demonstrate that complication rates are acceptably low and that laparoscopic hysterectomy is comparable to vaginal hysterectomy and allows for more precise surgery. A meta-analysis[5] that included only those studies with experienced surgeons demonstrated that total laparoscopic hysterectomy (TLH) was associated with fewer perioperative complications, less blood loss and shorter hospital stay but took longer to perform.

Many surgeons started out performing LAVH, but the majority of those with significant laparoscopic surgery experience have progressed to performing TLH. The most difficult part of any hysterectomy is usually the reflecting of the bladder, identification and division of the uterine arteries and excision of the cervix from the vaginal vault. In LAVH, all these steps are performed vaginally, but the experienced laparoscopic surgeon will usually develop the skills to perform these steps safely and without too much difficulty by use of the laparoscope. During an LAVH, the surgeon has to start all over again in a different position with a different orientation and it is not always easy to get the vaginal part of the dissection to meet up with the laparoscopic part of the dissection. If an operation has been started laparoscopically, it therefore seems logical and sensible to complete it laparoscopically providing this is not to the disadvantage of the woman undergoing the procedure. Those of us who routinely perform TLHs argue that there is no disadvantage to completing the surgery laparoscopically, but there are a few tricks that are helpful.

Technique

As with all laparoscopic surgery, a safe entry technique is important. An umbilical port for the camera is ideal and usually two further 5 mm ports are required for the surgical instruments. The author places the left port lateral to the inferior epigastric vessels and the right port just to the right of the midline

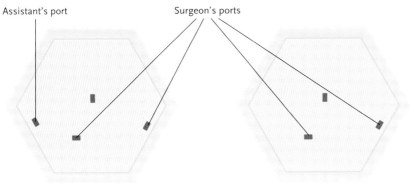

Assistant's port   Surgeon's ports

Three operating port technique   Two operating port technique
for more difficult cases

FIGURE 12.1 **Set-up for three- and two-port operating techniques**

but medial to the inferior epigastrics. While this makes the ports asymmetrical, it seems logical to me because the surgeon stands on the right side of the woman undergoing surgery and ergonomically this is better than placing the second port lateral to the inferior epigastrics and leaning over the woman to gain the correct angle. A third operating port may be required in difficult situations and this is placed lateral to the inferior epigastrics on the right. It is used by the assistant.

When only two operating ports are required, many surgeons will put in a left-sided port and then insert the second port where the assistant usually puts their port. This makes no sense to me except perhaps for symmetrical patterns being more pleasing to the eye (Figure 12.1).

Single-incision laparoscopic surgery is possible using adapted instruments, but the size of the incision at the umbilicus is much larger than that required using the techniques mentioned previously. In addition, the total size of the incisions is similar regardless of whether a single large one is used or a number of small ones.

Robotic surgery offers the novice laparoscopist the opportunity to perform laparoscopic surgery as the instruments can be more easily manipulated and suturing is similar to open surgery. However, the cost of the procedure is greatly increased. Additionally, more ports are required (a suction irrigator cannot be used through the robotic ports) and with some robots the size of those ports needs to be larger to accommodate larger instruments. The ports also need to be placed higher on the abdomen to accommodate the working angles of the robot. Nevertheless, large numbers of *da Vinci*® (Intuitive Surgical, Sunnyvale, CA, USA) robots have been sold and the successful marketing of this expensive facility has been a lesson to us all.

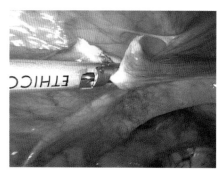

FIGURE 12.2 **Division of round ligament**

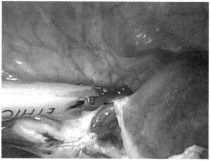

FIGURE 12.3 **Opening of broad ligament and creation of window**

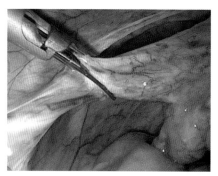

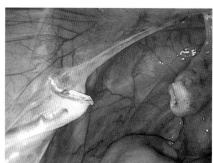

FIGURE 12.4 **Division of infundibulopelvic ligament**

TLH is performed in much the same way as a TAH. The round ligaments are divided and the ovarian blood supply identified. The ovarian ligament is then divided if conserving the ovaries, or the infundibulopelvic ligament is divided if removing the ovaries. Either way, the pedicle can be divided by bipolar diathermy, an ultrasonic scalpel, staples (which require a larger 12 mm port) or other energy sources (Figures 12.2–12.4). These pedicles can be sutured, but using the various energy sources for haemostasis is usually easier.

When removing the ovaries, the infundibulopelvic ligament needs to be identified as separate from the ureter, which is close by even in normal anatomy and can be closely applied where adhesions or ovarian masses are present.

The same process is repeated on the other side. Then, the peritoneum over the uterovesical fold is incised and the bladder reflected inferiorly (Figure 12.5). The uterine arteries are skeletalised, coagulated and divided (Figure 12.6).

Once the uterine arteries on one side are divided, the process is repeated on the other side. The junction between the cervix and the vagina is difficult to identify, but with insertion of the Lina McCartney Tube™ (Lina Medical,

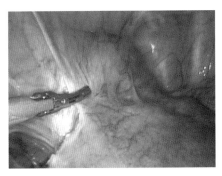 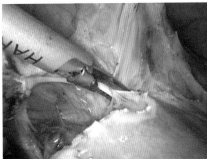

FIGURE 12.5 Incision of the uterovesical fold and bladder reflection

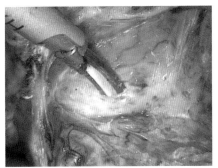 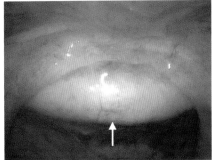

FIGURE 12.6 Skeletalised uterine arteries

FIGURE 12.7 Colpotomy tube distending the posterior fornix (arrow)

Cullompton, UK) or colpotomy cup (Figure 12.7), the top of the vagina is easily identified.

The vagina is incised and the colpotomy cup or tube becomes visible. This maintains the pneumoperitoneum that would otherwise be lost after the colpotomy (Figure 12.8). The template produced by the tube is followed and the cervix and uterus amputated from the vagina. The cervix is then grasped with vulsellum forceps and morcellated if necessary to remove the uterus (Figure 12.9).

In Figure 12.10, a monofilament dissolvable suture is used to suture the vault. Incorporation of the uterosacral ligaments in this suture ensures good haemostasis and closure of the vagina. The suture is then passed back through the vault into the tube and tied in the vagina (Figure 12.11).

At the end of the procedure, haemostasis is checked and the ports on the anterior abdominal wall closed.

Video 12.1 provides an example of total laparoscopic hysterectomy.

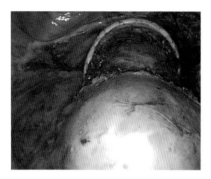

FIGURE 12.8 **Vagina opened and colpotomy cup visible**

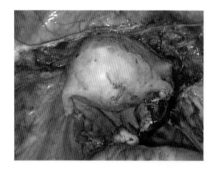

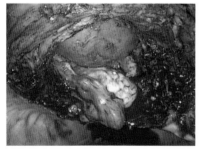

FIGURE 12.9 **Uterus delivered through the vagina**

Variations

The round ligament and vascular pedicles can be coagulated and divided using a variety of energy sources. The secret to being able to complete the whole procedure laparoscopically is being able to identify the edge of the vagina and to maintain the pneumoperitoneum once the colpotomy has been made. In the figures in this chapter, the McCartney Tube has been used, which is a simple disposable inert plastic tube. Any device placed in the vagina that fits over the cervix and otherwise fills the vagina will complete this task. Alternatives include the VCare® (ConMed Endosurgery, Utica, NY, USA), the RUMI® (CooperSurgical, Trumbull, CT, USA) uterine manipulator, the Koh Colpotomizer™ System[6] (CooperSurgical, Trumbull, CT, USA) and the modified manipulator described by Ramirez et al.[7] Whichever instrument is used, the principle is the same.

Recovery

The total complication rates for laparoscopic hysterectomies vary depending on how the information is gathered and how many surgeons contributed to the series; it lies somewhere between 1% and 11%.[3,8] Serious complications include bladder, bowel and ureteric injury, haemorrhage and conversion to laparotomy. These complications are highest in the early experience of any surgeon.

Overall, complication rates are relatively low. If wound infections are included, the complication rates are significantly lower in TLH than in TAH. Some surgeons have proposed that subtotal hysterectomy or supracervical hysterectomy is associated with even fewer complications. Certainly, Harmanli et al.[9] showed in a comparison study that there is less damage to the bladder, with 2.2% bladder damage in the TLH group versus 0.5% in the laparoscopic subtotal hysterectomy group. These statistics need to be compared against the morbidity of leaving the cervix and getting continuing cyclical bleeding.

Recovery from TLH is faster than recovery from open surgery. Comparison studies indicate that inpatient stay is 2.5 days shorter and analgesic requirements are decreased.[5]

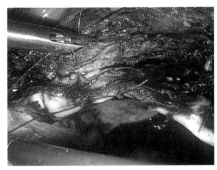

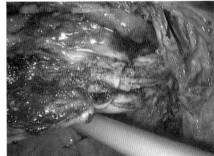

FIGURE 12.10 **Vaginal vault closure**   FIGURE 12.11 **Vault inspection**

As long as the uterosacral ligaments are included in the vaginal vault suture, there do not seem to be any long-term sequelae that are different from those with open hysterectomy, apart from incision-related complications such as hernias, of which there are obviously fewer, and cosmesis.

Learning the technique

The teaching of any surgery is a subject of much debate, especially in the current environment. The time taken to teach means that fewer operations can be performed on an operating list and the careful scrutiny of complications inevitably means that trained surgeons are more likely to say, 'I'll do this one myself'. Trainees gain significantly less training experience than in the past and therefore a smaller group of carefully trained surgeons will have to perform the vast majority of procedures in the future. However, difficulties in training everyone should not be used as an excuse for not training enough surgeons to provide the best possible service. TLH is an excellent example where this holds true.

References

1 Vessey M P, Villard-Mackintosh L, McPherson K, Coulter A, Yeates D. The epidemiology of hysterectomy: findings in a large cohort study. *Br J Obstet Gynaecol* 1992;99:402–7.

2 Johnson N, Barlow D, Lethaby A, Tavender E, Curr L, Garry R. Surgical approach to hysterectomy for benign gynaecological disease. *Cochrane Database Syst Rev* 2006;(2):CD003677.

3 Donnez O, Jadoul P, Squifflet J, Donnez J. A series of 3190 laparoscopic hysterectomies for benign disease from 1990 to 2006: evaluation of complications compared with vaginal and abdominal procedures. *BJOG* 2009;116:492–500.

4 Brummer T H, Seppälä T T, Härkki P S. National learning curve for laparoscopic hysterectomy and trends in hysterectomy in Finland 2000–2005. *Hum Reprod* 2008;23:840–5.

5 Walsh C A, Walsh S R, Tang T Y, Slack M. Total abdominal hysterectomy versus total laparoscopic hysterectomy for benign disease: a meta-analysis. *Eur J Obstet Gynecol Reprod Biol* 2009;144:3–7.

6 Keriakos R, Zaklama M. The RUMI manipulator and Koh colpotomiser system for total laparoscopic hysterectomy. *BJOG* 2000;107:274–7.

7 Ramirez P T, Frumovitz M, Dos Reis R, Milam M R, Bevers M W, Levenback C F, et al. Modified uterine manipulator and vaginal rings for total laparoscopic radical hysterectomy. *Int J Gynecol Cancer* 2008;18:571–5.

8 Garry R, Fountain J, Masons S, Hawe J, Napp V, Abbott J, et al. The eVALuate study: two parallel randomised trials, one comparing laparoscopic with abdominal hysterectomy, the other comparing laparoscopic with vaginal hysterectomy. *BMJ* 2004;328:129.

9 Harmanli O H, Tunitsky E, Esin S, Citil A, Knee A. A comparison of short-term outcomes between laparoscopic supracervical and total hysterectomy. *Am J Obstet Gynecol* 2009;201:536.e1–7.

13 Laparoscopic urogynaecology

Karen I Rose and Anthony RB Smith

Introduction

Urogynaecology is a growing specialty with increasing demands secondary to the global ageing of the population. Demographic studies have shown that for most nations, regardless of geographical location or developmental stage, the 80 years or over age group is the fastest growing segment of the older population.[1] The lifetime risk of undergoing a single operation for pelvic organ prolapse or urinary incontinence is 11.1% by the age of 80 years with a 29.2% risk of requiring further surgical intervention.[2] The growing demand for surgical treatment, significant failure rates and rapidly evolving technology have encouraged a constant adaptation of pelvic floor surgery.

Over the last three decades, laparoscopic surgery has become a widely accepted modality in various specialties. Traditional surgical procedures that previously relied on vaginal or abdominal access are now successfully being performed laparoscopically. The laparoscopic route uses smaller incisions with a possible reduction of postoperative pain, shorter hospital admissions and faster recovery. Advances in equipment and minimal access surgical skills have led to the introduction and development of new techniques that benefit from the enhanced visualisation of laparoscopic surgery.

Since the early 1990s, numerous laparoscopic techniques have been described for the treatment of urinary incontinence and pelvic organ prolapse. The large variation in practice and materials used makes it difficult to evaluate the results. This problem is compounded as most series contain small numbers and in addition pelvic floor defects frequently require concomitant surgery. This chapter provides an up-to-date literature review of the various laparoscopic urogynaecological techniques described.

Incontinence

Laparoscopic colposuspension

Open colposuspension, first described by Burch in 1961,[3] had long been considered the gold standard surgical procedure for treating stress urinary incontinence. Vancaillie and Schuessler[4] published the earliest series of laparoscopic colposuspensions in 1991, in which nine women were included. The authors described a modification of the original Marshall–Marchetti–Krantz procedure, using nonabsorbable sutures to attach the periurethral tissue to the symphysis pubis. The first series of laparoscopic modified Burch colposuspensions was published in 1993 by Liu and Paek,[5] who used absorbable sutures to suspend the paravaginal fascia to the ileopectineal ligaments (Cooper's ligament). Both procedures produced encouraging results, but the difficulty with laparoscopic suturing led to the development of faster alternative techniques such as the use of mesh and staples.

Video 13.1 provides an example of a laparoscopic colposuspension.

Combined laparoscopic and vaginal approach

In 1996, Breda et al.[6] devised and reported a laparoscopically assisted colposuspension technique that removed the need for intracorporeal laparoscopic suturing and therefore reduced the operating time. The space of Retzius was prepared by creating a pneumocavity using a single suprapubic port. Specially designed handle-needles loaded with nonabsorbable sutures were then passed through two small suprapubic incisions, and the colposuspension to Cooper's ligament was performed with extracorporeal knotting. Harewood[7] and Carter[8] described similar techniques using Stamey needles for suturing of the perivaginal tissue. Both Breda et al.[6] and Harewood[7] reported 70% success rates with shorter operating times.

Number of sutures

Persson et al.[9] randomised 161 consecutive women to either one double-bite suture or two single-bite sutures on either side of the urethra. Postoperative 'ultrashort' pad tests and interviews with the participating women were performed at 1-year follow-up. A significantly greater number of women reported being cured in the two-suture group (89%) compared with the one-suture group (65%) (relative risk [RR] 1.37, 95% CI 1.14–1.64). Objective findings were also in favour of the two-suture group because 83% of the women in this group who underwent a pad test were found to be cured compared with 58% in the one-suture group (RR 1.42, 95% CI 1.14–1.77). One woman in the two-suture group required repeat incontinence surgery.

The study revealed a low incidence of postoperative urge symptoms and voiding dysfunction, which were not significantly different between the two groups. Perioperative complication rates were similar in both groups (15 women in the two-suture group compared with 14 women in the one-suture group). One woman in the one-suture group suffered from postoperative pubic bone osteitis. The median hospital stay was 1.7 days using both techniques and the median operating time was 17 minutes longer among those allocated to two sutures.

Powers et al.[10] compared the open versus laparoscopic Burch colposuspension using a one-suture technique. Their results were consistent with those from Persson et al.[9] and the authors concluded that, compared with reported success rates for the two-suture technique, Burch colposuspension using a one-suture technique was associated with an unacceptably low objective cure rate at 1 year, in particular when performed laparoscopically.

Mesh

The challenges of laparoscopic suturing led to the development of sutureless techniques. The use of polypropylene mesh and titanium hernia staples in a laparoscopic colposuspension was first described in 1993 by Ou et al.[11] The mesh was placed along the paravaginal fascia and fixed to Cooper's ligaments with staples. Several publications[12–15] have since described sutureless techniques using staples, tacks and bone anchors, many of which report simplification of the operation and shorter operating times.

Studies comparing the use of sutures with mesh and staples found the former technique to be more effective. Ross[16] demonstrated similar cure rates in both groups (91% in the suture group compared with 94% in the mesh group); however, subsequent good-quality and larger studies favoured the use of sutures.[17,18] Despite the significantly improved subjective and objective outcomes, Ankardal et al.[18] demonstrated a higher perioperative complication rate in the suture group (mainly bladder perforations) and therefore the authors reported the overall analysis results in favour of the mesh for perioperative complications.

Complications such as mesh and staple erosion should be anticipated when applying the sutureless laparoscopic colposuspension technique. Several case reports[19,20] have described the presence of tacks in pelvic structures such as the vagina and bladder and Yesilli et al.[21] reported a stone formation on a surgical staple found in the bladder 6 years after a laparoscopic colposuspension. The use of bone anchors to secure suburethral slings has been associated with pubic osteomyelitis.[22]

Glue

To develop less invasive techniques, fibrin sealants have been used to perform sutureless endoscopic colposuspensions. Kiilholma et al.[23] reported their small case series of 17 women in whom a two-component fibrin sealant was used as a substitute for sutures. Fifteen women noted immediate benefit and 10 of the 12 women followed up after 6 months reported to be completely dry. Kjolhede et al.[24] published a prospective observational study evaluating the long-term efficacy and safety of abdominal urethrocystopexy through a minilaparotomy using solely fibrin sealant as the fixation glue. Despite using the same sealant, their long-term data were not as promising as Kiilholma's earlier study. The subjective cure rates of the 43 women were 72% and 55% at 1 and 3 years, respectively. The corresponding objective cure rates were 64% and 60%.

Transperitoneal versus extraperitoneal approach

Variations exist not only in the materials used. Two approaches to the cave of Retzius are commonly employed: trans- or extraperitoneal. The transperitoneal approach permits assessment of the intra-abdominal organs and offers the possibility of performing concomitant intraperitoneal procedures, such as hysterectomy. The extraperitoneal approach provides a shorter dissection time and reduces the risk of bladder and intra-abdominal viscera damage. Surgeons favouring the extraperitoneal approach commonly use sutureless techniques because of the reduced access and the high surgical skills required.

Two studies[25,26] comparing extraperitoneal and transperitoneal techniques revealed no statistically significant differences in the objective or subjective results. Both studies used sutures in the transperitoneal approach and mesh fixed with tacks in the extraperitoneal approach, making it impossible to compare the approaches alone.

Laparoscopic colposuspension versus open colposuspension

A Cochrane review[27] of laparoscopic colposuspension for urinary incontinence in women used ten trials to compare laparoscopic with open colposuspension. The results were difficult to compare because of large variation in the lengths of follow-up, outcome measures and definitions used. Subjective cure rates using women's observations within 18 months of follow-up ranged from 58% to 96% in the open group and from 62% to 100% in the laparoscopic group. Objective cure rates measured by urodynamics or pad tests performed within 18 months of surgery favoured the open colposuspension; however, no significant difference was found between 18 months and 5 years of follow-up. The risk of developing voiding dysfunction or de novo detrusor overactivity was similar in both groups, as were the results of various quality of life questionnaires.

Barr et al.[28] published long-term outcome data of 139 women who had undergone laparoscopic colposuspensions more than 10 years previously and compared the results with 52 women who had open colposuspensions in the same unit during a similar period of time. The women were routinely followed up at 6 months and a structured telephone interview was performed, which included the short-form Bristol Female Lower Urinary Tract Symptoms questionnaire. Ninety-six (69%) women from the laparoscopic group and 31 (60%) women from the open group responded to the 10-year questionnaire. Subjective cure rates deteriorated over time from 71% and 67% at 6 months to 52% and 36% at 10 years for the laparoscopic and open procedures, respectively.

Bladder, ureteric and vascular injuries are recognised complications of colposuspension. The Cochrane review[27] reported 21 bladder injuries among 521 laparoscopic procedures (compared with 10 among 507 open procedures) and two studies reported obturator vein lacerations. However, compared with the traditional open colposuspension, the laparoscopic group was found to have significantly fewer postoperative complications (RR 0.74, 95% CI 0.58–0.96) with lower estimated blood losses and shorter duration of catheterisation.

Longer operating times are a significant disadvantage of the laparoscopic approach; however, women have reported significantly less pain,[29,30] shorter hospital admissions, faster recoveries and quicker return to normal activities.[31–34] Although the laparoscopic approach was not cost-effective during the first 6 months following surgery, Dumville et al.[35] reported a favourable economic case for this approach at 24 months.

Tension-free vaginal tape versus laparoscopic colposuspension

Eight studies comparing laparoscopic colposuspension with tension-free vaginal tape (TVT) sling procedures were reviewed in the Cochrane review.[27] Despite the variations in techniques and material used, none of the studies found a significant difference in subjective cure rates within 18 months of follow-up. Even at longer-term follow-up (4–8 years), TVT was found to have similar results to laparoscopic colposuspension.

Objective cure rates within 18 months were higher for TVT than for laparoscopic colposuspension. Various definitions were used among the trials, including pad tests, clinical stress tests, urodynamic tests and urinary diaries. However, overall the laparoscopic colposuspensions had statistically significantly lower objective cure rates (RR 0.88, 95% CI 0.81–0.95).

Quality of life questionnaires demonstrated a significant improvement in both the laparoscopic group and the vaginal sling group with no disparity between them.[27] However, Valpas et al.[36] did find a significant difference in favour of TVT at 1-year follow-up. Although no significant variation was found in the rates of perioperative complications, the laparoscopic group required longer operating times (mean difference 20.31 minutes), hospital admissions (mean difference 1.01 days) and recovery times (mean difference 8.03 days).

Conclusions

Laparoscopic colposuspension performed with at least two sutures on each side of the urethra appears to be an acceptable alternative for the treatment of stress urinary incontinence and produces similar continence rates to the open procedure. The laparoscopic approach has the advantage over open colposuspension of faster recovery times, less analgesia requirement and fewer wound infections and does not have the risk of mesh erosion associated with TVT. It does, however, require the surgeon to learn laparoscopic suturing skills. Laparoscopic colposuspension is economically comparable to the open procedure and appears to produce a similar cure rate on longer-term follow-up.

Prolapse

Anterior wall

Laparoscopic paravaginal repair

In the early 19th century, Cooper[37] reported an association between the development of hernias and the tearing of the transversalis fascia, which was often found to have avulsed from its skeletal attachments. Although his discoveries led to the development of site-specific facial repairs, the paravaginal repair for cystocele described by White[38] in 1909 was soon abandoned for the central plication technique described by Kelly and Dumm[39] in 1914, and this approach became widely referred to as anterior vaginal colporrhaphy.

Although Richardson et al.[40] reintroduced the concept of site-specific vaginal repair in 1976, it was not widely accepted until the 1980s. This coincided with the development of laparoscopic surgery, which provided a clearer view of the white line and the detached pubocervical fascia. As laparoscopic colposuspensions developed and minimal access operative skills improved, surgeons instituted concomitant paravaginal repairs.

Procedure

Laparoscopic paravaginal repair can be performed trans- or extraperitoneally. The former provides easier access with a wider field of view. Both techniques involve attachment of the pubocervical fascia to either the arcus tendineus fasciae pelvis (white line) or the pectineal ligament (Cooper's ligament). After medial retraction of the bladder, the tissues are traditionally approximated using three to six sutures bilaterally, which are sequentially placed between the ischial spine and the urethrovesical junction. Suturing within the depths of the space of Retzius requires advanced surgical expertise and therefore variations of the technique have been developed including the use of mesh and staples.[41]

Outcomes

Few studies have looked at the outcome of laparoscopic paravaginal repairs without concomitant surgery. Washington and Somers[41] reported a small case series of 12 women who underwent a paravaginal repair using mesh and staples. A subjective and objective improvement in 10/11 and 9/11 women was found, respectively. To draw any meaningful conclusions about the value of laparoscopic paravaginal repair, robust studies are required that preferably compare alternative approaches.

Complications

Lower urinary tract injuries including cystotomies, ureteric obstruction and suture material within the bladder are recognised complications of paravaginal repair. Speights et al.[42] demonstrated a 2.3% bladder injury rate in their retrospective analysis of 171 women undergoing a laparoscopic Burch urethropexy and/or paravaginal repair. Comparable rates were found in the Demirci et al.[43] study looking at 42 women undergoing abdominal paravaginal repairs.

Dissection and suturing within the space of Retzius is associated with a risk of injury to the obturator neurovascular bundle. Although most studies report minimal median blood losses,[42,44] blood losses of greater than 1000 ml have been described.[45]

Both Behnia-Willison et al.[44] and Seman et al.[45] reported major complications in 4% of women who underwent laparoscopic paravaginal repairs with concomitant surgery. The complications included urinary tract or bowel injuries, conversion to laparotomy, anaesthetic complications and blood losses of more than 1000 ml. Minor complications such as infection, haematoma formation, prolonged catheterisation and deep vein thrombosis were also described.

The advantage of mesh and surgical tacks in the vagina and surrounding tissues was disputed in the Albright et al.[46] case report of a woman suffering from lower abdominal pain, dyspareunia and urinary symptoms following a laparoscopic Burch and paravaginal repair. Mesh, permanent suture material and 13 helical tacks were found among dense adhesions in the space of Retzius on exploratory laparotomy.

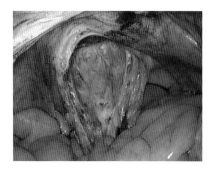

FIGURE 13.1 **The rectovaginal space is opened**

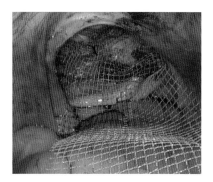

FIGURE 13.2 **Mesh is inserted**

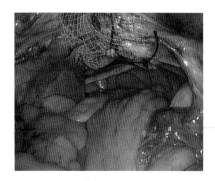

FIGURE 13.3 **Mesh is sutured to the full length of the posterior vaginal wall**

Vault

Laparoscopic sacrocolpopexy

Originally described by Ameline and Huguier in 1957,[47] the abdominal sacrocolpopexy is an effective treatment for vaginal vault prolapse. Endorsed by the National Institute for Health and Clinical Excellence (NICE),[48] abdominal sacrocolpopexy has reported objective and subjective failure rates of 0–6.1% and 3.3–31%, respectively, at an average follow-up of 2 years.[49]

The first laparoscopic sacrocolpopexy was described in 1994 by Nezhat et al.[50] and has since been suggested to match the gold standard of abdominal sacrocolpopexy in terms of efficacy.[51] Although numerous studies have described high success rates with the advantages of smaller incisions, faster recovery times and enhanced views of the anatomy, the large variations in methodology and frequent use of concomitant surgery make it difficult to compare and analyse the data.

Video 13.2 provides an example of laparoscopic sacrocolpopexy.

Techniques

Numerous techniques and materials have been described to interpose a suspensory hammock between the prolapsed vaginal vault and the anterior surface of the sacrum. Mesh, which was traditionally sutured to the vaginal apex, is frequently extended and secured along the full length of the rectovaginal septum. The rectovaginal space is opened (Figure 13.1), allowing for the mesh to be inserted and sutured to the posterior vaginal wall (Figures 13.2 and 13.3). The peritoneum is then opened over the sacral promontory (Figure 13.4), exposing the surface to which the mesh is attached (Figure 13.5). The mesh is often attached to both the anterior and the posterior vaginal wall by use of a folded, Y-shaped or divided piece of mesh that is individually attached to the vagina and then fixed to the sacrum. To reduce the incidence of intra-abdominal mesh-related complications, the mesh can be covered with peritoneum (Figure 13.6).

Time-consuming laparoscopic suturing has led to the development of several products, including staples, bone anchors and helical tacks, to secure mesh to the sacral promontory. However, little research has been performed

directly comparing these techniques. Absorbable vaginal staples have also been used to attach Mersilene® (Ethicon Endo-
Surgery, Cincinnati, OH, USA) mesh to the vaginal tissue.[52]

SYNTHETIC MESH

Various synthetic and biological meshes have been used in
both abdominal and laparoscopic sacrocolpopexies. Although
little evidence is available to support a particular mesh, Chen
et al.[53] provided Level I evidence indicating that repair of apical prolapse with abdominal sacrocolpopexy using synthetic
mesh resulted in improved outcomes.

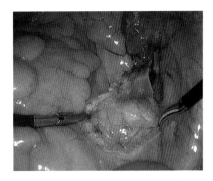

FIGURE 13.4 **Peritoneum opened over the sacral promontory**

Higgs et al.[54] reviewed 140 consecutive laparoscopic sacrocolpopexies performed over a 6-year period using polypropylene mesh, with 57 women requiring concomitant surgery.
In total, 103 women completed a postoperative questionnaire
after a median of 66 months (range 37–124 months) and
66 women attended an additional full pelvic organ prolapse
quantification (POP-Q) examination. Successful long-term
vault support was found in 92% of the women examined.
Eleven of the 103 women required further prolapse surgery
and recurrent vaginal vault prolapse was found in 42% of the
women. However, 79% felt that their symptoms of prolapse
were cured or improved following their surgery. Immediate
and long-term complications were rare. The only significant
long-term complication was mesh erosion, which occurred
in nine women. The technique was altered after the first 20
procedures from vaginal mesh insertion to laparoscopic mesh
insertion, which reduced the erosion rate from 20% to 6%.

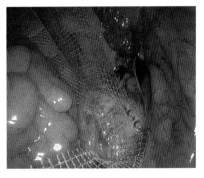

FIGURE 13.5 **Mesh is attached to the lower border of L5 with a tacker**

An Italian study[55] looked at 165 laparoscopic sacrocolpopexy procedures using polypropylene mesh that were
performed over an 8-year period. Several women required
concomitant surgery. Eighty-three per cent of the women were
followed up at a median follow-up of 43 months (range 6–96
months) and the authors reported success rates of 94.9%
with high satisfaction rates. Seven women (5%) were found
to have recurrent vaginal vault prolapse and one had evidence

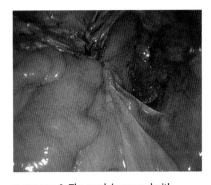

FIGURE 13.6 **The mesh is covered with peritoneum**

of mesh erosion in the vagina. Intraoperative complications included bladder
injuries (3%) and sigmoid perforations (2%).

BIOLOGICAL MESH

The use of biological mesh in sacrocolpopexies remains controversial. Although smaller studies have described promising outcomes, larger trials comparing the use of absorbable polypropylene with synthetic meshes have produced less favourable results. Culligan et al.[56] performed a randomised controlled trial comparing the use of cadaveric fascia lata and polypropylene mesh in sacrocolpopexies. In this study, 100 women were randomised in a double-blinded fashion and were followed up at regular intervals for 1 year. Objective outcomes were measured using the POP-Q system and anatomical failure was defined as POP-Q stage 2. Measurements of the anterior wall and vault at 1-year follow-up were significantly in favour of the polypropylene group.

Deprest et al.[57] prospectively studied 50 consecutive women who underwent a laparoscopic sacrocolpopexy with porcine mesh of small intestinal submucosa or dermal collagen and compared them with 100 consecutive controls in whom polypropylene mesh was used. The women underwent a functional (86%) and anatomical (67%) evaluation at a mean follow-up of 33 months. Although there were no differences in functional outcomes between the two groups, significant increases in failure rates were found in the xenograft group when comparing the vault (21% versus 3%, $P<0.01$) and the posterior compartment (36% versus 19%, $P<0.05$). All six women requiring further prolapse surgery were confined to the xenograft group and the use of xenografts did not decrease the number of mesh-related complications (11% in both groups).

Complications

Lower urinary tract and bowel injuries are recognised complications of the sacrocolpopexy. The risk of organ damage has been reported to be in the range of 0–7.9% (15 studies, $n=1723$).[58] Considerable haemorrhage secondary to trauma of the presacral venous plexus, middle sacral artery and common iliac veins has been described with blood transfusion rates in the range of 0–17% (19 studies, $n=2080$).[58]

Despite the use of modern meshes, mesh erosion remains a significant complication of sacrocolpopexy (0–17%). Concurrent hysterectomy was reported to be a modifiable risk for mesh erosion.[59] However, in a larger cohort study of 446 consecutive women who underwent laparoscopic sacrocolpopexy with a macroporous soft polypropylene mesh, no statistically significant increase in mesh-related complications was observed among women undergoing concurrent hysterectomies.[60] Debodinance et al.[61] suggested in their review that mesh rejections are proportional to the surface area of the synthetic tissue and the proximity of the vaginal scar.

Synthetic meshes have advanced considerably over the last few decades and recent studies have favoured lightweight macroporous soft polypropylene meshs.[60,62] Although these latest developments appear to be promising, mesh-related complications still occur, indicating that the perfect mesh has not yet been created.

SACROCOLPOPEXY VERSUS SACROSPINOUS COLPOPEXY

NICE carried out a meta-analysis[49] to compare the subjective and objective failure rates between sacrocolpopexy and sacrospinous colpopexy (without mesh) and reported no evidence of a statistically significant difference between the two operations. The subjective failure rates at 24–36 months of follow-up ranged from 7% to 22% in the sacrocolpopexy group (with mesh) compared with a range of 9–12% in the sacrospinous colpopexy group (no mesh). Maher et al.[63] studied 95 women who were randomly allocated to undergo abdominal sacrocolpopexy or vaginal sacrospinous colpopexy and described objective failure rates of 24% and 31%, respectively. The authors noted a lower rate of recurrent vault prolapse and dyspareunia in the abdominal sacrocolpopexy group. However, they felt that these benefits had to be balanced against a longer operating time, longer time to return to activities of daily living and increased cost of the abdominal approach.

In a retrospective study, Marcickiewicz et al.[64] compared vaginal sacrospinous colpopexy with laparoscopic sacrocolpopexy for the treatment of vaginal vault prolapse in 111 women. Both groups had low perioperative complication rates, but three women in the laparoscopic sacrocolpopexy group required conversion to laparotomy. The median time for the postoperative follow-up visit was 33.6 months (range 13–60 months) for the laparoscopic sacrocolpopexy group and 38.4 months (range 7–108 months) for the vaginal sacrospinous colpopexy group. Subjective success rates were comparable in both groups (78% in the laparoscopic sacrocolpopexy group versus 82% in the vaginal sacrospinous colpopexy group). However, seven of the 60 (11.7%) women undergoing laparoscopic sacrocolpopexy required surgery for the recurrence of vault prolapse compared with no woman in the vaginal sacrospinous colpopexy group. Although the lengths of inpatient stays were similar (3.7 days [range 1–18 days] in the vaginal sacrospinous colpopexy group and 4.0 days [range 2–21 days] in the laparoscopic sacrocolpopexy group), the operating time was significantly longer in the laparoscopic sacrocolpopexy group (median 129 minutes) than in the vaginal sacrospinous colpopexy group (median 62 minutes). It is possible that the length of postoperative stay was influenced by factors other than the need for hospital care since a substantial proportion of women are fit for discharge the day after laparoscopic sacrocolpopexy.[64]

Although the laparoscopic approach is commonly associated with prolonged operating times, Akladios et al.[65] demonstrated a steady decrease in the duration of surgery as the surgeons progressed up the laparoscopic sacrocolpopexy learning curve. They observed a turning point after 18–24 procedures, but no change in morbidity was noted throughout.

Uterus

Laparoscopic hysteropexy
An increasing number of women in the reproductive age group are seeking surgical treatment for pelvic floor prolapse. These women regularly request preservation of their fertility, rapid return to daily activities and good cosmetic results. Uterine preservation is often felt to be favourable in sexually active women because of the suggested physiological and psychological roles of the uterus in sexual function. Several uterus-conserving laparoscopic procedures have been described for the treatment of uterovaginal prolapse, including uterine suspension to the round ligaments, uterosacral ligaments and the anterior longitudinal ligament of the sacral promontory.

Round ligament suspension/plication
Uterine ventrosuspension, more frequently described for the treatment of deep dyspareunia, pelvic pain and infertility, is a long-standing procedure that has steadily declined in use because of its high reported failure rate in both treating symptoms and maintaining uterine suspension. Since the introduction of laparoscopic surgery, the use of laparoscopic round ligament suspension as an alternative treatment for uterine prolapse has been described.

Shalev et al.[66] performed laparoscopic ventrofixations in 34 women, 15 of whom received concomitant cystocele repairs. Follow-up ranged from 6 to 36 months and the procedure was described as successful in 100% of women, who all reported to be content and symptom-free. O'Brien and Ibrahim[67] presented a case series of nine postmenopausal women who underwent laparoscopic round ligament ventrosuspension for the treatment of genital prolapse. Segments of the round ligament were laparoscopically advanced through the rectus sheath and fixed. Their results were not as promising as those by Shalev et al. because one of the procedures had to be abandoned secondary to tearing and bleeding of the round ligament, and at 3-month follow-up eight of the nine women were found to have recurrent prolapse requiring further surgery.

Two studies looking at the use of laparoscopic ventrosuspension for the treatment of chronic pelvic pain and dyspareunia also reported poor outcomes. Yoong[68] operated on 72 women and described an 18–45% success rate at 6 months of follow-up. By the time of their 2-year follow-up, 28% of the women had undergone a hysterectomy. Halperin et al.[69] studied the long-term outcome of 82 women undergoing open or laparoscopic ventrosuspensions. Despite the initial symptomatic improvement noted in 70.7% of the women, only 46.3% reported improvement at long-term follow-up (mean 12 years, range 5–20 years). No significant difference was found between the open and laparoscopic groups.

Laparoscopic uterosacral ligament suspension

Vaginal and abdominal uterosacral ligament suspension has been successfully performed for the treatment of uterine and vault prolapse. Several laparoscopic techniques have since been described and favoured because of the improved visualisation of the pelvic anatomy.

Wu[70] presented a case series of seven women who underwent laparoscopic uterine suspensions with high McCall colpopexy. Three nonabsorbable Gore-Tex® (WL Gore and Associates, Newark, DE, USA) sutures were used at various levels of the uterosacrals to purse-string the ligaments to the posterior vagina, cervix, peritoneum of the pararectal spaces and the serosal layer of rectosigmoid. No recurrent prolapses were reported at 9–17 months of follow-up.

Maher et al.[71] published a prospective evaluation of 43 women with symptomatic uterine prolapse who underwent a laparoscopic suture hysteropexy. Polydioxalone sutures were used to close the pouch of Douglas before plicating the uterosacral ligaments and reattaching them to the cervix with interrupted Gore-Tex sutures. The mean operating time of the laparoscopic suture hysteropexy alone was 42 ± 15 minutes (range 22–121 minutes). The mean blood loss was less than 50 ml, but one woman acquired a left uterine artery laceration, which required conversion to laparotomy, oversewing of the uterine artery and a two-unit blood transfusion. At a mean follow-up of 12 ± 7 months (range 6–32 months), 81% of the women reported no symptoms of prolapse and 79% had no objective evidence of prolapse. However, seven (16%) women required additional pelvic floor surgery including hysterectomies, sacrocolpopexies and sacrospinous fixations. Two women subsequently completed term pregnancies without prolapse and delivered their infants by elective caesarean section.

Medina and Takacs[72] used the International Continence Society pelvic POP-Q examination to determine the stage of prolapse and the immediate postoperative results in 23 women undergoing laparoscopic uterosacral uterine suspension for the treatment of symptomatic prolapse. A significant improvement of cervical and posterior vaginal fornix support (POP-Q points

C and D) was noted (–0.6 versus –7.8 and –5.0 versus –8.6, respectively; $P<0.01$) and none of the women reported symptomatic prolapse at their mean follow-up of 15.9 months.

Several studies have assessed the value of laparoscopic uterosacral ligament suspension for the treatment of symptomatic uterine retroflexion rather than symptoms and signs of prolapse. Ostrzenski[73] randomised 62 women to either a laparoscopic retroperitoneal uterine suspension group or a diagnostic laparoscopy group and followed them up for at least 24 months. Neither group reported intraoperative complications and 87.5% described symptomatic relief following surgery. Although the statistical analysis demonstrated a significant improvement of symptoms in the hysteropexy group ($P<0.0001$), a large proportion of the women were excluded from the final analysis.

Gargiulo et al.[74] described a variation of laparoscopic hysteropexy for the treatment of pelvic pain, deep dyspareunia and infertility. Fifty women in the reproductive age group with uterine retroversion underwent three-stitch laparoscopic uterine suspension. The round ligaments were secured bilaterally to the anterior horns of the uterus by use of nonabsorbable sutures. The uterosacral ligaments were then approximated behind the cervix by use of a third suture. No intraoperative complications were reported, but one woman reported postoperative abdominal pain. Of the 40 women seen at 1 year of follow-up, 33 described symptomatic improvement.

Laparoscopic sacrohysteropexy
Sacrohysteropexy has become increasingly popular in the literature over the last couple of decades, but the number of studies and case reports remains small, providing limited data regarding its efficacy and safety. Both abdominal and laparoscopic approaches have been described as well as a variety of techniques that broadly fall into two categories: suture sacrohysteropexy or mesh sacrohysteropexy.

Krause et al.[75] published a prospective review of 81 women who underwent laparoscopic sacral suture hysteropexy over the course of 2 years. Their technique involved the placement of two monofilamentous nonabsorbable continuous sutures, which were run from the posterior cervix along the length of the uterosacral ligament to the anterior longitudinal ligament of the sacral promontory and back along the other uterosacral ligament to the cervix. Care was taken to avoid the ureters and postoperative cystoscopies were performed to exclude ureteric obstruction. Only two perioperative complications were reported, which included a thromboembolic event and a small bowel perforation. One woman developed a small bowel obstruction 17 months postoperatively secondary to entanglement of the bowel between the ligaments and the exposed suture. The woman required a bowel resection and anastomosis.

Cutner et al.[76] used Mersilene tape to suspend the uterus to the sacral promontory (Video 13.3). The peritoneum over the sacral promontory was incised and a retroperitoneal tunnel was created from the sacral promontory to the insertion of the uterosacral ligament complex into the cervix bilaterally. A 5 mm Mersilene tape was sutured through the cervix at the isthmic–cervical junction and passed through the uterosacral ligaments laterally to avoid bowel obstruction. The tape was then retroperitoneally tunnelled towards the sacral promontory bilaterally and affixed with tacks (Protack™; Covidien, Mansfield, MA, USA). Care was taken to reperitonealise and completely cover the tape. The technique was employed in eight women and had a median duration of 125 minutes. Perioperative complications included one conservatively managed surgical emphysema and two urinary retentions, which resolved following 7 days of catheterisation. The length of follow-up ranged between 6 and 12 months. However, the authors did not publish their results.

The use of various techniques and meshes has been described in both abdominal and laparoscopic sacrohysteropexies, although the numbers of women in each study remain small.

In 2001, Leron and Stanton[77] described their prospective observational study of 13 women who had undergone abdominal sacrohysteropexy with the use of Teflon® (DuPont, Wilmington, DE, USA) mesh to secure the uterine isthmus to the anterior longitudinal ligament of the first or second sacral vertebra in a tension-free fashion. A range of concomitant surgeries was performed and no intraoperative or postoperative complications were reported. Uterine descent was detected in only one woman at a mean follow-up of 15.6 months (range 4–49 months).

In 2004, Seracchioli et al.[78] reported on 15 women of reproductive age with genital prolapse who had laparoscopic sacrohysteropexy with concomitant laparoscopic Burch colposuspension, paravaginal repair or prosthetic reconstruction. A V-shaped polypropylene mesh was sutured to the anterior vaginal wall and isthmus before being passed through a window created on the right side of the broad ligament and secured behind the isthmus and onto the sacral promontory. All of the women were followed up for 24 months and none were reported to have recurrence of their apical prolapse.

Rosenblatt et al.[79] published a retrospective case series of 40 consecutive women who had a laparoscopic sacrocervicopexy with synthetic mesh. The mesh was attached from the distal uterosacral ligaments and posterior endopelvic fascia to the anterior longitudinal ligament of the sacral promontory. Serial POP-Q measurements were taken and the mean value for POP-Q point C changed from −1.13 (range +9 to −4) preoperatively to −5.28 (range −3 to −13) at 6 weeks, −5.26 (range −3 to −8) at 6 months and −4.84 (−3 to −7) at 1 year postoperatively.

Price et al.[80] recently reported a prospective observational study of 51 women who underwent a laparoscopic sacrohysteropexy for uterovaginal prolapse. A bifurcated polypropylene mesh was used to suspend the uterus from the sacral promontory. Two arms of the mesh were introduced through bilateral windows in the broad ligaments and sutured anteriorly to the cervix. The mesh was then tacked to the anterior longitudinal ligament over the sacral promontory to elevate the uterus. No major intraoperative complications were reported, although two women were admitted with lower abdominal discomfort and subsequently underwent laparoscopies for division of small bowel and sigmoid colon from mesh. Following these incidences, the technique was amended to include complete peritonisation of the mesh to avoid bowel adhesions. Concomitant vaginal repair was performed and TVT was inserted if necessary. All 51 women were examined using the POP-Q and the Baden–Walker halfway system at 10 weeks of follow-up and 39 women completed the vaginal symptoms module of the International Consultation on Incontinence Questionnaire (ICIQ-VS) 4–6 months postoperatively. Both subjective and objective improvements were noted in 50 of the 51 women (98%).

NICE published a guideline[81] in January 2009 on the insertion of mesh uterine suspension sling (including sacrohysteropexy) for uterine prolapse repair. Their literature review of sacrohysteropexy revealed subjective and objective failure rates of 0–39% and 0–8%, respectively. Reported complications of mesh sacrohysteropexy included mesh erosion (0–3% at 2–4-year follow-up), mesh infection requiring surgery (5%), postoperative vault abscess (5%), postoperative pyrexia of unknown origin (7%) and perivesical haematoma or voiding dysfunction (13%). Owing to the limitations of the available data, NICE concluded that mesh for uterine prolapse repair should be used only in the context of audit and research.

Posterior wall

The repair of posterior vaginal wall prolapse has been described using vaginal, transanal and laparoscopic approaches. The decision to employ a certain technique is often multifactorial. However, the choice is frequently influenced by the surgeon's preference and skills. A number of laparoscopic techniques for the treatment of posterior vaginal defects have been described in the literature. Most studies include small numbers, compare a variety of methods and often involve concomitant surgery, making it difficult to evaluate the results. Both laparoscopic enterocele and laparoscopic rectocele repairs have been described using either sutures or mesh.

Sutures

Cadeddu et al.[82] described a transperitoneal laparoscopic enterocele repair using a modified Moschcowitz technique. The cul-de-sac was obliterated by approximating the posterior vaginal fascia to the anterior wall of the rectum with a running suture. Only three women were included in the series, all of whom underwent concomitant surgery. All women were asymptomatic and had no objective enterocele recurrence at a mean follow-up of 10.5 months (range 7–15 months). Seman et al.[45] also described enterocele sac invagination or excision in combination with laparoscopic supralevator repair, laparoscopic vaginal vault suspension and transvaginal posterior repair for the treatment of posterior compartment defects.

Thornton et al.[83] compared 40 women who underwent laparoscopic suture repair of a rectocele using nonabsorbable Ethibond® (Ethicon Endo-Surgery, Cincinnati, OH, USA) sutures with 40 women who underwent transanal repair by a colorectal surgeon. Significantly fewer women in the laparoscopic group reported bowel symptom alleviation ($P<0.002$) and satisfaction with the procedure ($P<0.003$) at a median of 44 months of follow-up. Only 28% in the laparoscopic group reported more than 50% improvement in their bowel symptoms compared with 63% in the transanal group. However, higher rates of faecal incontinence and dyspareunia were found following the transanal approach.

Mesh

Weng and Liu[84] described the use of polypropylene mesh combined with uterosacral ligament suspension to treat 40 women with advanced vaginal vault prolapse and concurrent enteroceles. Half the group had undergone previous prolapse surgery. No recurrence was observed in either group at a mean follow-up of 26.6 months. Complications included two intraoperative bladder perforations and five mesh erosions. Mesh-related pain syndromes and dyspareunia were reported in 21.4% of women in the recurrent prolapse group and in 6.3% of women in the nonrecurrent group.

Lyons and Winer[85] prospectively studied 20 women undergoing laparoscopic treatment of rectocele defect by use of a polyglactin mesh graft and reported low morbidity rates with an 80% resolution of prolapse symptoms at 1-year follow-up.

Seracchioli et al.[78] reported a small series of women who underwent laparoscopic sacrohysteropexies and described the use of prosthetic reconstruction of the rectovaginal support structure in those with posterior compartment defects. None of the 15 women in this series had undergone further prolapse surgery at 24 months of follow-up.

The role of laparoscopic repair of posterior vaginal compartment defects is still unclear. The limited studies suggest feasibility, promising results and the ability to perform concomitant surgery. The technique requires a high level of laparoscopic skill and is therefore unlikely to become a common surgical choice. Further larger studies are required to compare the various approaches.

Conclusions

There seems little doubt that laparoscopic surgery can achieve all that can be accomplished by open surgery with respect to the repair of pelvic organ prolapse. It is probable that the laparoscopic approach confers some advantages over the open approach with respect to visualisation, particularly deep in the pelvis. While colposuspension has been studied in robust randomised controlled trials, prolapse repair surgeries have been reported in varied depth by committed enthusiasts, which makes assessment of their value more difficult. The recent addition of robotics has further complicated the assessment but does seem to make some of the laparoscopic surgery techniques easier to learn. Whether the additional cost involved is merited will be judged in time.

Given the evidence from randomised controlled trials comparing laparoscopic and open colposuspension, there is no reason to believe that a laparoscopic sacrocolpopexy, performed in a manner similar to the open procedure, should not produce similar results with respect to pelvic floor support. In addition, the laparoscopic approach will be accompanied by reduced postoperative morbidity and earlier return to normal activity.

References

1 United Nations Population Division. Demographic profile of the older population. In: *World Population Ageing 1950–2050*. New York, NY: United Nations; 2010; p. 23–7 [www.un.org/esa/population/publications/worldageing19502050/].

2 Olsen A L, Smith V J, Bergstrom J O, Colling J C, Clark A L. Epidemiology of surgically managed pelvic organ prolapse and urinary incontinence. *Obstet Gynecol* 1997;89:501–6.

3 Burch J C. Urethrovaginal fixation to Cooper's ligament for correction of stress incontinence, cystocele and prolapse. *Am J Obstet Gynecol* 1961;81:281–90.

4 Vancaillie T G, Schuessler W. Laparoscopic bladderneck suspension. *J Laparoendosc Surg* 1991;1:169–73.

5 Liu C Y, Paek W. Laparoscopic retropubic colposuspension (Burch procedure). *J Am Assoc Gynecol Laparosc* 1993;1:31–5.

6 Breda G, Silvestre P, Gherardi L, Xausa D, Tamai A, Giunta A. Correction of stress urinary incontinence: laparoscopy combined with vaginal suturing. *J Endourol* 1996;10:251–3.

7 Harewood L M. Laparoscopic needle colposuspension for genuine stress incontinence. *J Endourol* 1993;7:319–22.

8 Carter J E. Laparoscopic Burch procedure for stress urinary incontinence: the Carter modification. *Keio J Med* 1996;45:168–71.

9 Persson J, Wølner-Hanssen P. Laparoscopic Burch colposuspension for stress urinary incontinence: a randomized comparison of one or two sutures on each side of the urethra. *Obstet Gynecol* 2000;95:151–5.

10 Powers K, Lazarou G, Connell K. Greston W. Mikhail M. One-suture Burch colposuspension: laparotomy versus laparoscopy. *J Pelvic Med Surg* 2005;11:235–8.

11 Ou C S, Presthus J, Beadle E. Laparoscopic bladder neck suspension using hernia mesh and surgical staples. *J Laparoendosc Surg* 1993;3:563–6.

12 Henley C. The Henley staple-suture technique for laparoscopic Burch colposuspension. *J Am Assoc Gynecol Laparosc* 1995;2:441–4.

13 Newcomer J. Vaginal pain caused by laparoscopic colposuspension with tacks. *Obstet Gynecol* 2000;96:823–4.

14 Das S, Palmer JK. Laparoscopic colpo-suspension. *J Urol* 1995;154:1119–21.

15 Batislam E, Germiyanoglu C, Erol D. Simplification of laparoscopic extraperitoneal colposuspension: results of two-port technique. *Int Urol Nephrol* 2000;32:47–51.

16 Ross J. Two techniques of laparoscopic Burch repair for stress incontinence: a prospective, randomized study. *J Am Assoc Gynecol Laparosc* 1996;3:351–7.

17 Zullo F, Palomba S, Piccione F, Morelli M, Arduino B, Mastrantonio P. Laparoscopic Burch colposuspension: a randomized controlled trial comparing two transperitoneal surgical techniques. *Obstet Gynecol* 2001;98:783–8.

18 Ankardal M, Milsom I, Stjerndahl J H, Engh M E. A three-armed randomized trial comparing open Burch colposuspension using sutures with laparoscopic colposuspension using sutures and laparoscopic colposuspension using mesh and staples in women with stress urinary incontinence. *Acta Obstet Gynecol Scand* 2005;84:773–9.

19 Kenton K, FitzGerald M P, Brubaker L. Multiple foreign body erosions after laparoscopic colposuspension with mesh. *Am J Obstet Gynecol* 2002;187:252–3.

20 Washington J L. Staple erosion into the bladder after mesh and staple laparoscopic colposuspension. A case report. *J Reprod Med* 2002;47:325–6.

21 Yesilli C, Seckiner I, Mungan N A, Akduman B. Stone formation on surgical staple in the bladder: a long-term complication of laparoscopic colposuspension. *Surg Laparosc Endosc Percutan Tech* 2007;17:568–9.

22 Glowacki C A, Wall L L. Bone anchors in urogynecology. *Clin Obstet Gynecol* 2000;43:659–69.

23 Kiilholma P, Haarala M, Polvi H, Mäkinen J, Chancellor MB. Sutureless endoscopic colposuspension with fibrin sealant. *Tech Urol* 1995;1:81–3.

24 Kjolhede P, Rydén G, Hewardt P. Abdominal urethrocystopexy using fibrin sealant. A prospective study of long-term efficacy. *Int Urogynecol J Pelvic Floor Dysfunct* 2000;11:93–6.

25 Bulent Tiras M, Sendag F, Dilek U, Guner H. Laparoscopic Burch colposuspension: comparison of effectiveness of extraperitoneal and transperitoneal techniques. *Eur J Obstet Gynecol Reprod Biol* 2004;116:79–84.

26 Wallwiener D, Grischke E M, Rimbach S, Maleika A, Bastert G. Endoscopic retropubic colposuspension: "Retziusscopy" versus laparoscopy—a reasonable enlargement of the operative spectrum in the management of recurrent stress incontinence? *Endosc Surg Allied Technol* 1995;3:115–8.

27 Dean N M, Ellis G, Wilson P D, Herbison G P. Laparoscopic colposuspension for urinary incontinence in women. *Cochrane Database Syst Rev* 2006;(3):CD002239.

28 Barr S, Reid F M, North C E, Hosker G, Smith A R. The long-term outcome of laparoscopic colposuspension: a 10-year cohort study. *Int Urogynecol J Pelvic Floor Dysfunct* 2009;20:443–5.

29 Carey M, Rosamilia A, Maher C, Cornish A, Murray C, Ugoni A. Laparoscopic versus open colposuspension: a prospective multi-centre randomised single-blinded comparison. *Neurol Urodyn* 2000;19:389–91.

30 Burton G. A three year prospective randomised urodynamic study comparing open and laparoscopic colposuspension. *Neurol Urodyn* 1997;16:353–4.

31 Cheon W C, Mak J H, Liu J Y. Prospective randomised controlled trial comparing laparoscopic and open colposuspension. *Hong Kong Med J* 2003;9:10–4.

32 Fatthy H, El Hao M, Samaha I, Abdallah K. Modified Burch colposuspension: laparoscopy versus laparotomy. *J Am Assoc Gynecol Laparosc* 2001;8:99–106.

33 Kitchener H C, Dunn G, Lawton V, Reid F, Nelson L, Smith A R; COLPO Study Group. Laparoscopic versus open colposuspension – results of a prospective randomised controlled trial. *BJOG* 2006;113:1007–13.

34 Su T H, Wang K G, Hsu C Y, Wei H J, Hong B K. Prospective comparison of laparoscopic and traditional colposuspensions in the treatment of genuine stress incontinence. *Acta Obstet Gynecol Scand* 1997;76:576–82.

35 Dumville J C, Manca A, Kitchener H C, Smith A R, Nelson L, Torgerson D J; COLPO Study Group. Cost-effectiveness analysis of open colposuspension versus laparoscopic colposuspension in the treatment of urodynamic stress incontinence. *BJOG* 2006;113:1014–22.

36 Valpas A, Kivelä A, Penttinen J, Kujansuu E, Haarala M, Nilsson CG. Tension-free vaginal tape and laparoscopic mesh colposuspension for stress urinary incontinence. *Obstet Gynecol* 2004;104:42–9.

37 Cooper A. *The Anatomy and Surgical Treatment of Inguinal Congenital Hernia*. London: JT Cox; 1804.

38 White G R. Cystocele: a radical cure by suturing lateral sulci of vagina to white line of pelvic fascia. *JAMA* 1909;LIII:1707–10.

39 Kelly H A, Dumm W M. Urinary incontinence in women without manifest injury to the bladder: a report of cases. *Surg Gynec Obstet* 1914;18:444–50.

40 Richardson A C, Lyon J B, Williams N L. A new look at pelvic relaxation. *Am J Obstet Gynecol* 1976;126:568–73.

41 Washington J L, Somers K O. Laparoscopic paravaginal repair: a new technique using mesh and staples. *JSLS* 2003;7:301–3.

42 Speights S E, Moore R D, Miklos J R. Frequency of lower urinary tract injury at laparoscopic burch and paravaginal repair. *J Am Assoc Gynecol Laparosc* 2000;7:515–8.

43 Demirci F, Ozdemir I, Somunkiran A, Gul OK, Gul B, Doyran G D. Abdominal paravaginal defect repair in the treatment of paravaginal defect and urodynamic stress incontinence. *J Obstet Gynaecol* 2007;27:601–4.

44 Behnia-Willison F, Seman E I, Cook J R, O'Shea R T, Keirse M J. Laparoscopic paravaginal repair of anterior compartment prolapse. *J Minim Invasive Gynecol* 2007;14:475–80.

45 Seman E I, Cook J R, O'Shea R T. Two-year experience with laparoscopic pelvic floor repair. *J Am Assoc Gynecol Laparosc* 2003;10:38–45.

46 Albright T S, Garlich C L, Iglesia C B. Complications after laparoscopic burch with hernia mesh and surgical tacks. *Obstet Gynecol* 2006;108:718–20.

47 Ameline A, Huguier J. [Posterior suspension to the lumbo-sacral disk; abdominal method of replacement of the utero-sacral ligaments]. *Gynecol Obstet (Paris)* 1957;56:94–8. Article in French.

48 National Institute for Health and Clinical Excellence. *Sacrocolpopexy Using Mesh for Vaginal Vault Prolapse Repair.* Interventional Procedure Guidance 283. London: NICE; 2009 [www.guidance.nice.org.uk/IPG283].

49 Jia X, Glazener C, Mowatt G, Jenkinson D, Fraser C, Burr J. *Systematic Review of the Efficacy and Safety of Using Mesh or Grafts in Surgery for Uterine or Vaginal Vault Prolapse.* London: NICE; 2008 [www.guidance.nice.org.uk/IPG284/Scope/pdf/English].

50 Nezhat C H, Nezhat F, Nezhat C. Laparoscopic sacral colpopexy for vaginal vault prolapse. *Obstet Gynecol* 1994;84:885–8.

51 Ganatra A M, Rozet F, Sanchez-Salas R, Barret E, Galiano M, Cathelineau X, et al. The current status of laparoscopic sacrocolpopexy: a review. *Eur Urol* 2009;55:1089–103.

52 Villet R. [Treatment of prolapse using the abdominal approach]. *Acta Urol Belg* 1992;60:61–6. Article in French.

53 Chen C C, Ridgeway B, Paraiso M F. Biologic grafts and synthetic meshes in pelvic reconstructive surgery. *Clin Obstet Gynecol* 2007;50:383–411.

54 Higgs P J, Chua H L, Smith A R. Long term review of laparoscopic sacrocolpopexy. *BJOG* 2005;112:1134–8.

55 Granese R, Candiani M, Perino A, Romano F, Cucinella G. Laparoscopic sacrocolpopexy in the treatment of vaginal vault prolapse: 8 years experience. *Eur J Obstet Gynecol Reprod Biol* 2009;146:227–31.

56 Culligan P J, Blackwell L, Goldsmith L J, Graham C A, Rogers A, Heit M H. A randomized controlled trial comparing fascia lata and synthetic mesh for sacral colpopexy. *Obstet Gynecol* 2005;106:29–37.

57 Deprest J, De Ridder D, Roovers J P, Werbrouck E, Coremans G, Claerhout F. Medium term outcome of laparoscopic sacrocolpopexy with xenografts compared to synthetic grafts. *J Urol* 2009;182:2362–8.

58 Maher C, Feiner B, Baessler K, Adams E J, Hagen S, Glazener C M. Surgical management of pelvic organ prolapse in women. *Cochrane Database Syst Rev* 2007;(4):CD004014.

59 Cundiff G W, Varner E, Visco A G, Zyczynski H M, Nager C W, Norton P A, et al. Pelvic Floor Disorders Network. Risk factors for mesh/suture erosion following sacral colpopexy. *Am J Obstet Gynecol* 2008;199:688 e1–5.

60 Stepanian A A, Miklos J R, Moore R D, Mattox T F. Risk of mesh extrusion and other mesh-related complications after laparoscopic sacral colpopexy with or without concurrent laparoscopic-assisted vaginal hysterectomy: experience of 402 patients. *J Minim Invasive Gynecol* 2008;15:188–96.

61 Debodinance P, Delporte P, Engrand J B, Boulogne M. [Development of better tolerated prosthetic materials: applications in gynecological surgery]. *J Gynecol Obstet Biol Reprod (Paris)* 2002;31:527–40. Article in French.

62 Agarwala N, Hasiak N, Shade M. Laparoscopic sacral colpopexy with Gynemesh as graft material–experience and results. *J Minim Invasive Gynecol* 2007;14:577–83.

63 Maher C F, Qatawneh A M, Dwyer P L, Carey M P, Cornish A, Schluter P J. Abdominal sacral colpopexy or vaginal sacrospinous colpopexy for vaginal vault prolapse: a prospective randomized study. *Am J Obstet Gynecol* 2004;190:20–6.

64 Marcickiewicz J, Kjöllesdal M, Engh M E, Eklind S, Axén C, Brännström M, et al. Vaginal sacrospinous colpopexy and laparoscopic sacral colpopexy for vaginal vault prolapse. *Acta Obstet Gynecol Scand* 2007;86:733–8.

65 Akladios C Y, Dautun D, Saussine C, Baldauf J J, Mathelin C, Wattiez A. Laparoscopic sacrocolpopexy for female genital organ prolapse: establishment of a learning curve. *Eur J Obstet Gynecol Reprod Biol* 2010;149:218–21.

66 Shalev E, Bustan M, Peleg D. Laparoscopic ventrofixation: an alternative treatment approach for uterine prolapse. *J Gynecol Surg* 1996;12:105–7.

67 O'Brien P M, Ibrahim J. Failure of laparoscopic uterine suspension to provide a lasting cure for uterovaginal prolapse. *Br J Obstet Gynaecol* 1994;101:707–8.

68 Yoong A F. Laparoscopic ventrosuspensions. A review of 72 cases. *Am J Obstet Gynecol* 1990;163:1151–3.

69 Halperin R, Padoa A, Schneider D, Bukovsky I, Pansky M. Long-term follow-up (5–20 years) after uterine ventrosuspension for chronic pelvic pain and deep dyspareunia. *Gynecol Obstet Invest* 2003;55:216–9.

70 Wu M P. Laparoscopic uterine suspension for the treatment of uterovaginal prolapse. *Int J Gynaecol Obstet* 1997;59:259–60.

71 Maher C F, Carey M P, Murray C J. Laparoscopic suture hysteropexy for uterine prolapse. *Obstet Gynecol* 2001;97:1010–4.

72 Medina C, Takacs P. Laparoscopic uterosacral uterine suspension: a minimally invasive technique for treating pelvic organ prolapse. *J Minim Invasive Gynecol* 2006;13: 472–5.

73 Ostrzenski A. Laparoscopic retroperitoneal hysteropexy. A randomized trial. *J Reprod Med* 1998;43:361–6.

74 Gargiulo T, Leo L, Gomel V. Laparoscopic uterine suspension using three-stitch technique. *J Am Assoc Gynecol Laparosc* 2000;7:233–6.

75 Krause H G, Goh J T, Sloane K, Higgs P, Carey M P. Laparoscopic sacral suture hysteropexy for uterine prolapse. *Int Urogynecol J Pelvic Floor Dysfunct* 2006;17:378–81.

76 Cutner A, Kearney R, Vashisht A. Laparoscopic uterine sling suspension: a new technique of uterine suspension in women desiring surgical management of uterine prolapse with uterine conservation. *BJOG* 2007;114:1159–62.

77 Leron E, Stanton S L. Sacrohysteropexy with synthetic mesh for the management of uterovaginal prolapse. *BJOG* 2001;108:629–33.

78 Seracchioli R, Hourcabie J A, Vianello F, Govoni F, Pollastri P, Venturoli S. Laparoscopic treatment of pelvic floor defects in women of reproductive age. *J Am Assoc Gynecol Laparosc* 2004;11:332–5.

79 Rosenblatt P L, Chelmow D, Ferzandi T R. Laparoscopic sacrocervicopexy for the treatment of uterine prolapse: a retrospective case series report. *J Minim Invasive Gynecol* 2008;15:268–72.

80 Price N, Slack A, Jackson S R. Laparoscopic hysteropexy: the initial results of a uterine suspension procedure for uterovaginal prolapse. *BJOG* 2010;117:62–8.

81 National Institute for Health and Clinical Excellence. *Insertion of Mesh Uterine Suspension Sling (Including Sacrohysteropexy) for Uterine Prolapse Repair.* Interventional Procedure Guidance 282. London: NICE; 2009 [www.guidance.nice.org.uk/IPG282].

82 Cadeddu J A, Micali S, Moore R G, Kavoussi L R. Laparoscopic repair of enterocele. *J Endourol* 1996;10:367–9.

83 Thornton M J, Lam A, King D W. Laparoscopic or transanal repair of rectocele? A retrospective matched cohort study. *Dis Colon Rectum* 2005;48:792–8.

84 Weng S S, Liu C Y. Laparoscopic pelvic floor repair using polypropylene mesh. *Taiwan J Obstet Gynecol* 2008;47:312–7.

85 Lyons T L, Winer W K. Laparoscopic rectocele repair using polyglactin mesh. *J Am Assoc Gynecol Laparosc* 1997;4:381–4.

14 Minimal access surgery in paediatric and adolescent gynaecology

Lina Michala, Sarah M Creighton and Alfred S Cutner

Introduction

Minimal access surgery is becoming increasingly popular in all disciplines of paediatric surgery. This is supported by a growing body of evidence on the laparoscopic management of gynaecological pathology in children and adolescents, both by paediatric surgeons and by gynaecologists.

Less postoperative pain, reduced hospitalisation and shorter recovery time are important advantages of minimal access surgery because they reduce anxiety associated with treatment and enable the child or adolescent to return to schooling and other activities sooner. Minimal access surgery is associated with better visualisation of the pelvis and abdomen and this can be of great benefit when dealing with a complex and distorted anatomy, as in the case of müllerian anomalies. It is also associated with less bleeding and adhesion formation, leading to better preservation of future fertility.

Operating on children and adolescents

There are clear guidelines for surgeons operating on children and these apply to gynaecologists as well as to paediatric surgeons.[1] The team caring for the girl should be skilled in looking after children. Appropriate paediatric anaesthetic and pain management support should be available and the child or young person should be managed in age-appropriate in- and outpatient surroundings. Surgeons should have the correct skills in obtaining consent and communicating with children, paediatric life support training and awareness of child protection issues. Gynaecologists operating on children with complex pathology should be part of a multidisciplinary team.

Planning minimal access surgery in children and adolescents

Adequate preoperative assessment and preparation are essential when dealing with children or adolescents. In the case of complex anomalies, accurate imaging is of the utmost importance before surgery. Ultrasound may be less useful as vaginal scans are not possible and magnetic resonance imaging (MRI) may be required. Performing a diagnostic laparoscopy without the means of treating pathology should be discouraged because it increases the risks to the girl undergoing surgery through multiple anaesthetics and operations.

It is also important to assess the suitability of the girl for laparoscopic surgery, especially in cases of children and adolescents with extensive prior surgery, who are likely to have adhesions and are therefore more at risk of sustaining a bowel injury. If an extensive operation is planned, bowel preparation should be undertaken, taking into account that people of this age group are more vulnerable to dehydration and should receive adequate maintenance intravenous hydration preoperatively.

Gynaecologists more used to dealing with adult women should bear in mind the particular needs of children and adolescents. Girls under the age of 16 years are not legally able to consent; this is the responsibility of their parent or guardian. It is nevertheless good practice to involve the young person in the decision making, by informing in plain language and using visual material where possible to explain the procedure to be undertaken.

Laparoscopic techniques / instruments

Positioning of the child or adolescent is similar to that of older individuals. The Lloyd–Davies position is the preferred one, although special consideration and adjustments should be made to the smaller body size. Paediatric-sized stirrups are available. The bladder should be catheterised to decrease the risk of bladder injury and improve visualisation of the pelvis.

Vaginal examination and uterine manipulation is avoided in girls who are not sexually active unless uterine surgery is anticipated or manipulation is required to aid visualisation of pelvic structures. This should be discussed with the parents and the girl undergoing surgery beforehand.

Children and adolescents are more susceptible to vascular injury during the initial entry for the creation of a pneumoperitoneum because of their small size and the relatively small distance between the anterior abdominal wall and the aorta, inferior vena cava and iliac vessels. To minimise this risk, it is usually advised to use the Hasson entry technique.[2]

The volume of gas introduced should be adjusted to the girl's size. This means introducing enough gas to reach a preset pressure of 20 mmHg for adolescents and 12–15 mmHg for younger children. Smaller children may require even lower settings of 8–12 mmHg. Skin closure is best performed with absorbable sutures or glue to avoid the extra stress of suture removal.

Minimal access surgery procedures in paediatric and adolescent gynaecology

MAS procedures can be broadly divided into common gynaecological procedures that happen to be required in a child or adolescent, such as ovarian cystectomy and treatment of endometriosis, and those that are unique to this age group, such as procedures that relate to the treatment of congenital anomalies.

Procedures to treat common gynaecological pathologies

Benign functional ovarian cysts are common among older children and adolescents. These cysts often regress spontaneously and should therefore be managed conservatively, unless they cause considerable pain. Nevertheless, ovarian accidents such as torsion, haemorrhage and rupture can occur and will require immediate medical attention.

Ovarian torsion in particular is more common among younger girls because the infundibulopelvic pedicle is longer, and so can be the mesovaria and fallopian tubes.[3] An ovary containing a small cyst can tort and lead to necrosis. Ovarian torsion has also been described in normal ovaries.[4] A high index of suspicion is required among treating clinicians, often paediatricians and paediatric surgeons, who should investigate the pelvis with an ultrasound before any surgery, so that a gynaecologist can be involved early in the management of the girl if an ovarian cyst accident is diagnosed. At laparoscopy, the ovary should be untwisted and every effort should be made to preserve it if it is deemed viable. Whether the affected and contralateral ovaries should be fixed (Figure 14.1) is an issue of debate. Recurring torsion in the affected or contralateral ovary has been described in the literature,[5] with devastating effects on fertility. Fixation of the ovary is not without risks because it may potentially affect the function of the fallopian tube and therefore interfere with future fertility.[5] It may be more appropriate to consider fixing the remaining ovary as an interval procedure, allowing clear discussion of the risks and benefits. It does, however, increase the risks involved with a second operation. Benign and malignant ovarian tumours do occur in this age group.

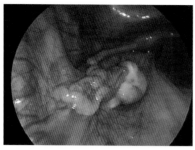

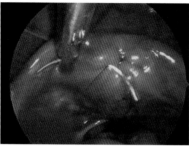

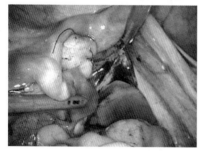

FIGURE 14.1 **Fixation of an ovary after the other one has been removed owing to torsion**

The diagnosis can be suspected on ultrasound imaging, Doppler examination and MRI or from tumour marker elevations. Investigated tumour markers should include human chorionic gonadotrophin and alphafetoprotein because ovarian malignancies in young women are more likely to be of germ cell origin. If a malignant tumour is suspected, an appropriate referral to a gynaecological oncologist should be made. Treatment of ovarian malignancies should be fertility-sparing, with preservation of the uterus and contralateral ovary where possible.

Endometriosis in adolescence is much more common than previously thought, affecting up to 73% of adolescents with chronic pelvic pain. The diagnosis should be suspected in girls with severe dysmenorrhoea refractory to nonsteroidal analgesics and the combined oral contraceptive pill. In such situations, a diagnostic laparoscopy is warranted to investigate the condition further. If endometriosis is found, it is at an early stage in the majority of adolescents, although extensive endometriosis (revised American Fertility Society stages III and IV) has been described. The treatment modalities are similar to those in older women, with surgical excision appearing to be a safe treatment option with good short-term results.[6] There is little information on the long-term impact on either recurrent symptoms or fertility in adolescents diagnosed with endometriosis.

Procedures to treat congenital anomalies

Laparoscopic gonadectomy

Gonadectomy is required in girls with a 46,XY disorder of sex development either to prevent virilisation where the sex of rearing is female or because of the malignancy potential of the gonad. The timing of the procedure depends on the condition and indication. In partial androgen insensitivity syndrome or in virilising conditions where there is a defect in the androgen synthesis pathway, the gonads will need to be removed in childhood before puberty to prevent permanent virilisation changes, such as clitoral enlargement or deepening of the voice.

Dysgenetic gonads, such as those found in Swyer syndrome or in mosaic Turner syndrome (45,X/46,XY), have a high risk of malignancy that is estimated to be at the level of 40% and should be removed early, as soon as the diagnosis is made. In these situations, the uterus and fallopian tubes are often present. The procedure is technically similar to performing a laparoscopic oophorectomy (Video 14.1).[7] However, the fallopian tube is usually excised at the time of gonadectomy because the gonad can be a streak gonad making the definition of planes between gonad and tube difficult. In addition, leaving the tube behind confers no advantages to fertility, whereas if hydrosalpinges form, these may negatively interfere with fertility treatment by affecting embryo implantation.

In complete androgen insensitivity syndrome (CAIS), the gonads are structurally normal testes. However, they still hold a malignancy risk of approximately 5%, similar to that seen in cryptorchidism. At present, it is recommended that the gonads in women with CAIS are removed in late adolescence, after completion of pubertal development. In CAIS, there are no müllerian structures and the gonads can lie anywhere in the line of testicular descent, from high in the abdomen to low down in the inguinal area or labia majora. MRI or ultrasound is necessary preoperatively to locate the gonads and plan for the route of surgery. If the gonads are in the inguinal canal, exploration of the groin may be required, which would usually be carried out by a urologist. Laparoscopic gonadectomy is performed in those situations where the gonads are located within the abdominal cavity.

Laparoscopic creation of a neovagina
Vaginal agenesis is most commonly associated with Mayer–Rokitansky–Küster–Hauser syndrome and CAIS. In both conditions, the vagina is blind-ending and short and in the majority of affected people treatment is required before sexual intercourse. Conservative management in the form of vaginal dilation is usually recommended first, with good results. However, in about 20% of individuals this will not be adequate and surgical treatment will be required.[8]

Surgical intervention rather than dilation will also be required in women who have had prior unsuccessful reconstructive surgery (usually in childhood), leaving a scarred perineum unsuitable for dilation. In some women, dilation is not possible because the perineum is flat, without a dimple, such as in women with partial androgen insensitivity syndrome and in those with vaginal agenesis associated with bladder or rectal congenital anomalies.

Any intervention should ideally be planned for late adolescence or early adulthood, as procedures performed in infancy and childhood have a high rate of failure and a repeat procedure is likely to be required.[9] Furthermore, deferring treatment until later allows the affected person to be involved with decision making and consent and increases compliance with postoperative vaginal dilation, which is invariably required to prevent restenosis.

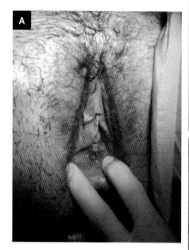

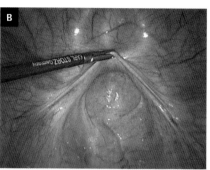

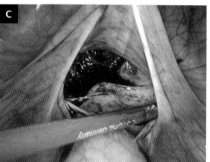

FIGURE 14.2 **Laparoscopic Vecchietti procedure**

(A) Perineum before surgery

(B) Laparoscopic view of pelvis

(C) Vesicorectal space opened

(D) First suture passed

(E) Both sutures passed

(F) Peritoneal defect closed

(G) Traction device placed on abdomen

In women whose external genitalia are normal, who have a vaginal dimple and who have not had previous genital surgery, the operation of choice is the laparoscopic Vecchietti procedure (Figure 14.2 and Video 14.2). This was first described as an open operation but has been modified with great success to the laparoscopic route.[10] An acrylic olive is threaded and positioned in the vaginal dimple. The threads are then passed into the pelvis and onto the abdominal wall laparoscopically and attached to a special traction device that is positioned on the anterior abdominal wall. The device holds the threads under tension and has a small screw that, when turned, pulls the vaginal bead and the vault upwards by a centimetre. The vagina is gradually dilated in the space of 1 week, at which point the traction device and bead are removed. Postoperative dilation is necessary to maintain the vaginal length.[11]

In women whose external genitalia are scarred and who have no vaginal dimple, a different surgical approach is recommended. In those situations, the space between rectum and bladder is dissected both from the perineum below and laparoscopically from above. The neovaginal space created is lined with peritoneum that is mobilised from the pelvis. The procedure is called a laparoscopic Davydov procedure and is also a modification of an open operation (Video 14.3).[12] The procedure is feasible only where there have been no previous major surgical procedures to the abdomen.

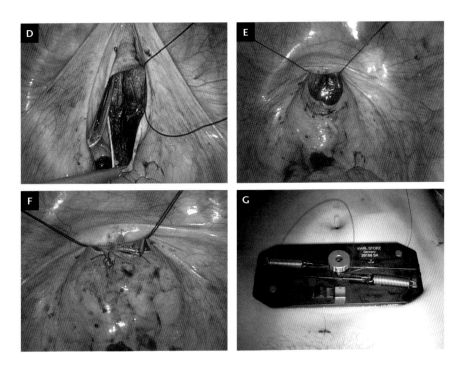

With the advent of minimal access anastomotic devices, intestinal vagino-plasty can now be performed laparoscopically.[13] However, there are no clear clinical indications for such surgery. Intestinal vaginoplasty is indicated in women unsuitable for a laparoscopic Davydov procedure. The reason they are unsuitable is usually because they have had major complex abdominal surgery such as bladder reconstruction for cloacal anomalies and so may also not be suitable for a laparoscopic procedure.

Choosing who should undergo surgery and, if surgery is chosen, which operation is not always easy. The woman must be motivated and psychologi-cally ready. It is an advantage if the referral unit can offer all of the surgical options so that the best choice is made on an individual basis. A surgical algorithm has been developed at University College Hospital in London to aid the decision-making process (Figure 14.3).[14]

Obstructive müllerian anomalies

In embryonic life, the müllerian ducts grow in a caudal and medial direction and fuse in the midline by 9 weeks to form the right and left fallopian tubes, the uterus, the cervix and the proximal two-thirds of the vagina. Failure of reabsorption of the vaginal septum or failure of canalisation will lead to mül-lerian anomalies. The most widely used classification is that proposed by the

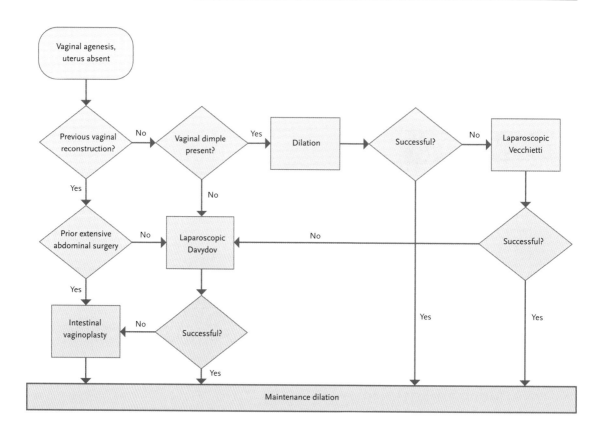

American Fertility Society[15] and the most common presentation among adolescent girls is type IIb from that classification. In this situation, the diagnosis is often delayed because the girls menstruate normally from the communicating uterus, whereas the noncommunicating uterus distends with blood, causing increasingly severe menstrual pain.

FIGURE 14.3 **University College Hospital London algorithm for the treatment of vaginal agenesis**

American Fertility Society[15] and the most common presentation among adolescent girls is type IIb from that classification. In this situation, the diagnosis is often delayed because the girls menstruate normally from the communicating uterus, whereas the noncommunicating uterus distends with blood, causing increasingly severe menstrual pain.

A much rarer diagnosis causing müllerian obstruction is cervical agenesis, with an estimated incidence of 1/80 000–100 000 births. Clinical examination and MRI will differentiate this from an imperforate hymen and a transverse vaginal septum. The vagina may be of normal length or shortened.

In both situations, although the adolescent may present acutely, there is no need to treat this as an emergency. Pain can be alleviated by suppressing menstruation using gonadotrophin-releasing hormone analogues, depot medroxyprogesterone acetate, continuous progesterone or the combined oral contraceptive pill. This allows for appropriate preoperative imaging and preparation. Management of these anomalies should be undertaken in tertiary referral centres because the conditions are relatively rare and require a team approach including adolescent gynaecologists, radiologists for image interpretation and surgeons with advanced laparoscopic skills. It is also important

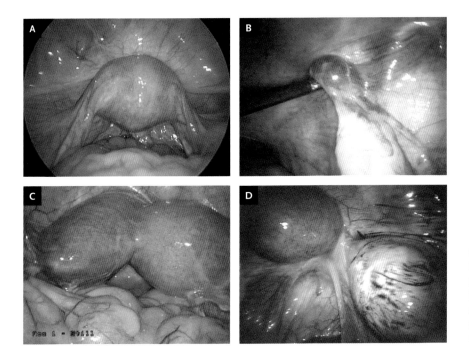

FIGURE 14.4
(A) Normal uterus;
(B) Unicornuate uterus;
(C) Communicating accessory uterus;
(D) Noncommunicating accessory uterus

to perform imaging of the renal tract preoperatively to identify potentially related renal and ureteric anomalies. Up to 30% of these adolescents will have associated renal tract abnormalities.

Treatment of an obstructed uterine horn

Treatment is by surgical removal of the obstructed horn. The ipsilateral fallopian tube must also be removed to prevent an ectopic pregnancy. Although traditionally this surgery was performed open, it is ideal for the laparoscopic approach.[16] If the obstructed horn lies completely separate, the laparoscopic procedure is a relatively easy one (Figures 14.4 and 14.5). It can nevertheless be challenging if the obstructed horn is adjacent to a functioning uterus, especially if the two horns are covered by myometrium. In such situations, the laparoscopic appearance should be correlated with the one obtained from MRI to avoid damaging the uterine wall of the unicornuate uterus. In addition, the accessory uterus may have a rudimentary cervix. Failure to remove all endometrial tissue can result in recurrent symptoms. The use of an electronic morcellator enables easy tissue extraction (Video 14.4).

Long-term follow-up data on women who have undergone such procedures are not yet available. It is likely that the remaining unicornuate horn will lead to increased risks of preterm labour, late miscarriage and malposition, but longer-term fertility and pregnancy outcome data would help with counselling.

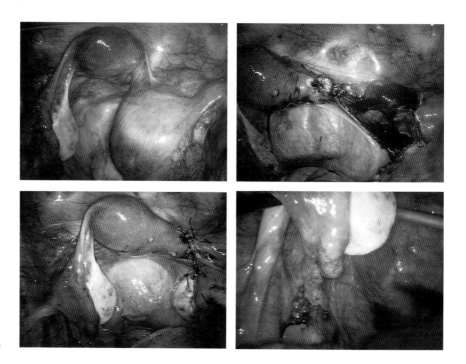

FIGURE 14.5 **Removal of an accessory uterine horn**

Cervical agenesis

In the past, hysterectomy was advocated by many as the procedure of choice for cervical agenesis. Canalisation of the cervical region has a high stenosis rate and there are case reports of sepsis and death in the literature following this procedure.[17] However, a case series [18] of open uterovaginal anastomosis with long-term follow-up indicates that maintaining fertility is a viable option for these girls.

Uterovaginal anastomosis is now feasible laparoscopically (Video 14.5).[19] During the procedure, the distal end of the obstruction is canalised from the perineum with a combination of sharp and blunt dissection. The uterovesical pouch is dissected down laparoscopically and the uterine body is sounded from the uterine fundus to identify the level of obstruction. The fibromuscular tissue at the level of the obstruction is then resected and the distal end of the uterine cavity is sutured to the upper vagina in a combined laparoscopic and perineal approach. A Foley catheter is left within the uterine cavity to prevent adhesion formation and re-obstruction. This is then removed under anaesthetic at an examination approximately 1 month following the initial operation. There are currently case series reported in the literature with encouraging short-term results, such as return of menstruation and good sexual function.[20] However, there are no data yet on fertility. There has been some debate on

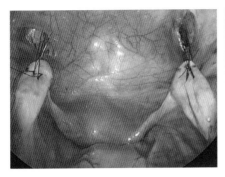 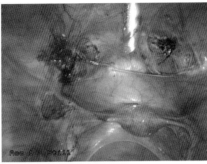

FIGURE 14.6 **Ovarian transposition to the ileopectineal ligament and then releasing after radiation is completed**

whether insertion of an abdominal suture around the anastomosis either at the time of the primary procedure or at a later date would improve competence of the uterine isthmus. However, women undergoing the same procedure during a laparotomy have successful term pregnancies without suture insertion.

Ovarian transposition

As childhood cancer survival improves, more and more women will be facing the consequences of cancer treatment in their adult life, including loss of fertility. Ovarian transposition is a surgical procedure that is used to protect the ovary from the risk of ovarian failure during pelvic irradiation. The ovaries are fixed outside the field of radiation. A radiopaque clip is usually positioned at the lower edge of the ovary to enable demarcation of the ovarian position on X-ray.[21] After radiation is completed, the ovaries are released back into their normal position to allow for resolution of the anatomical relation to the fallopian tube (Figure 14.6).[22] Short-term data on fertility preservation are encouraging, with spontaneous pregnancies being described after completion of radiation treatment.

In situations where the ovaries need to be moved out of the pelvis, the ovarian pedicle is transected and the ovary and fallopian tube are divided. The ovary, fallopian tube and infundibulopelvic ligament are then mobilised and the ovary is attached by use of polypropylene sutures at the level of the xiphisternum. In this situation, a second laparoscopy to release the ovary is not carried out.

Conclusion

Minimal access surgery has huge advantages in the management of children and adolescents with gynaecological conditions. Complex operations are performed with precision and safety and with the added advantage of a quicker recovery. However, it is essential that, as well as possessing the required laparoscopic skills, gynaecologists operating on children have appropriate clinical skills including training in communication with children and families and in child protection. Children and adolescents should also be cared for in an age-appropriate setting. The team approach is essential in the management of these rare challenging conditions.

References

1 The Royal College of Surgeons of England. *Surgery for Children; Delivering a first class service.* London: RCS; 2007 [www.rcseng.ac.uk/publications/docs/CSF.html].

2 Royal College of Obstetricians and Gynaecologists. *Preventing Entry-related Gynaecological Laparoscopic Injuries.* Green-top Guideline No. 49. London: RCOG; 2008 [www.rcog.org.uk/womens-health/clinical-guidance/preventing-entry-related-gynaecological-laparoscopic-injuries-green-].

3 Breech L L, Hillard P J. Adnexal torsion in pediatric and adolescent girls. *Curr Opin Obstet Gynecol* 2005;17:483–9.

4 Davis A J, Feins N R. Subsequent asynchronous torsion of normal adnexa in children. *J Pediatr Surg* 1990;25:687–9.

5 Crouch N S, Gyampoh B, Cutner A S, Creighton S M. Ovarian torsion: to pex or not to pex? Case report and review of the literature. *J Pediatr Adolesc Gynecol* 2003;16:381–4.

6 Stavroulis A I, Saridogan E, Creighton S M, Cutner A S. Laparoscopic treatment of endometriosis in teenagers. *Eur J Obstet Gynecol Reprod Biol* 2006;125:248–50.

7 Esegbona G, Cutner A, Cuckow P, Creighton S. Laparoscopic gonadectomy in paediatric and adolescent girls with intersex disorders. *BJOG* 2003;110:210–2.

8 Ismail-Pratt I S, Bikoo M, Liao L M, Conway G S, Creighton S M. Normalization of the vagina by dilator treatment alone in Complete Androgen Insensitivity Syndrome and Mayer-Rokitansky-Kuster-Hauser Syndrome. *Hum Reprod* 2007;22:2020–4.

9 Creighton S M, Minto C L, Steele S J. Objective cosmetic and anatomical outcomes at adolescence of feminising surgery for ambiguous genitalia done in childhood. *Lancet* 2001;358:124–5.

10 Fedele L, Bianchi S, Zanconato G, Raffaelli R. Laparoscopic creation of a neovagina in patients with Rokitansky syndrome: analysis of 52 cases. *Fertil Steril* 2000;74:384–9.

11 Ismail I S, Cutner A S, Creighton S M. Laparoscopic vaginoplasty: alternative techniques in vaginal reconstruction. *BJOG* 2006;113:340–3.

12 Giannesi A, Marchiole P, Benchaib M, Chevret-Measson M, Mathevet P, Dargent D. Sexuality after laparoscopic Davydov in patients affected by congenital complete vaginal agenesis associated with uterine agenesis or hypoplasia. *Hum Reprod* 2005;20:2954–7.

13 Cai B, Zhang J R, Xi X W, Yan Q, Wan X P. Laparoscopically assisted sigmoid colon vaginoplasty in women with Mayer-Rokitansky-Kuster-Hauser syndrome: feasibility and short-term results. *BJOG* 2007;114:1486–92.

14 Michala L, Cutner A, Creighton S M. Surgical approaches to treating vaginal agenesis. *BJOG* 2007;114:1455–9.

15 The American Fertility Society classifications of adnexal adhesions, distal tubal occlusion, tubal occlusion secondary to tubal ligation, tubal pregnancies, mullerian anomalies and intrauterine adhesions. *Fertil Steril* 1988;49:944–55.

16 Strawbridge L C, Crouch N S, Cutner A S, Creighton S M. Obstructive mullerian anomalies and modern laparoscopic management. *J Pediatr Adolesc Gynecol* 2007;20:195–200.

17 Maciulla G J, Heine M W, Christian C D. Functional endometrial tissue with vaginal agenesis. *J Reprod Med* 1978;21:373–6.

18 Deffarges J V, Haddad B, Musset R, Paniel B J. Utero-vaginal anastomosis in women with uterine cervix atresia: long-term follow-up and reproductive performance. A study of 18 cases. *Hum Reprod* 2001;16:1722–5.

19 Creighton S M, Davies M C, Cutner A. Laparoscopic management of cervical agenesis. *Fertil Steril* 2006;85: 1510–5.

20 Fedele L, Bianchi S, Frontino G, Berlanda N, Montefusco S, Borruto F. Laparoscopically assisted uterovestibular anastomosis in patients with uterine cervix atresia and vaginal aplasia. *Fertil Steril* 2008;89:212–6.

21 Tulandi T, Al-Took S. Laparoscopic ovarian suspension before irradiation. *Fertil Steril* 1998;70:381–3.

22 Visvanathan D K, Cutner A S, Cassoni AM, Gaze M, Davies M C. A new technique of laparoscopic ovariopexy before irradiation. *Fertil Steril* 2003;79:1204–6.

15 Laparoscopic treatment of mild to moderate endometriosis

Adam Moors and Sameer Umranikar

Introduction

Endometriosis is a unique and sometimes devastating clinical condition in which tissue similar to endometrium is present outside the uterus, affecting up to 10% of women of reproductive age. The pathogenesis is multifactorial and the risk of developing the disease is increased seven-fold if a first-degree relative is affected. Superficial peritoneal endometriosis is probably the result of retrograde menstruation and governed by factors affecting cell adhesion, growth and differentiation. The immunological and hormonal environment will dictate development of the disease.[1,2] It commonly affects the peritoneal lining of the pelvic viscera (Figure 15.1) and the ovaries, but it can also be present in distant organs including the lungs, intestines and surgical skin incisions. Endometriosis is more common on the left with stasis of menstrual debris above the sigmoid colon and is more common with congenital uterine anomalies and outflow obstruction.

The result of endometriosis is a chronic inflammatory process causing extensive fibrosis and adhesion formation with distortion of the pelvic anatomy. This leads to various forms of pelvic pain and infertility, causing considerable morbidity. Treatment of endometriosis is increasingly surgically based. Current drug-based treatments offer temporary relief, but after discontinuation there is a high rate of relapse and the treatments are unsuitable in women who want to conceive.

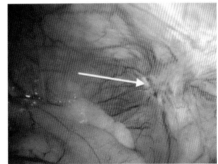

FIGURE 15.1 **Pelvic sidewall endometriosis (arrow)**

Classification of endometriosis

A diverse array of classification systems has been recommended for endometriosis because the pathological and clinical presentation of the disease is variable. Endometriosis may exist superficially on the pelvic peritoneum and ovaries or be deeply invasive, infiltrating the rectovaginal septum and uterosacral ligaments. Hence, it has been suggested that the various presentations of endometriosis should be classified as separate disease entities with different aetiologies.[3]

The revised American Society for Reproductive Medicine classification[4] gives a numerical score and classifies endometriosis into minimal, mild, moderate and severe disease based on the site, depth of endometriotic lesions and adhesions in the pelvis. However, the prognostic value of this classification system is limited with poor correlation to both pelvic pain and fertility.[5]

The more recently proposed ENZIAN scoring system[6] is pain based and focused on deeply invasive endometriosis, particularly retroperitoneal disease. This is more analogous to an oncological staging system and not readily applicable to superficial mild disease.

As the aetiology and presentation of endometriosis are variable and uncertain, no single classification system fits all. Hence, Garry[7] suggested the classification of endometriosis on the basis of clinical findings, using symptoms or signs or a combination of both.

Vercellini et al.[8] looked at over 1000 women with endometriosis using the rAFS system and addressed the association between the stage of endometriosis, the lesion type, demographic characteristics and the severity of pelvic pain symptoms. They found a significant inverse relationship between the age of the woman at surgery and the severity of symptoms of dysmenorrhoea, dyspareunia and nonmenstrual pain. The stage of endometriosis correlated poorly with the severity of symptoms and there was only a marginal nonsignificant association with dysmenorrhoea and nonmenstrual pain. There was, however, a strong association between posterior cul-de-sac lesions and dyspareunia (odds ratio 2.64, 95% CI 1.68–4.24).

Characteristics of mild / moderate endometriotic lesions

Endometriotic lesions may have different appearances based on the evolution of the disease. Early stages of the disease can be subtle, giving appearances such as vesicular (Figures 15.2 and 15.3), petechial, haemorrhagic and polypoidal lesions with sometimes simply mild scarring (Figure 15.4). However, as the disease evolves with bleeding within the implants, the nature of the lesions changes. Older lesions are described as having a typical 'powder burn' (Figure 15.5) or 'gunshot' appearance because of the presence of dark haemosiderin pigment within them (Figures 15.6 and 15.7). The appearance is of black or brown puckered nodular lesions. In view of the chronic inflammatory process, there are associated adhesions around these lesions. These

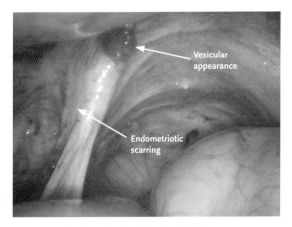

FIGURE 15.2 **Endometriosis with vesicular lesions and scarring**

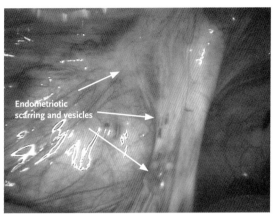

FIGURE 15.3 **Vesicular endometriotic lesion on the left uterosacral ligament**

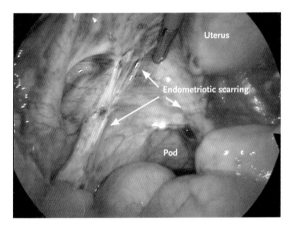

FIGURE 15.4 **Scarring caused by endometriosis**

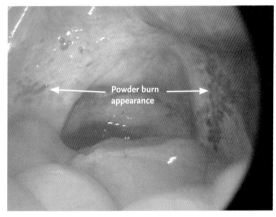

FIGURE 15.5 **Powder burn appearance of endometriosis**

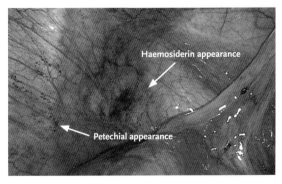

FIGURE 15.6 **Haemosiderin staining of the peritoneum**

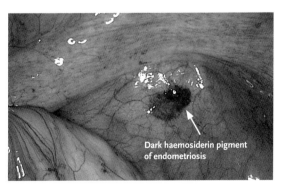

FIGURE 15.7 **Haemosiderin deposition in the pouch of Douglas**

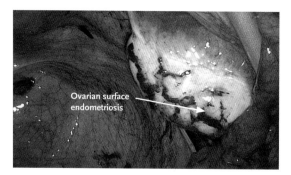

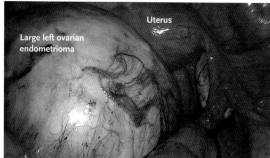

FIGURE 15.8 **Endometriosis on the surface of the right ovary**

FIGURE 15.9 **Large ovarian endometrioma**

adhesions can become dense between the various pelvic organs, causing marked distortion of the pelvic anatomy. Endometriosis affecting the ovaries can present as superficial disease (Figure 15.8) on the surface of the ovary or as endometriomas, which contain old dark blood giving them the common name of 'chocolate cysts' (Figure 15.9).

Laparoscopic treatment of mild to moderate endometriosis

The main indication for laparoscopic treatment of mild to moderate endometriosis is to improve symptoms of pain and infertility. The aim of surgical treatment is to excise or destroy the endometriotic implants.

Pelvic pain and endometriosis

Pain related to endometriosis is difficult to quantify and there is poor correlation between the location and severity of the disease and pain. Indeed, endometriosis may be found incidentally in asymptomatic women undergoing surgery for other reasons. Sometimes, the pain may be excruciating and significantly affect quality of life even though the disease may be staged as minimal or mild.

Endometriotic pain is multifactorial with several possible aetiologies. It is suggested that endometriotic implants respond to hormonal changes in a similar way to the endometrium, resulting in small amounts of bleeding within the implants. This leads to an inflammatory process and fibrosis, which are demonstrated by an increase in inflammatory markers in peritoneal fluid. The presence of blood itself may cause pelvic irritation and pain. Alternatively, the involvement of nerve fibres in deep endometriosis may account for the severe degree of pain associated with them, rationalising a strategy of removing these implants but also explaining persistent pelvic pain associated with inevitable neural damage. In general, there would seem to be sufficient evidence in the medical literature to support a surgical approach to treating endometriosis.[5]

Abbott et al.[9] conducted a randomised placebo-controlled trial to look at the effect of laparoscopic treatment on pain and quality of life. In their study, 39 women with diagnosed endometriosis were randomised to either having a diagnostic laparoscopy (delayed surgery group) or having primary laparoscopic excision (immediate surgery group) for their endometriosis. The women underwent a further laparoscopy 6 months later and any disease noted then was completely treated in both groups. The main outcomes were changes in the visual analogue pain score, validated quality of life questionnaires score and sexual activity questionnaire score. There was a significant improvement in symptoms in women who had undergone excisional surgery compared with the women who had had a diagnostic laparoscopy (80% versus 32%). However, a placebo effect was noted in 30% of the women who had undergone only the diagnostic procedure, which was not related to the severity of the disease.

Another novel randomised placebo-controlled study[10] investigated the effect of anti-tumour necrosis factor alpha treatment for pain associated with deep endometriosis. In this study, 21 women with a rectovaginal endometriotic nodule were randomised to have an infusion of infliximab (5 mg/kg) or placebo. All women then underwent surgery 3 months later. There was a significant placebo effect with improvement in pain symptoms and pelvic tenderness in 30% of the untreated women. The placebo effect can probably be explained by the women's perception of having an important intravenous infusion and observation following the infusion, and of the enthusiasm of the researchers who felt that infliximab was likely to be effective. After subsequent surgery, the pain symptoms in these women were reduced to less than 20%. This study showed that infliximab does not affect the pain associated with deep endometriosis and the placebo effect is clearly a factor in some women's response to treatment, which is difficult to quantify.

In a Cochrane review, Jacobson et al.[11] described a study by Sutton and colleagues[12] in which 63 women were randomised to having either a diagnostic laparoscopy or laser treatment of their endometriosis, adhesiolysis and uterine nerve transection. Relief of pain was the primary outcome and pain scores at 3 and 6 months were measured postoperatively using a visual analogue scale. The authors of this study found a significant improvement in pain symptoms in women who were treated by laser laparoscopic surgery for minimal, mild or moderate endometriosis (OR 4.97; 95% CI 1.85–13.39).

The same team undertook a prospective, randomised, double-blind controlled trial of laparoscopic uterine nerve ablation (LUNA) in the treatment of pelvic pain associated with endometriosis.[13] In total, 51 women underwent laparoscopic laser ablation of their endometriosis and were then randomised to having or not having the LUNA procedure. The main outcomes were symptoms of dysmenorrhoea, dyspareunia and chronic nonmenstrual pain as assessed by visual analogue scales. There was a significant improvement in pain scores at 6 months in all women, indicating that surgical treatment of endometriosis is beneficial. Women who did not have the LUNA procedure at the time of surgery fared better at 3 and 6 months for symptoms of dysmenorrhoea and at 6 months for chronic nonmenstrual pain. The conclusion was that treatment of endometriosis was safe and effective in improving different types of pain symptoms, and that undertaking the LUNA procedure at the same time did not confer any further benefits.

In a further Cochrane review, Jacobson et al.[14] undertook a meta-analysis of five studies that looked at laparoscopic surgery for pelvic pain associated with endometriosis. The studies compared different laparoscopic surgical techniques with diagnostic laparoscopy with the addition of medical treatment in one study. The studies evaluated pain outcomes at 6 and 12 months following surgery. The results from all studies showed a significant improvement in pain symptoms after surgical treatment compared with diagnostic laparoscopy.

Therefore, surgical treatment of endometriosis does seem to be of some benefit to the woman. This has been highlighted by the Royal College of Obstetricians and Gynaecologists (RCOG) in its evidence-based Green-top Guideline on the investigation and management of endometriosis.[15] The RCOG recommends that laparoscopy should be used to diagnose and treat endometriosis at the same time with appropriate preoperative counselling and consent.

Infertility and endometriosis

In mild to moderate peritoneal endometriosis, the fallopian tubes are usually not affected and commonly maintain their normal anatomical relationship to the ovaries. However, in more severe disease and in the presence of a large endometrioma or severe pelvic sidewall disease (rAFS stage III–IV), the fallopian tubes can be affected owing to the inflammation, scarring and tethering of the tubes over the enlarged ovaries. In women with isolated rectovaginal disease, fertility rates do not seem to be significantly reduced. The presence of ovarian endometriomas does, however, often affect fertility. Frequently, rectovaginal endometriosis co-exists with pelvic sidewall disease and ovarian endometriomas, leading to a significant risk of subfertility.

In a recent Cochrane review, Hart et al.[16] looked at the effect of surgical treatment of ovarian endometriomas and found the pregnancy rates in women with infertility improved after surgery. The authors looked at two randomised studies where ovarian endometriomas greater than 3 cm were treated. There was an increased spontaneous conception rate in women with prior subfertility (OR 5.21; CI 2.04–13.29). In a further randomised study, there was an increase in the ovarian follicular response in women who required gonadotrophin stimulation for their subfertility.

The relationship between minimal disease and infertility in women with no tubal or ovarian pathology is unclear and the subject of heated debate. The issue is addressed by Akande et al.,[17] who conducted a retrospective case series to assess spontaneous conception in 117 women with unexplained subfertility and 75 infertile women with minimal/mild endometriosis without adhesions. The women were followed up for 3 years after laparoscopy and both groups were managed conservatively. The infertile women with endometriosis had a lower probability of pregnancy (36%) than the women with unexplained subfertility (55%), with the difference being statistically significant. The monthly conception rate (fecundity) was reduced in the women with mild endometriosis.

In a similar study with a multicentre prospective cohort design, Bérubé et al.[18] looked at the fecundity of 168 infertile women with minimal or mild endometriosis and 262 women with unexplained infertility who underwent diagnostic laparoscopy. Both groups were managed expectantly and were followed up for 36 weeks; pregnant women were followed up until week 20 of gestation. The authors found a fecundity of 18.2% and a fecundity rate of 2.52/100 person-months in infertile women with minimal to mild endometriosis compared with a fecundity of 23.7% and a fecundity rate of 3.48/100 person-months in those without endometriosis.

Treatment of mild to moderate endometriosis and outcomes in infertility

Although there seems to be convincing evidence linking mild endometriosis with infertility, does surgical resection or ablation of the deposits improve natural fertility?

This question was addressed in a Cochrane meta-analysis[19] that included two randomised studies, one by Marcoux et al.[20] and the other by Parazzini et al.[21]

Marcoux et al.[20] studied 341 infertile women between 20 and 39 years of age with minimal or mild endometriosis. The women were randomised to undergo resection or ablation of the visible endometriosis or a diagnostic laparoscopy only. These women were followed up for 36 weeks after their surgery. In women who became pregnant, follow-up was until week 20 of pregnancy. The pregnancy rate in the women in whom the endometriosis was treated was 30.7% compared with 17.7% in the nontreated group. The corresponding rates of fecundity were 4.7 and 2.4/100 person-months. Overall, the fecundity rate in women who underwent laparoscopic treatment of the endometriosis was 6.7/100 person-months, which was noted to be much lower than would be expected in fertile women. In the pregnant women, fetal losses occurred in approximately 20% in both groups. The conclusion was that treatment of minimal and mild endometriosis by laparoscopic resection or ablation improves fecundity in women with infertility.

However, these results were not reproduced in the randomised study by Parazzini et al.[21] In this study, 51 women underwent resection/ablation of their endometriosis versus 45 women in the diagnostic group. Follow-up was for a period of 1 year. Overall, 24% of women in the resection/ablation group and 29% in the nontreatment group conceived. The birth rate at the end of 1 year was 19.6% in the treatment group versus 22.2% in the nontreatment group and the difference was not significant. It should be noted that 42% of the women with endometriosis were treated with gonadotrophin-releasing hormone (GnRH) analogues postoperatively, confusing interpretation of this study.

Combining the results from these two studies in their meta-analysis, Jacobson et al.[19] found the combined pregnancy and live birth rates were significantly improved in women who underwent laparoscopic surgical treatment of minimal and mild endometriosis (OR 1.64; 95% CI 1.05–2.57).

In a large cohort study of 1268 women, Paulson et al.[22] found a significant difference between laser laparoscopy and laparotomy compared with expectant, medical and laparoscopic cautery in women with mild to moderate endometriosis with infertility. In women with mild endometriosis, pregnancy rates were 81% after treatment with laser laparoscopy and 84% after conservative laparotomy, compared with 54% after expectant treatment. Similarly, in women with moderate disease, pregnancy rates were 70% after laser laparoscopy compared with 39% in women who had previously received medical treatment. However, this study was observational and it is difficult to compare the interventions without proper randomisation.

Tulandi et al.[23] evaluated the reproductive outcomes in 101 women treated by laparoscopic excision and ablation. They found a pregnancy rate of 57.1% in the ablation group versus 53.5% in the excision group with a median time interval between surgery and conception of 10.7 months. The difference between the two groups was not significant, indicating that treatment with either modality was equally effective.

Vercellini et al.[24] took a pragmatic look at surgery related to endometriosis. The authors pointed out that there are very few randomised studies that investigated the benefits of surgery related to endometriosis. Most of the studies in this area are nonrandomised and observational and it may be that the benefits of surgery have been overestimated as a result. The authors also highlighted that surgery may eliminate the physical lesions but would not have any effect on the biomolecular changes associated with endometriosis. Similarly, staging of the disease is difficult as there is no obvious natural progression of the disease.

In contrast to the more severe forms of the disease, laparoscopic resection/ablation of mild endometriosis is safe and within the ability of most laparoscopic and reproductive surgeons. A small benefit in terms of improved fertility is usually demonstrated and this has led both the European Society of Human Reproduction and Embryology[5] and the RCOG[15] to recommend surgical treatment.

According to the fertility guidelines issued by the National Institute of Clinical Excellence,[25] women with moderate to severe disease should be offered surgical treatment. This recommendation is based on a few observational studies in which the pregnancy rates were similar or improved after laparoscopic treatment of endometriosis compared with laparotomy (54–66% versus 36–45%).[25]

Stage of endometriosis and fertility outcome

There are no randomised controlled trials looking at fertility related to treatment of the different stages of endometriosis. Treatment of rAFS stage I disease when no other cause for infertility has been found has been a subject of great debate. The two previously mentioned randomised trials by Marcoux et al.[20] and Parazzini et al.[21] have addressed this issue. However, their findings were contradictory. The study by the Italian group can be criticised for its small numbers. In the study by Marcoux et al.,[20] substantially more women with minimal and mild endometriosis were randomised to treatment and these authors found a pregnancy rate of 30.7% after treatment.

Other retrospective studies analysed women with different stages of endometriosis based on the rAFS classification and found similar pregnancy rates across the different stages of endometriosis.[26]

Chang et al.[27] studied 176 women with stage I disease who were divided into four groups undergoing carbon dioxide laser treatment, electrocoagulation, diagnostic laparoscopy or diagnostic laparoscopy and postoperative danazol for 3 months. No differences in the pregnancy rates were observed between the different groups after 3 years of follow-up.

Treatment of moderate to severe endometriosis is usually surgical because the ovaries are commonly affected with associated pelvic sidewall disease and tubal distortion. In several case series[28–30] that included over 200 women, pregnancy rates were found to be 52–60% for moderate disease and 42–47% for severe disease after treatment. In these women, the surgical treatment was combined with medical therapy either before or after surgery. Few prospective studies have shown that treatment of moderate to severe endometriosis is effective at improving pregnancy rates. In one such study,[31] 309 women with stage III/IV disease underwent surgery in the form of laparoscopic carbon dioxide laser ablation, laparoscopic electrocoagulation or laparotomy. The pregnancy rates between the groups were fairly similar, ranging from 32% to 41%, thus emphasising the fact that surgical treatment either laparoscopically or through laparotomy improves the outlook for infertile women with significant endometriosis. In a further randomised study[32] of 141 women, the cumulative pregnancy rate after 24 months was 57%. A greater benefit was seen in women with stage III disease (51%) than in those with stage IV disease (16%). The authors of this study questioned the discrepancy in outcome between the two stages and felt that a larger series of stage IV disease would be useful to see the actual benefits in treating these women surgically.

The cumulative pregnancy rate following reoperation for rAFS stage III/IV endometriosis has been quoted at between 5.9% and 24.4 %.[33] This compares unfavourably with assisted conception, where success rates of 33.3–69.6% were achieved in a similar group of women.[33] The inference is that assisted conception techniques would be a suitable alternative and that surgery would not confer any further benefits in women who are asymptomatic.

In more recent studies, fertility outcomes in women undergoing treatment for deeply infiltrative bowel disease have been more promising. In a retrospective analysis,[34] 187 women with refractory small or large bowel endometriosis underwent laparoscopic shaving of the endometriotic implant, disc resection or segmental resection of the affected bowel. In this cohort, 58 women had impaired fertility and the pregnancy rate among these women was 34% after treatment.

Segmental resection of colorectal endometriosis when associated with extensive pelvic disease may improve fertility rates, as demonstrated by Darai et al.[35] In this prospective study, 83 women underwent surgery for colorectal endometriosis (77 had laparoscopic treatment, with a conversion to laparotomy in six women). Over 95% of the women had multiple deposits of deep infiltrating endometriosis, with over half of them having three different anatomical locations of the endometriosis (95% uterosacral, 50% ovarian) in

TABLE 15.1 **Pregnancy outcomes by stage of endometriosis after laparoscopic surgical treatment of the endometriosis**

Author	Year of publication	Type of study	Stage I	Stage II	Stage III	Stage IV
Donnez et al.[28,29]	1987	Prospective			52–60%	42–47%
Pagidas et al.[33]		Retrospective analysis				
	1996			6–24%		
Marcoux et al.[20]	1997	Randomised controlled trial	31%			
Soong et al.[31]	1997	Prospective			32–41%	
Guzick et al.[26]	1997	Retrospective analysis	39%	31%	30%	25%
Chapron et al.[59]	1999	Cohort	47%		46.1%	
Busacca et al.[32]	1999	Prospective			51%	16%
Mohr et al.[34]	2005	Retrospective			34%	
Darai et al.[35]	2010	Prospective			46%	

addition to the colorectal disease. The pregnancy rate following surgery in this series was 46%. The mean follow-up of the women was 34 months and the median time in which the women conceived was 11 months. Furthermore, 40% of the women who had had a failure of assisted conception before surgery conceived after treatment. This study showed some promising results, but it has to be borne in mind that a significant number of women had disease in other areas of the pelvis, which could have some bearing on fertility rates.

Pregnancy rates following treatment of endometriosis are summarised in Table 15.1.

Ovarian endometriomas

Ovarian endometriotic cysts are present in about 16% of women presenting with endometriosis.[36] These cysts are characterised by their viscous chocolate-like contents, are usually confidently diagnosed with ultrasound, are associated with a modestly raised level of serum CA125 and, although frequently presenting with pelvic pain and/or infertility, may be asymptomatic.

The origin of ovarian endometriomas is still the subject of much debate, but the majority accept the view that endometriotic glands or stroma proliferate on the surface of the invaginated ovarian cortex.[1,2,37] The endometrioma is usually fused to the pelvic sidewall, but the disease remains superficial to the ovarian cortex. The alternative view expressed by Nisolle and Donnez[3] is that the endometrioma originates within the ovarian cortex and results from metaplasia of invaginated coelomic epithelium. This is supported by the fact that 12% of endometriomas are not fused to the pelvic sidewall and by the demonstration of epithelial invaginations in continuum with endometriotic tissue. The perceived origin of these ovarian cysts will influence the surgical choice of ablation or resection of the cyst capsule.

It is now firmly established that surgery for ovarian endometriomas should be conducted laparoscopically. What is less certain is whether the cyst lining should be ablated with thermal energy or excised in the manner of an ovarian cystectomy. Simple fenestration and drainage of the cyst is inadequate and will lead to high rates of recurrence. Endometriotic cysts of the ovary usually coexist with deeply invasive endometriosis elsewhere in the pelvis and intestinal involvement is common. For these reasons, surgical management should be carried out in specialist centres with the necessary laparoscopic expertise to excise severe endometriosis.

The question of whether to excise or ablate the lining of an ovarian endometrioma has been scrutinised in a Cochrane review.[16] The review included results from two randomised studies of the laparoscopic management of ovarian endometriomas of more than 3 cm in diameter and concluded that excision of the cyst wall was associated with a reduced recurrence rate of the symptoms of dysmenorrhea, dyspareunia and nonmenstrual pain. A reduced rate of endometrioma recurrence and necessity for further surgery was also noted in the excision group.

Where the ovarian endometrioma is large (more than 5 cm in diameter), surgical excision or stripping of the lining can pose significant problems (Figure 15.10). The excision may become ragged and piecemeal, requiring abundant use of diathermy to control bleeding, which in turn results in damage to ovarian tissue and function. Donnez et al.[38] have proposed a two-stage procedure with initial drainage of the endometrioma (Video 15.1) followed by the use of GnRH analogues for 12 weeks and then a second procedure with carbon dioxide laser vaporisation of the cyst and excision of extra-ovarian endometriosis. This results in a reduction of endometrioma diameter of up to 50% and recurrence rates of only 8%.[38] The other advantage of a two-stage approach is that it allows accurate counselling of the extent and situation of deeply invasive endometriosis prior to laparoscopic excisional surgery. By contrast, Canis et al.[39] demonstrated that cystectomy can be effective even for the larger cyst, with recurrence rates of 8% at second-look laparoscopy.

Where ablation of the cyst lining is considered, it is preferably performed with a carbon dioxide or potassium–titanyl–phosphate (KTP) laser. The KTP laser has the advantage that it functions well in the presence of blood on the cyst surface. Bipolar diathermy is commonly used, but there are concerns over thermal spread and damage to potentially healthy ovarian tissue. Monopolar diathermy is avoided because of the risk of thrombosis of the ovarian vessels in the infundibulopelvic ligament.

Hart et al.[16] concluded in their Cochrane review that excisional surgery for ovarian endometriomas results in increased spontaneous pregnancy rates in women with documented

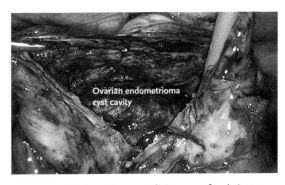

FIGURE 15.10 **Endometrioma cyst lining seen after drainage of the endometrioma**

prior subfertility (odds ratio 5.21; CI 2.04–13.29). In a randomised study, Alborzi et al.[40] demonstrated an increased ovarian follicular response to gonadotrophin stimulation for women who had undergone excisional surgery compared with ablative surgery (mean difference 0.6, 95% CI 0.04–1.16 favouring excision). However, Vercellini et al.[24] pointed out that the benefit of excision of ovarian endometriomas is difficult to define because of methodological drawbacks in the studies. Their concern is that, although the laparoscopic management of endometriosis-associated infertility is gaining in popularity, this approach is mostly supported by uncontrolled trials and may be overvalued.

It is common practice to treat ovarian endometriomas surgically before in vitro fertilisation (IVF), although there are only few data comparing laparoscopic excision with no treatment before IVF. The RCOG[15] recommends ovarian cystectomy if an ovarian endometrioma is more than 4 cm in diameter to confirm the histopathological diagnosis, reduce the risk of infection, improve access to follicles and, possibly, improve ovarian response and prevent endometriosis progression. Demirol et al.[41] have reported on the first randomised controlled trial in this debate, in which they compared 49 women allocated to conservative surgery before intracytoplasmic sperm injection and 50 women who underwent immediate intracytoplasmic sperm injection without surgery. No significant differences were noted in the rates of fertilisation (86% compared with 88%), implantation (16.5% compared with 18.5%) and pregnancy (34% compared with 38%). The consensus seems to be to recommend treatment of a larger endometrioma before assisted conception.

If long-standing ovarian endometriomas are untreated, there may be a small risk of malignant transformation. In a retrospective cohort study, Brinton et al.[42] looked at nearly 21 000 women with endometriosis over a period of 11.4 years. The records of these women were identified through the Swedish

Inpatient Register and linked to the National Swedish Cancer Registry. The authors found an increased risk of ovarian cancer (standardised incidence ratio 1.9; 95% CI 1.3–2.8) and this risk was considerably higher in women with long-standing endometriosis (standardised incidence ratio 4.2; 95% CI 2.0–7.7). The authors also found an increased risk of breast and haemato-poetic cancers in this group of women, which indicates a link with hormonal or immunological factors. However, this was a retrospective observational study and further research needs to be done to explore these links. Most endometriosis-associated ovarian malignancies are endometrioid or clear cell tumours, which represent about 25% of all ovarian malignancies.[43] In animal studies using mice, there is evidence of a genetic predisposition for malignant transformation.[44] Where the decision is taken not to treat an asymptomatic endometrioma, these figures could provide useful counselling material. However, during the counselling it should be highlighted that these studies are observational and there is active research being undertaken in this field.

Resection or ablation of endometriosis

Both superficial and deep deposits of endometriosis can be resected or ablated laparoscopically (Video 15.2) using different energy sources, but there is uncertainty over the relative merits of each technique. The general aim must be to completely remove all endometriotic deposits so that normal tissue is exposed with minimal collateral damage. The laparoscopic purists usually opt for the greater precision of resection, although complete clearance can be achieved with carbon dioxide laser vaporisation as well. The concern with resection in less experienced hands is of possible damage or injury to underlying structures. On the other hand, with ablation techniques, particularly where diathermy is used, the treatment may remain incomplete if the lesions extend more deeply than can be visualised. Ablation may lead to further problems with carbonisation, inflammation, superficial tissue damage and adhesion formation.

There is little guidance from the published literature on this matter and with mild disease, positive benefits are marginal whichever technique is used. In a small randomised study, Wright et al.[45] compared excision with ablation in 24 women with mild endometriosis. The women were randomised at laparoscopy if rAFS stage I/II endometriosis was found, with 12 women in each group. There were improvements in pain scores and reduction in pelvic tenderness in both groups at 6 months, but the differences between the groups did not reach statistical significance. The women with a higher pain score before surgery showed a more marked response.

Adjuvant medical therapy

Medical therapy for endometriosis will improve symptoms of pain, but recurrence is common after stopping the therapy.[15] However, in women who want to conceive, medical treatments are contraindicated because they are all contraceptive. Is there any benefit in initiating medical therapy before and/or after surgery? The rationale is to suppress the endometriotic implants and the associated inflammation, which may confer some benefit at the time of the surgery or prolong the symptom-free interval in women after surgery. This was demonstrated in a randomised study by Hornstein et al.,[46] in which 109 women were given a GnRH analogue or placebo for 6 months after their surgery. Approximately one-third (31%) of the women on GnRH analogues needed alternative therapy after 24 months compared with 57% of those who had the placebo. In a subsequent randomised controlled trial, Busacca et al.[47] demonstrated no difference in outcomes in women with stage III/IV disease who did or did not receive postoperative GnRH analogue therapy. Thus, the evidence in the literature has been conflicting, until 2004, when a Cochrane review was published that addressed this question.

The Cochrane meta-analysis[48] looked at 11 randomised controlled trials in which medical therapy was given before and/or after surgical treatment of endometriosis. The effectiveness with regard to eradication of the disease, improvement in symptoms, pregnancy rates, tolerability and adverse effects was addressed. The conclusion was that there was insufficient evidence of a beneficial effect. The National Institute for Health and Clinical Excellence also concluded that postoperative treatment with medical therapies does not improve pregnancy rates in women with moderate to severe disease and should not be recommended.[25]

In women with pelvic pain, however, use of the levonorgestrel-releasing intrauterine system has been found to reduce the recurrence of painful periods after surgical treatment of endometriosis.[49]

Large ovarian endometriomas can be treated with aspiration followed by a short course of medical ovarian suppression with GnRH analogues.[50,51] This would aid complete surgical treatment of the ovarian endometriomas without excessively destroying normal ovarian tissue.

Health economics and the treatment of endometriosis

Endometriosis is often perceived as a chronic debilitating condition. From diagnosis to treatment, women may need several medical and surgical interventions. Data on the actual costs of treatment of endometriosis are limited.

Gao et al.[52] looked at the economic burden of endometriosis. They reviewed published studies from 1990 onwards and conducted an analysis of available national databases. The hospital length of stay had declined from 1993 to 2002, but the direct and indirect costs of endometriosis per patient had increased by 61%. The number of adolescents requiring hospitalisation had increased and over half of the 600 000 endometriosis-related visits during the study period required specialist care.

In another study[53] in the USA, the average length of stay and cost related to endometriosis was 3.8 days and US$ 6,597 in 1991 and 3.5 days and US$ 7,450 in 1992. The total estimated hospitalisation charges were US$ 504 million in 1991 and US$ 579 million in 1992, indicating major cost implications related to endometriosis.

In a more recent study,[54] the annual cost associated with endometriosis was estimated to be around US$ 2,801 with a cost of productivity loss of US$ 1,023 per affected woman. Using these estimates, the calculated annual cost of endometriosis would be US$ 22 billion in 1 year assuming a prevalence of endometriosis in the population of 10%. This reflects the magnitude of the problem and has major implications in healthcare economics because the costs of treatment have become significantly more over the years.

In mild to moderate endometriosis, surgery is the most cost-effective treatment, whereas IVF is more cost-effective in women with severe tubal factors and endometriosis.[55] In 2009, the World Endometriosis Research Foundation launched the prospective EndoCost Study.[56] The aim of the study was to calculate the direct and indirect/hidden cost of endometriosis from a societal and personal perspective. It involved 12 centres in 10 countries and ran until the end of 2009. At the time of writing, the results had not yet been published.

See and treat: the death of diagnostic laparoscopy

In the investigation and treatment of pelvic pain, a 'see and treat' policy using resection or ablation is preferable for minor and moderate presentations of endometriosis and this should be within the repertoire of all surgeons performing laparoscopy. The concept of laparoscopy as a purely diagnostic tool should be relegated to the archives. Where severe endometriosis is diagnosed, referral to a centre with the necessary expertise to perform radical excision is required.

The situation with regard to fertility investigation is not so clear. There is an increasing tendency to bypass laparoscopy in favour of less invasive options such as hysterosalpingo contrast sonography (HyCoSy) and hysterosalpingo-gram. Compared with laparoscopy, transvaginal ultrasound has limited value in diagnosing peritoneal endometriosis, but it is a useful tool both to make and to exclude the diagnosis of an ovarian endometrioma.[57] Laparoscopy and dye is the favoured investigation if endometriosis or pelvic adhesions are suspected, but how many women are asymptomatic and does it matter? The answer is probably affirmative since laparoscopy has been shown to change treatment decisions in 25% of women scheduled for assisted conception.[58] In addition, evidence has previously been presented demonstrating a beneficial impact on infertility if pelvic endometriosis and/or adhesions are surgically treated and this is a recommendation in both the European Society of Human Reproduction and Embryology[5] and the RCOG[15] guidelines.

References

1 Sampson J A. Peritoneal endometriosis due to the menstrual dissemination of endometrial tissue into the peritoneal cavity. *Am J Obstet Gynecol* 1927;14:422–69.

2 Sampson J A. Perforating hemorrhagic (chocolate) cysts of the ovary. Their importance and especially their relation to pelvic adenomas of endometrial type ("adenomyoma" of the uterus, rectovaginal septum, sigmoid, etc.). *Arch Surg* 1921;3:245–323.

3 Nisolle M, Donnez J. Peritoneal endometriosis, ovarian endometriosis and adenomyotic nodules of the rectovaginal septum are three different entities. *Fertil Steril* 1997;68: 585–96.

4 Revised American Society for Reproductive Medicine classification of endometriosis: 1996. *Fertil Steril* 1997;67:817–21.

5 Kennedy S, Bergqvist A, Chapron C, D'Hooghe T, Dunselman G, Greb R, et al. ESHRE guideline for the diagnosis and treatment of endometriosis. *Hum Reprod* 2005;20:2698–704.

6 Tuttlies F, Keckstein J, Ulrich U, Possover M, Schweppe KW, Wustlich M, et al. [ENZIAN-score, a classification of deep infiltrating endometriosis]. *Zentralbl Gynäkol* 2005;127:275–81. Article in German.

7 Garry R. The endometriosis syndromes: a clinical classification in the presence of aetiological confusion and therapeutic anarchy. *Hum Reprod* 2004;19:760–8.

8 Vercellini P, Fedele L, Aimi G, Pietropaolo, Consonni D, Crosignani PG. Association between endometriosis stage, lesion type, patient characteristics and severity of pelvic pain symptoms: a multivariate analysis of over 1000 patients. *Hum Reprod* 2007;22:266–77.

9 Abbott J, Hawe J, Hunter D, Holmes M, Finn P, Garry R. Laparoscopic excision of endometriosis: a randomized, placebo-controlled trial. *Fertil Steril* 2004;82:878–84.

10 Koninckx P R, Craessaerts M, Timmerman D, Cornillie F, Kennedy S. Anti-TNF-alpha treatment for deep endometriosis-associated pain: a randomized placebo-controlled trial. *Hum Reprod* 2008;23:2017–23.

11 Jacobson T Z, Barlow D H, Garry R, Koninckx P. Laparoscopic surgery for pelvic pain associated with endometriosis. *Cochrane Database Syst Rev* 2001; (4):CD001300.

12 Sutton C J G, Ewen S P, Whitlaw N, Haines P. Prospective randomized, double blind, controlled trial of laser laparoscopy in the treatment of pelvic pain associated with minimal, mild and moderate endometriosis. *Fertil Steril* 1994;62:696–700.

13 Sutton C, Pooley A, Jones K, Dover R, Haines P. A prospective, randomized, double-blind controlled trial of laparoscopic uterine nerve ablation in the treatment of pelvic pain associated with endometriosis. *Gynaecol Endosc* 2001;10:217–22.

14 Jacobson T Z, Duffy J M N, Barlow D, Koninckx, Garry R. Laparoscopic surgery for pelvic pain associated with endometriosis. *Cochrane Database Syst Rev* 2009; (4):CD001300.

15 Royal College of Obstetricians and Gynaecologists. *The Investigation and Management of Endometriosis*. Green-top Guideline No. 24. London: RCOG; 2006 [www.rcog.org.uk/womens-health/clinical-guidance/investigation-and-management-endometriosis-green-top-24].

16 Hart R J, Hickey M, Maouris P, Buckett W. Excisional surgery versus ablative surgery for ovarian endometriomata. *Cochrane Database Syst Rev* 2008;(2):CD004992.

17 Akande V A, Hunt L, Cahill D, Jenkins J. Differences in time to natural conception between women with unexplained infertility and infertile women with minor endometriosis. *Hum Reprod* 2004;19:96–103.

18 Bérubé S, Marcoux S, Langevin M, Maheux R. Fecundity of infertile women with minimal or mild endometriosis and women with unexplained infertility. The Canadian Collaborative Group on Endometriosis. *Fertil Steril* 1998;69:1034–41.

19 Jacobson T Z, Duffy J M, Barlow D, Farquhar C, Koninckx P R, Olive D. Laparoscopic surgery for subfertility associated with endometriosis. *Cochrane Database Syst Rev* 2010;(1):CD001398.

20 Marcoux S, Maheux R, Bérubé S. Laparoscopic surgery in infertile women with minimal or mild endometriosis. The Canadian Collaborative Group on Endometriosis. *N Engl J Med* 1997;337:217–22.

21 Parazzini F. Ablation of lesions or no treatment in minimal–mild endometriosis in infertile women: a randomized trial. Gruppo Italiano per lo Studio dell" Endometriosi. *Hum Reprod* 1999:14;1332–4.

22 Paulson J D, Asmar P, Saffan D. Mild and moderate endometriosis. Comparison of treatment modalities for infertile couples. *J Reprod Med* 1991;36:151–5.

23 Tulandi T, Al-Took S. Reproductive outcome after treatment of mild endometriosis with laparoscopic excision and electrocoagulation. *Fertil Steril* 1998;69:229–31.

24 Vercellini P, Somigliana E, Viganò P, Abbiati A, Barbara G, Crosignani PG. Surgery for endometriosis-associated infertility: a pragmatic approach. *Hum Reprod* 2009;24:254–69.

25 National Collaborating Centre for Women's and Children's Health. *Fertility: Assessment and Treatment for People with Fertility Problems*. London: RCOG Press; 2004 [www.guidance.nice.org.uk/CG11].

26 Guzick D S, Silliman N P, Adamson G D, Buttram V C Jr, Canis M, Malinak L R, Schenken R S. Prediction of pregnancy in infertile women based on the American Society for Reproductive Medicine's revised classification of endometriosis. *Fertil Steril* 1997;67:822–9.

27 Chang F H, Chou H H, Soong Y K, Chang M Y, Lee C L, Lai Y M. Efficacy of isotopic CO_2 laser laparoscopic evaporation in the treatment of infertile women with minimal to mild endometriosis: a life table cumulative pregnancy rates study. *J Am Assoc Gynecol Laparosc* 1997;4:219–23.

28 Donnez J. CO_2 laser laparoscopy in infertile women with endometriosis and women with adnexal adhesions. *Fertil Steril* 1987;48:390–4.

29 Donnez J, Lemaire-Rubbers M, Karaman Y, Nisolle-Pochet M, Casanas-Roux F. Combined hormonal and microsurgical therapy in infertile women with endometriosis. *Fertil Steril* 1987;48:239–42.

30 Donnez J, Nisolle-Pochet M, Casananas-Roux F. Endometriosis-associated infertility: evaluation of preoperative use of danazol, gestrinone, and buserelin. *Int J Fertil* 1990;35:297–301.

31 Soong Y K, Chang F H, Chou H H, Chang M Y, Lee C L, Lai Y M, et al. Life table analysis of pregnancy in women with moderate or severe endometriosis comparing danazol therapy after carbon dioxide laser laparoscopy plus electrocoagulation or laparotomy plus electrocoagulation versus danazol therapy only. *J Am Assoc Gynecol Laparosc* 1997;4:225–30.

32 Busacca M, Bianchi S, Agnoli B, Candiani M, Calia C, De Marinis S, et al. Follow-up of laparoscopic treatment of stage III/IV endometriosis. *J Am Gynecol Laparosc* 1999;6:55–8.

33 Pagidas K, Falcone T, Hemmings R, Miron P. Comparison of reoperation for moderate (stage III) and severe (stage IV) endometriosis-related infertility with in vitro fertilization-embryo transfer. *Fertil Steril* 1996;65:791–5.

34 Mohr C, Nezhat F, Nezhat C, Seidman D, Nezhat C. Fertility considerations in laparoscopic treatment of infiltrative bowel endometriosis. *JSLS* 2005;9:16–24.

35 Darai E, Carbonnel M, Dubernard G, Lavoue V, Coutant C, Bazot M, et al. Determinant factors of fertility outcomes after laparoscopic colorectal resection for endometriosis. *Eur J Obstet Gynecol Reprod Biol* 2010;149:210–4.

36 Donnez J, Donnez O, Squiffet J, Nisolle M. The concept of retroperitoneal adenomyotic disease is born. In: Donnez J, Nisolle M, editors. *An Atlas of Operative Laparoscopy and Hysteroscopy.* New York, NY: Parthenon; 2001. p. 113–20.

37 Hughesdon P E. The structure of the endometrial cysts of the ovary. *J Obstet Gynaecol Br Emp* 1957;44:481–7.

38 Donnez J, Nisolle M, Gillet N, Smets M, Bassil S, Casanas-Roux F. Large ovarian endometriomas. *Hum Reprod* 1996;11:641–6.

39 Canis M, Mage G, Wattiez A, Chapron C, Pouly J-L, Bassil S. Second-look laparoscopy after laparoscopic cystectomy of large ovarian endometriomas. *Fertil Steril* 1992;58;3:617–9.

40 Alborzi S, Ravanbakhsh R, Parsanezhad M E, Alborzi M, Alborzi S, Dehbashi S. A comparison of follicular response of ovaries to ovulation induction after laparoscopic ovarian cystectomy or fenestration and coagulation versus normal ovaries in patients with endometrioma. *Fertil Steril* 2007;88:507–9.

41 Demirol A, Guven S, Baykal C, Gurgan T. Effect of endometrioma cystectomy on IVF outcome: a prospective randomised study. *Reprod Biomed Online* 2006;12:639–3.

42 Brinton L A, Gridley G, Persson I, Baron J, Berquist A. Cancer risk after a hospital discharge diagnosis of endometriosis. *Am J Obstet Gynecol* 1997;176:572–9.

43 Ness R. Endometriosis and Ovarian cancer. Thoughts on shared pathophysiology. *Am J Obstet Gynecol* 2003;189:280–94.

44 Dinulescu D, Ince T A, Quade B, Shafer S, Crowley D, Jacks T. Role of K-ras and Pten in the development of mouse models of endometriosis and endometrioid ovarian cancer. *Nature Med* 2004;11:63–70.

45 Wright J, Lotfallah H,Jones K, Lovell D. A randomized trial of excision versus ablation for mild endometriosis. *Fertil Steril* 2005;83:1830–6.

46 Hornstein M, Hemmings R, Yuzpe A. Use of nafareline versus placebo after reductive laparoscopic surgery for endometriosis. *Fertil Steril* 1997;68:860–4.

47 Busacca M, Somigliana E, Bianchi S, Marinis A De, Calia C, Candiani, Vignali M. Post-operative GnRh analogue treatment after conservative surgery for symptomatic endometriosis stage III-IV a randomized controlled trial. *Hum Reprod* 2001;16:2399–402.

48 Yap C, Furness S, Farquhar C. Pre and post operative medical therapy for endometriosis surgery. *Cochrane Database Syst Rev* 2004;(3):CD003678.

49 Abou-Setta A M, Al-Inany H G, Farquhar C. Levonorgestrel-releasing intrauterine device (LNG-IUD) for symptomatic endometriosis following surgery. *Cochrane Database Syst Rev* 2006;(4):CD005072.

50 Donnez J, Pirard C, Smets M, Jadoul P, Squifflet J. Surgical management of endometriosis. *Best Pract Res Clin Obstet Gynaecol* 2004;18:329–48.

51 McVeigh E. The surgical management of endometriosis. *Womens Health Med* 2005;2:29–33.

52 Gao X, Outley J, Botteman M, Spalding J, Simon J A, Pashos CL. Economic burden of endometriosis. *Fertil Steril* 2006;86:1561–72.

53 Zhao S Z, Wong J M, Davis M B, Gersh G E, Johnson K E. The cost of inpatient endometriosis treatment: an analysis based on the Healthcare Cost and Ultilization Project Nationwide Inpatient Sample. *Am J Manag Care* 1998;4:1127–34.

54 Simoens S, Hummelshoj L, D'Hooghe T. Endometriosis: cost estimates and methodological perspective. *Hum Reprod Update* 2007;13:395–404.

55 Philips Z, Barraza-Llorens M, Posnett J. Evaluation of the relative cost-effectiveness of treatments for infertility in the UK. *Hum Reprod* 2000;15:95–106.

56 EndoCost Study [www.endometriosisfoundation.org/endocost].

57 Moore J, Copley S, Morris J, Lindsell D, Golding S, Kennedy S. A systematic review of the accuracy of ultrasound in the diagnosis of endometriosis. *Ultrasound Obstet Gynecol* 2002;20:630–4.

58 Tanahatoe S, Hampes PGA, Lambalk C B. Should diagnostic laparoscopy be performed in the infertility work up programme in patients undergoing intrauterine insemination. *Hum Reprod* 2003;18:8–11.

59 Chapron C, Fritel X, Dubuisson J B. Fertility after laparoscopic management of deep endometriosis infiltrating the uterosacral ligaments. *Hum Reprod* 1999;14:329–32.

16 Laparoscopic treatment of advanced and rectovaginal endometriosis

Jim English

Introduction

As a result of advances in laparoscopic equipment and the development of technical skills, more gynaecologists are now undertaking radical surgery to treat severe endometriosis involving the bowel and urinary tract.

Severe endometriosis in the cul-de-sac may be an extension of a large adenomyoma in the posterior wall of the cervix with continuity of disease between the cervix and the vagina and rectum. Such disease has been demonstrated as early as 1920.[1]

Disease spread/extension

Apart from growing by direct expansion, endometriosis may spread either along lymphatic channels or by means of vascular invasion. The former is probably a fairly common event and explains the presence of disease in pararectal lymph nodes and in the groin following passage along the round ligaments. Vascular spread would explain the presence of disease at distal and otherwise inexplicable sites. Unfortunately, the natural course taken by such distal deposits is entirely unclear.

Although the aim of surgery may be the complete extirpation of all disease, the role of preoperative determination of the extent of disease, particularly lymphatic spread or spread to a distal site, has not been established. It would, however, seem logical to remove all evident disease at the time of surgery so long as the risks involved are not disproportionate to the benefit.

Diagnosis and preoperative investigation

Preoperative planning aims to determine the extent of disease so that adequate surgical time is allowed for and to ensure that the personnel with the necessary skills are available. Because of the inherent surgical risks, it is

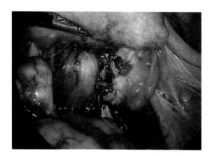

FIGURE 16.1 **Stage IV endometriosis** (laparoscopic view)

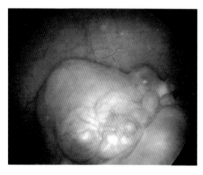

FIGURE 16.2 **Bladder endometriosis** (cystoscopic view)

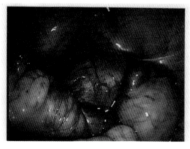

FIGURE 16.3 **Obliterated pelvis**

imperative to know what surgery is to be undertaken and to counsel the woman appropriately. This may be achieved in several ways.

Staging surgery by means of laparoscopy (Figure 16.1), cystoscopy (Figure 16.2) and sigmoidoscopy may be sufficient to establish the extent of disease. However, when the pelvis is obliterated (Figure 16.3), laparoscopic visualisation is probably suboptimal and the depth and even the presence of deep rectal disease may be difficult to determine.

Improvements in transvaginal ultrasound have made it possible to diagnose deep rectal disease. Preoperative scanning with transvaginal ultrasound has been shown to have high levels of sensitivity and specificity (91% and 98%, respectively),[2] making the planning of surgery easier. In Figures 16.4 and 16.5, a large bladder nodule protruding into the posterior wall of the bladder is seen. In Figures 16.6 and 16.7, a 3 cm rectal nodule is seen after excision and on a transvaginal scan. Thus, transvaginal ultrasound scanning may be used to plan surgery, particularly in complex disease when surgeons from different specialties may be required to work collaboratively.

Magnetic resonance imaging (MRI) has also been used to try to identify rectovaginal disease preoperatively to plan surgery. However, Fallioli et al.[3] demonstrated that unenhanced MRI may be able to detect only 71% of all deep rectal lesions, whereas the use of double-contrast barium enema may increase the detection rate to 84%. Other authors[4] have demonstrated that MRI jelly detects rectovaginal lesions with a sensitivity of 90.9% and a specificity of 77.8%. Thus, transvaginal ultrasound may be superior to MRI in the diagnosis of rectovaginal endometriosis with much lower costs.

When to operate and on whom?

Surgery to excise severe endometriosis is not only extremely complex and time-consuming but may also carry substantial risk, not just of morbidity but even of mortality. It has been demonstrated that endometriosis of the cul-de-sac may result in severe pain, particularly dyschesia, and a diminished quality of life.[5] Medical treatment is reasonably effective in the short term in the management of superficial disease,[6] but seems to be less effective in the

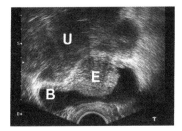

FIGURE 16.4 **Bladder nodule seen on transvaginal ultrasound** B = bladder; E = endometriotic lesion; U = uterus

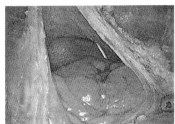

FIGURE 16.5 **Bladder nodule from Figure 16.4 visualised through the open bladder**

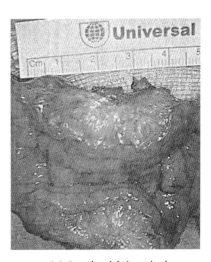

FIGURE 16.6 **Rectal nodule in excised specimen**

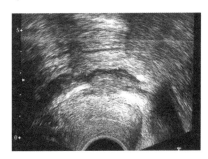

FIGURE 16.7 **Rectal nodule (transvaginal ultrasound)**

treatment of deep disease (especially in the cul-de-sac) even when used in conjunction with surgery.[7,8]

Some women with severe disease may be relatively asymptomatic. In addition, correlation of specific symptoms with the site or extent of disease is often poor. Thus, it is often difficult to identify those women who should be offered radical surgery and those in whom surgical intervention should not be considered.

Notwithstanding these caveats, endometriosis is associated with pain and removal of disease is associated both with a reduction in pain scores and an improvement in the quality of life. For these reasons, many surgeons base the decision to offer radical surgery on the severity of the woman's pain and its effect on her quality of life. Although not diagnostic, symptoms such as rectal bleeding, dyschesia, altered bowel function and pain experienced on sitting may point to the likelihood of rectal involvement and, if so, removal of disease may be associated with an amelioration in the severity of such symptoms.

On relatively rare occasions, severe endometriosis may provide a near absolute indication for radical surgery. Such circumstances include hydro-ureteronephrosis secondary to an endometriosis-related ureteric stricture and bowel obstruction or perforation.

Women with fertility issues present a further dilemma with regard to the benefits of surgical excision. Although ablation of mild endometriosis and excision of ovarian endometriomas has been shown to be associated with an increase in fertility rates,[9,10] the association between radical surgery and fertility is much less clear. While the effects of endometrioma removal on ovarian reserve have been well documented, there is no evidence pertaining to the effects of radical surgery on ovarian function and reserve. Furthermore, radical surgery is liable to result in adhesion formation in the pelvis with resultant implications for fertility. At present, the evidence to support radical surgery for severe endometriosis in subfertile women is unclear.

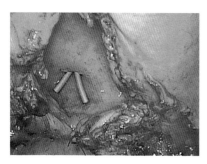

FIGURE 16.8 **Double J stents inserted following hemicystectomy**

Surgical techniques

Ureteric catheterisation/stenting

Some surgeons routinely insert catheters or stents into the ureters immediately before surgery to better visualise the ureters, to protect them during dissection and to enable insertion of double J stents postoperatively. However, this practice relates to the subjective preference of the surgeon rather than being evidence based. Indications for ureteric catheterisation include: identification of double ureters, which can then be catheterised individually, facilitation of ureteric dissection and facilitation of postoperative double J stenting if required (Figure 16.8).

If catheters are being employed, it is advisable to use a type through which a guide wire may be inserted in case a double J stent is required later. The ureter may become oedematous following surgery and, unless a guide wire is in place, it may become impossible to insert a double J stent. Insertion of stents is straightforward using an operating cystoscope, through which the ureteric catheter is passed over a soft-tipped guide wire. It is usually possible to insert a 6F catheter without undue difficulty to a depth of 20 cm from the ureteric orifice. The catheters are marked with bands corresponding to 1 cm and 5 cm intervals. If difficulty is encountered, a 4F Stamey catheter may be employed. However, if significant resistance is met, force should not be used because ureteric damage is more likely. In some instances, it is possible to leave just the guide wire in place for the course of the operation.

Some surgeons advocate the primary insertion of double J stents on the basis that, if stenting is required postoperatively, less ureteric trauma will ensue. However, the drawback is that the stenting procedure is slower and, in most cases, requires the use of radiographic image intensification to ensure the correct placement of the coiled stent tail within the renal pelvis.

Postoperative use of double J stents is desirable if the ureter has been opened or reanastomosed or reimplanted into the bladder. In these circumstances, there is a significant risk of ureteric leakage and fistula formation, especially if stents are not left in place postoperatively. Double J stents left in place postoperatively may give rise to significant discomfort owing to irritation either of the renal pelvis or of the bladder. The latter is often more prominent at the end of micturition. If possible, double J stents should be left in place for 6 weeks; however, earlier removal may be necessitated by discomfort. Removal may readily be performed under sedation and a check intravenous urogram is performed routinely afterwards.

Energy sources and instrumentation

Many different types of energy source have been employed for vaporisation (carbon dioxide and potassium–titanyl–phosphate [KTP] lasers) and excisional techniques (ultrasonic scalpels, monopolar current, KTP laser). The available literature is not capable of demonstrating the superiority of one energy source over another. The potential advantages and disadvantages of each energy source have been described in chapter 5 and will not be covered here. Although lasers are conventionally considered to cause tissue destruction through vaporisation, a laser may equally well be used as an energy source for haemostatic excision. Therefore, it is not possible to be prescriptive in terms of energy source selection and this chapter describes operative techniques that may be applied regardless of the choice of instrument.

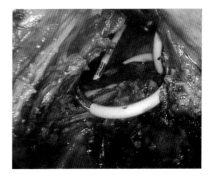

FIGURE 16.9 **Double J stents in duplex system**

Port placement

The author favours the use of a 10 mm umbilical port for the laparoscope and paired 5 mm ports low in the iliac fossae, inserted under direct vision lateral to the inferior epigastric arteries. A convertible 5–12 mm port is also inserted low suprapubically to the right of the midline. This allows for the introduction of sutures and Endo GIA® (US Surgical Corporation, Norwalk, CT, USA) staple guns as required.

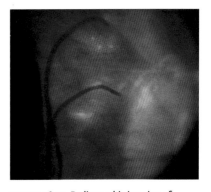

FIGURE 16.10 **Radiographic imaging of stents seen in Figure 16.9**

Bladder and ureteric endometriosis

Ureteric catheterisation or stenting as described is used by many to facilitate ureterolysis and to protect the ureters from damage during and after surgery. It also facilitates the recognition of ureteric duplication (Figures 16.9 and 16.10).

If the bladder disease is relatively superficial, or at least not evident at cystoscopy, it may be possible to shave the disease from the pelvic surface of the bladder. This may be facilitated by distension of the bladder with a few 100 ml of methylene blue dye. This will also render more visible any significant defect in the bladder wall requiring repair.

In cases of deep infiltration of the bladder wall, it is useful to mobilise the bladder first by opening the peritoneum in the uterovesical fold and dissecting the bladder caudally. Next, the dome of the bladder may be opened to reveal the extent of the lesion, which can then be excised fully. The bladder should be closed using a double row of interrupted absorbable sutures such as 2.0 Vicryl® (polyglactin 910; Ethicon Endo-Surgery, Cincinnati, OH, USA) and checked for any leak by distension with methylene blue dye. Although a continuous suture may be employed, the establishment of an appropriate degree of tension in the suture is more difficult to achieve laparoscopically. Postoperatively, a freely draining Foley catheter should be left in place for at least 7 days. If the excision margin is close to a ureteric orifice, consideration should be given to the insertion of double J stents.

Where the surgery required a large defect to be closed, it is advisable to obtain a cystogram to ensure that there is no leak before removal of the Foley catheter. If a hysterectomy is being performed at the same time, consideration may be given to the mobilisation of an omental pad, which should be interposed between bladder and vagina to reduce the risk of fistula formation.

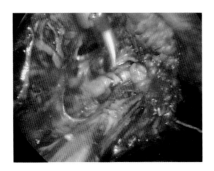

FIGURE 16.11 **Ureterolysis showing left ureter crossed by uterine artery**

Ureterolysis

It is not uncommon for endometriosis to affect the distal ureter at or just above its entry into the ureteric tunnel and junction with the bladder. Actual infiltration of the muscularis of the ureter is much less common. Nonetheless, what is commonly described as ureterolysis (Figure 16.11) seems to encompass everything from peritoneal stripping of the ureter to complete release and resection of all periureteric tissue in the region of the ureteric tunnel.

It is frequently more difficult to identify the left ureter and it may be necessary to trace it caudally from the level of the pelvic brim, where it may normally be identified crossing the bifurcation of the common iliac artery.

Ureterolysis, or at least resection of the pelvic peritoneum overlying the ureter, is frequently performed as part of a procedure increasingly referred to as radical resection of endometriosis or an extended arcus taurinus procedure. Most authors describe commencement of the resection anterolateral to the ureters. If possible, it is preferable to leave the ureters attached to the pelvic sidewall as this should reduce the risk of devascularisation.

If there is significant stricture formation in the ureter with proximal dilatation (Figure 16.12), ureterolysis alone may not be adequate because periureteric scarring may ensue with failure of resolution of the obstruction. In such instances, consideration should be given to the need for ureteric reimplantation. If so, the new orifice is best created in the midline directly opposite the urethral opening to facilitate its cystoscopic visualisation. Regardless of whether ureteric reimplantation has been performed, it would appear sensible to obtain an intravenous urogram 6 weeks following surgery to confirm that the stricture is no longer present. Rarely, very severe ureteric constriction may lead to hydronephrosis with silent destruction of the affected kidney.

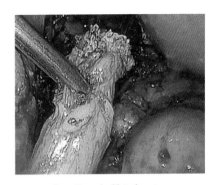

FIGURE 16.12 **Grossly dilated ureter transected proximal to obstruction**

If moderate to severe hydronephrosis is evident on preoperative urography or ultrasound, a mercaptoacetyltriglycine (MAG3) or dimercaptosuccinic acid (DMSA) scan should be performed to determine the proportion of overall renal function contributed by the diseased kidney. If renal function is markedly reduced in the hydronephrotic kidney, consideration should be given to its removal because of its poor function and the likelihood of recurrent infection in that kidney. Removal of the kidney may be performed laparoscopically at the same time as the surgery for endometriosis.

Resection of the pelvic peritoneum

The technique described for this procedure is demonstrated as part of the technique employed for anterior rectal resection. As already mentioned, most authors describe the commencement of dissection anterolateral to the evident disease and carry it caudally and medially with the aim of either resecting all disease en bloc or leaving all disease contracted and attached to the anterior rectum. This usually entails resection of the uterosacral ligaments. If there is no evidence of rectal involvement, surgery is usually complete at this stage.

As in the case of ureterolysis, great care must be taken in the case of perirectal dissection to avoid and recognise thermal injury and the risk of delayed bowel perforation.

When the cul-de-sac is found to be obliterated with the rectum adherent to the back wall of the cervix and posterior uterine wall, it becomes necessary to separate the bowel from the uterus. It may be possible to achieve this by means of a blunt dissection using a Lahey swab attached to a claw forceps. However, this may not be possible in the presence of a large adenomyoma that is entirely continuous with the cervix, vagina and rectum. In such a situation, there are options: one may cut down through the adenomyoma where one would normally anticipate the plane to be or one may dissect anterior to the adenomyoma leaving it attached to the rectum. In the first instance, the cervical adenomyoma will need to be excised independently.

The dissection of the cul-de-sac may be handled in this way regardless of whether the uterus is being conserved or not. If the latter is the case, en bloc resection of uterus and rectum (when required) may be facilitated by laparoscopic hysterectomy, in which, following division of all ligamentous and vascular attachments of the uterus, the anterior vagina is opened to expose the nodule in the posterior vaginal wall.

This permits easy identification of the caudal extent of the nodule of endometriosis in the posterior fornix and allows the surgeon to open the posterior vaginal wall from its vaginal side. Being caudal to the nodule permits the easy opening of the rectovaginal septum, whose dissection may then be continued as far distally as required.

Entry into the rectovaginal septum may be very difficult when approaching it through a large nodule obliterating the cul-de-sac. Identification of the septum may be made easier in one of two ways. The posterior fornix may be opened, the vaginal wall thus examined and the inferior extent of the nodule determined as described. Alternatively, it may prove possible to identify and enter the septum through a lateral approach and thereby open it below the limit of the disease.

Rectal disease

The management of disease involving the rectum remains highly contentious with proponents advocating anything from debulking surgery to segmental rectal resection, in some instances regardless of the extent of involvement. Because of the perceived inadequacy of medical treatment, many authors have recommended the complete excision of all endometriosis in rectovaginal disease even if it involves extensive surgery to the rectum.[11-13] Others have favoured a more conservative approach.[5,8] Evidence suggests that 5–10% of women with endometriosis – equating to 150 000–300 000 women in the UK – have rectal disease.[14,15] The lack of any suitable staging or scoring system for rectal disease makes comparison among studies difficult and this difficulty is in turn made all the greater by the lack of uniformity in the analysis of outcome measures. The very lack of adequate staging techniques and the lack of histological confirmation of rectal disease in women treated by debulking effectively render any direct comparison impossible.

The complications associated with segmental anterior rectal resection have been well documented.[16] However, most data pertain to surgery carried out for cancer and in a much older age group than is customary for endometriosis surgery.

So, how ought rectal endometriosis be treated? Unfortunately, there are no randomised controlled trials that seek to answer the question and what information exists is derived from retrospective audit of results.

Superficial endometriosis arouses the least debate as most surgeons will attempt to strip or ablate peritoneal or rectal serosal disease. Although such disease may be relatively straightforward to treat, this does not mean that such treatment is risk free. It is evident that accidental enterotomy and delayed perforation resulting from thermal injury are risks. Clearly, if such rectal shaving to remove disease is extensive and over a large distance, the risk of rectal perforation may be relatively high. If such extensive disease is recognised in the first instance, it may be safer to opt for segmental resection rather than extensive shaving.

Some surgeons have advocated disc resection of the rectum to remove isolated nodules on the grounds that the ensuing rectal repair is less likely to leak postoperatively and that the woman may avoid many of the symptoms and complications associated with segmental resection. The rectum is repaired in one or two layers using an absorbable suture. Rectal integrity should be assessed by means of an air test, in which the pelvis is filled with saline and the rectum insufflated with air via a sigmoidoscope.

Although the reported outcome of disc resection is very good, there remain a number of limitations to the technique. It may not be suitable if there are a number of 'skip lesions' rather than an isolated nodule. In addition, the size of the nodule may be prohibitive as the resultant size of the deficit in the rectal wall may prevent closure without tension. The size of nodule that may safely be removed by disc resection varies from surgeon to surgeon but – depending on technique and skill – is probably in the region of 3 cm in diameter. Perhaps the greatest limitations placed on the use of disc resection are the levels of training and practice of colorectal surgeons, the majority of whom do not otherwise employ disc resection in their practice and for whom segmental resection remains the standard surgical management for rectal pathology.

Indications for segmental anterior rectal resection
What, then, are the indications for segmental rectal resection? These include a single large nodule, multiple nodules or extensive superficial disease. Deep rectal disease has been shown to result in stenosis and occasionally perforation and disease of this degree will require treatment regardless of chronic pain or fertility needs. Severe disease may present at a very early age, as seen

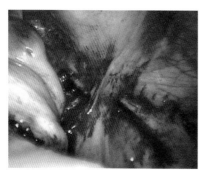

FIGURE 16.13 **Severe cul-de-sac disease in a 14-year-old girl**

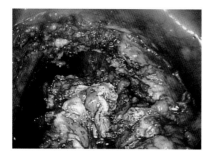

FIGURE 16.14 **Nodule left on rectum in preparation for resection**

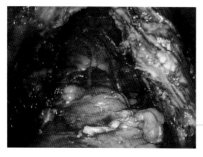

FIGURE 16.15 **Rectum following reanastomosis**

in Figure 16.13. At present, there is no consensus regarding what treatment should be offered to such women.

Technique

Having completed the resection of pelvic endometriosis and having left the residual disease attached to the rectum as described (Figure 16.14), the surgeon must decide on the need to resect a segment of rectum (Figure 16.15 and Video 16.1). Sometimes, preoperative assessment by MRI or transvaginal ultrasound scanning (Figure 16.7) may have given sufficient indication of the need to perform segmental resection. On other occasions, the need may become apparent only during the course of the operation. However, even at laparoscopy, the extent of rectal disease may be difficult to determine. As with disc resection, the presence of deep disease may become apparent only during the course of an attempted shaving of the disease from the rectal surface.

The first step in segmental resection must be the establishment of the likely extent of resection. Since deep disease is not always readily visible and is not infrequently identified for the first time by palpation following mobilisation and exteriorisation of the diseased segment of rectum, the resection margins can be difficult to determine. Whereas the standard mode of segmental anterior rectal resection for cancer requires the resection of the mesorectum with invariable disruption of the pelvic nerves, this is rarely required for the resection for endometriosis. This should result in less damage to the pelvic nerves.

The operation to remove the rectal segment may often commence at the level of the pelvic brim, even though the nearest disease may be some distance caudal, because this allows adequate mobilisation of the rectum so as to carry out reanastomosis without undue tension. Most surgeons now use either an ultrasonic scalpel or monopolar diathermy to perform the operation. The posterior rectal attachment to the mesorectum is opened from the right side at or below the level of the pelvic brim and the dissection is carried through to the left side to create a window in the mesorectum directly below the rectal wall. Following this, close dissection of the rectal tube may be continued distally as far as the pelvic floor if required, but certainly at least 2 cm caudal to the disease to ensure adequacy of excision by means of an Endo GIA® staple gun.

Once the rectum has been separated from the cervix and vagina anteriorly, the distal rectum may be transected below the level of the disease. The area of the rectum to be transected should be stripped of perirectal fat, exposing the rectal serosa to allow exclusion of fat from the anastomosis. Transection may be performed by means of a reticulating Endo GIA® 60 staple gun, which both staples and cuts having inserted three parallel rows of titanium staples on either side of the division. It is unusual to be able to transect the rectum completely with a single set of staples; one or two reloads are frequently required. Guns of less than 60 mm are available but will be associated with the need to perform more reloads. This increases the risk of creating a 'stellate' division and, through the insertion of multiple rows of staples at a single point, the potential to cause devascularisation of the distal rectum in the line of the anastomosis with resultant risk of anastomotic breakdown.

If more than 15 cm of rectum is being removed, it is frequently necessary to carry out further mobilisation of the rectum. This is achieved by division of the mesorectum on the left side from the level of the pelvic brim to the splenic flexure. During this procedure, it is necessary to be observant for the left ureter, which runs close by the rectum as it enters the pelvis. Once the rectum has been mobilised, it will then need to be exteriorised and the ultimate extent of the resection determined. An entirely laparoscopic technique for anterior rectal resection without such need for exteriorisation has previously been described, but this does not permit palpation of the rectum with the associated potential for overlooking nonvisible deep disease in the process. The rectum may be exteriorised through a hole provided by an extension of the 12 mm suprapubic port. To facilitate this, the author employs a wound protector, which serves as a retractor.

The proximal extent of disease may now be established by palpation and inspection and the necessary level for transection determined. Reanastomosis of the rectum may be end to end or end to side. The former allows for less tension in the anastomosis by using the maximum rectal length available, whereas the latter may result in less devascularisation of the anastomotic line. For end to end reanastomosis, the traditional use of crushing and noncrushing clamps has been superceded and the procedure facilitated by use of a purse-string device, which is applied at the site of intended transection. Prior to transection, a purse-string device may be used to facilitate the insertion of a 2.0 polypropylene purse-string proximal to the site of division. The rectum may then be divided and the purse-string device removed leaving the polypropylene suture in place. Most authors now recommend the use of a circular anastomosis gun that fires titanium staples into the rectal wall to secure union. A detachable anvil needs to be inserted into the proximal rectum and secured with a purse-string suture before assembling the gun and firing the staples. To prepare to perform an end-to-side anastomosis, the rectum must be divided with a scalpel proximal to the disease and the anvil of the reanastomosis gun introduced with its shaft pushed through the left side of the rectal wall a few centimetres proximal to the end. The rectum may then be closed using a staple gun such as the PI™ 30 (Autosuture™, Covidien, Mansfield, MA, USA) stapler or the Endo GIA® stapler as described. The rectum can then be restored to the abdominal cavity and the suprapubic port closed.

For reanastomosis, the circular anastomosis gun is then inserted into the rectum. Some degree of anorectal dilatation may be required beforehand to

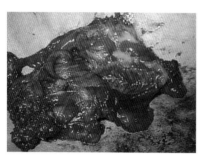

FIGURE 16.16 **Rectal specimen following excision**

facilitate this. The point of the anastomosis gun is advanced by the anticlockwise rotation of its handle until it has pierced the distal rectum. Some surgeons favour piercing the distal rectum in the staple line provided by the Endo GIA® stapler employed earlier, whereas others, for reason of avoiding devascularisation, favour a more posterior placement. Once the spike has been fully introduced, the shaft of the anvil may be slid down over it until firmly locked in position. Before activation of the anastomosis gun, it is vital to ensure that the rectum and sigmoid colon are not rotated in any way for this will lead to obstruction and breakdown of the anastomosis. Next, the spike of the anastomosis gun is withdrawn by rotating the handle of the gun in a clockwise direction, thereby drawing the opposing ends of the rectum together. Anastomosis guns have a marker – usually in the form of a green bar that becomes visible – to indicate adequate closure before firing. The gun is fired by apposition of the handles, which may be held in place for up to 10 seconds. To either loosen the anvil from the anastomosis or tilt it to facilitate its removal, it is again necessary to rotate the handle four half-turns in an anticlockwise direction. The gun may then be withdrawn gently while the surgeon gently rocks it from side to side. Figures 16.14 and 16.15 (page 260), 16.16 and 16.17, respectively, show the disease left on the

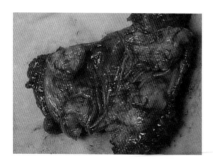

FIGURE 16.17 **Large nodules of endometriosis in the rectum not identifiable at laparoscopy**

rectum before resection, the rectum following reanastomosis and the rectal nodule removed.

A good-quality anastomosis should produce two complete donuts from either side of the anastomosis. These may be inspected to ensure the quality of the anastomosis. An incomplete donut ring may point to a potential inadequacy of the anastomosis. The donuts should be sent for histopathological examination to ensure the absence of endometriosis at the site of reanastomosis.

Integrity of the anastomosis may be tested by filling the pelvis with saline and distending the distal rectum with air insufflated via a rigid sigmoidoscope. Any evidence of air escaping through the anastomosis points to its inadequacy and the defect must be sealed if a defunctioning stoma is not to be performed. This may be achieved by use of a fine absorbable suture. Many surgeons would elect to cover an anastomosis of doubtful integrity with a defunctioning ileostomy.

Some surgeons advocate the use of a rectal drain to reduce postoperative distension of the bowel. This may be in the form of a 30F Foley catheter with a 30 ml balloon that is inflated proximal to the anal sphincter. Such a drain is usually passed spontaneously between days 3 and 6 after surgery. Many surgeons routinely drain the pelvis by means of a nonsuction drain such as a Robinson drain. These are usually removed after 24 hours as there is some evidence that late removal may be associated with an increased rate of anastomotic breakdown.[17]

Endometriosis in the terminal ileum (Figure 16.18), caecum and appendix may coexist with rectal disease and, if present, should be treated at the same time. Such treatment is likely to involve partial or full caecal resection (Video 16.2), appendicectomy and segmental resection of the terminal ileum.

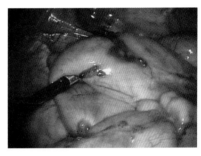

FIGURE 16.18 **Ileal endometriosis**

Clinical results

It is generally difficult to compare the results of different published series because different parameters are measured, and most series do not give specific results pertaining to those women who have undergone an anterior rectal resection. To date, all of the published reports deal with case series rather than randomised trials. Despite this, several authors[11,18,19] have achieved similar results in terms of pain relief. All reported improvement in pelvic pain, dysmenorrhoea, dyspareunia and dyschesia in women who had undergone segmental anterior rectal resection. Redwine and Wright[20] similarly found improvement in all symptoms relating to the cul-de-sac. Interestingly, when the results of English et al.[11] are compared with earlier work[21] conducted in the same unit and using the same surgical technique, it seems that anterior rectal resection achieved much better results than debulking surgery did (clinical cure rate 83%[11] versus 53%[21]). It is impossible to know if this was related to a more complete excision of disease or to denervation. However, the latter is less likely because the investigators used the technique entailing close dissection of the rectal tube, as described previously, and no woman complained of symptoms suggestive of wider neural damage. Although debulking surgery will not remove disease within the bowel or relieve a stricture, disc resection may not be sufficient to remove multifocal or microscopic disease as identified by Kavallaris[22] in 62% of rectal specimens.

Complications

Complications may be significant in terms of both severity and frequency. The most serious complications relate to either bowel or bladder. Anastomotic leakage is a relatively common complication with an incidence of up to 8% for ultra-low anastomosis;[23] the risk is also increased by contemporaneous gynaecological surgery.[17] Morbidity and mortality associated with anastomotic leakage may be reduced by prompt diagnosis and corrective surgery. Leaks most commonly happen once the bowel function has returned between days 3 and 10 after surgery. Any woman who, during this time, develops signs of sepsis or of an acute abdomen should be investigated by means of a Urografin® (Bayer Schering Pharma, Berlin, Germany) enema or a computed tomography scan. If a leak has occurred, the woman should be taken back to theatre, the abdomen washed out and a defunctioning stoma performed. A repeat Urografin enema is then advisable before reversal of the stoma. Fistula formation involving any of the bowel, bladder, ureters and vagina is also a potential complication because all of these organs are very closely approximated. Avoidance of infection, haematoma formation and devascularisation all serve to reduce the risk, as does the deployment of an omental fat pad mobilised and interposed between the different organs.

Radical surgery for advanced and rectovaginal endometriosis carries a significant risk of morbidity but does not appear to protect against further intervention. English et al.[11] reported a cumulative reoperation rate of 19%. Varol et al.[24] identified a reoperation rate of 36% and a recurrence of endometriosis in 15% of women after a 35-month follow-up.

Hysterectomy

The role of hysterectomy performed in conjunction with the resection of severe endometriosis remains in doubt. Hysterectomy does not affect the clinical cure rate but is more likely to be associated with a complete resolution of pain.[11] The presence of adenomyosis or discrete adenomyomas may well be the determining factor in the persistence of significant dysmenorrhoea in women whose severe endometriosis has been resected. The incidence of adenomyosis associated with severe endometriosis is 50%.[21] Although the desire for the retention of fertility may in many instances be the primary factor determining whether hysterectomy is performed, it would seem logical to also advocate hysterectomy if retention of fertility is not required.

Thus, to best advise the individual woman as to what operation is optimal, preoperative determination of the presence of adenomyosis or adenomyomas is recommended. If discrete adenomyomas are identified and if fertility is to be retained, consideration should be given to removal of the adenomyomas at the time of surgery for the endometriosis.

Conclusions

Surgery for severe endometriosis is usually highly complex and carries a real risk of serious morbidity. It is best carried out in centres with multidisciplinary teams of surgeons and others with an interest in the disease and in pain management. Considerable further work is required to determine the most appropriate management of severe disease, particularly in relation to its effect on fertility and ovarian reserve, for which no data are currently available.

References

1 Cullen T S. The distribution of adenomyomas containing uterine mucosa. *Arch Surg* 1920;1:215–83.

2 Hudelist G, English J, Thomas A, Tinelli A, Singer C F, Keckstein J. Diagnostic accuracy of transvaginal ultrasound for non-invasive diagnosis of bowel endometriosis: systematic review and meta-analysis. *Ultrasound Obstet Gynecol* 2011; 37:257–63.

3 Faccioli N, Foti G, Manfredi R, Minardi P, Spoto E, Ruffo G, et al. Evaluation of colonic involvement in endometriosis: double-contrast barium enema vs. magnetic resonance imaging. *Abdom Imaging* 2010;35:414–21.

4 Takeuchi H, Kuwatsura R, Kitade M, Kikuchi I, Shimanuki H, Kiroshita K. A novel technique using magnetic resonance imaging jelly for evaluation of rectovaginal endometriosis. *Fertil Steril* 2005;83:442–7.

5 Garry R, Clayton R, Hawe J. The effect of endometriosis and its radical laparoscopic excision on quality of life indicators. *BJOG* 2000;107:44–54.

6 Farquhar C. Endometriosis. *BMJ* 2007;334:249–53.

7 Donnez J, Nisolle M, Smoes P, Gillet N, Beguin S, Casanas-Roux F. Peritoneal endometriosis and "endometriotic" nodules of the rectovaginal septum are two different entities. *Fertil Steril* 1996;66:362–8.

8 Donnez J, Nisolle M, Gillerot S, Smets M, Bassil S, Casanas-Roux F. Rectovaginal septum nodules: a series of 500 cases. *Br J Obstet Gynaecol* 1997;104:1914–8.

9 Yeung P P, Schwayder J, Pasic R P. Laparoscopic management of endometriosis. *J Minim Invasive Gynecol* 2009;16:269–81.

10 Hart R J, Hickey M, Maouris P, Buckett W. Excisional surgery versus ablative surgery for ovarian endometriomata. *Cochrane Database Syst Rev* 2008;(2):CD004992.

11 English J, Kenney N, Edmonds S, Baig MK, Miles A. Limited segmental anterior rectal resection for the treatment of rectovaginal endometriosis: pain and complications. *Gynecol Surg* 2007;4:107–10.

12 Urbach D R, Reedijk M, Richard C S, Lie K I, Ross T M. Bowel resection for intestinal endometriosis. *Dis Colon Rectum* 1998;41:1158–64.

13 Jerby B L, Kessler H, Falcone T, Milsom J W. Laparoscopic management of colorectal endometriosis. *Surg Endosc* 1999; 13:1125–8.

14 Bailey H R, Ott M T, Hartendorp P. Aggressive surgical management for advanced colorectal endometriosis. *Dis Colon Rectum* 1994;37:747–53.

15 Redwine D B. Laparoscopic en bloc resection for the treatment of the obliterated cul-de-sac in endometriosis. *J Reprod Med* 1992;37:695–8.

16 Paun B C, Cassie S, MacLean A R, Dixon E, Bule W D. Postoperative complications following surgery for rectal cancer. *Ann Surg* 2010;251:807–18.

17 Boccola M A, Buettner P G, Rozen W M, Siu S R, Stetz R, Ho Y H. Risk factors and outcomes for anastomotic leakage in colorectal surgery: a single-institution analysis of 1576 patients. *World J Surg* 2011;35:186–95.

18 Keckstein J, Ulrich U, Kandolf O, Wiesinger H, Wustlich M. [Laparoscopic therapy of intestinal endometriosis and the ranking of drug treatment]. *Zentralbl Gynäkol* 2003;125: 259–66. Article in German.

19 Thomassin I, Bazot M, Detchev R, Barranger E, Cortez A, Darai E. Symptoms before and after surgical removal of colorectal endometriosis that are assessed by magnetic resonance imaging and rectal endoscopic sonography. *Am J Obstet Gynecol* 2004;190:1264–71.

20 Redwine D B, Wright J T. Laparoscopic treatment of complete obliteration of the cul-de-sac associated with endometriosis: long-term follow-up of en bloc resection. *Fertil Steril* 2001;76:358–65.

21 Ford J, English J, Miles W A, Giannopoulos T. Pain, quality of life and complications following the radical resection of rectovaginal endometriosis. *BJOG* 2004;111:353–6.

22 Kavallaris A, Köhler C, Kühne-Heid R, Schneider A. Histopathological extent of rectal invasion by rectovaginal endometriosis. *Hum Reprod* 2003;18:1323–7.

23 Platell C, Barwood N, Dorfman G, Makin G. The incidence of anastomotic leaks in patients undergoing colorectal surgery. *Colorectal Dis* 2007;9:71–9.

24 Varol N, Maher P, Healey M, Woods R, Wood C, Hill D, et al. Rectal surgery for endometriosis – should we be aggressive? *J Am Assoc Gynecol Laparosc* 2003;10:182–9.

17 Bowel surgery

Sanjay Wijeyekoon, George Pandis and Alastair Windsor

Introduction

The discipline of pelvic surgery has historically been divided into three areas, with colorectal surgeons being principally concerned with conditions of the posterior compartment containing the rectum and anus, gynaecologists managing conditions of the middle compartment and urologists managing the anterior compartment. Despite these artificial divisions, pelvic pathology crosses boundaries such that each specialty must have a working knowledge of inter-disciplinary pathologies that may be encountered outside the artificial specialty confines.

The anatomically close proximity of the rectosigmoid and anus to the fallopian tubes, ovaries and posterior surface of the uterus has consequences for both the diagnosis and the treatment of pelvic pathology regardless of the structure of origin. Colorectal inflammatory conditions such as Crohn's disease or diverticulitis can closely mimic the presentation of pelvic inflammatory disease or endometriosis both clinically and radiologically. Regardless of aetiology, any pelvic inflammation can lead to obliteration of the plane between the colorectum and vagina and the formation of adhesions between pelvic organs. The distortion of the normal anatomy may compromise any operative approach, necessitating at least partial excision of the reproductive organs when performing an anterior resection or proctocolectomy for a primary colorectal pathology. Unfamiliarity with both anatomy and techniques between specialties may thus compromise outcomes, such as adequate resection margins when tackling pelvic pathology originating from an organ managed primarily by another specialty.

This dilemma is particularly well demonstrated with the example of intestinal endometriosis, where colorectal surgeons have had to adapt and modify their generally radical surgical approach to the colorectum and gynaecologists are faced with disease extending into the unfamiliar territory within the intestine. Although two reports indicate that gynaecologists alone can satisfactorily perform the advanced laparoscopic procedures required to treat intestinal endometriosis,[1,2] most would accept that the collaboration between gynaecologist and colorectal surgeon is also essential during the pre-, intra- and postoperative management of this disease. In fact, the gynaecologist may lack experience in resecting structures such as the bowel, particularly the lower rectum, which could lead to incomplete disease excision. On the other hand, the colorectal surgeon may not encounter endometriosis frequently enough to obtain sufficient experience to adequately manage the condition and its complications. Adhesion and retraction of the rectosigmoid colon in the cul-de-sac can often obscure endometriotic nodules underneath and the actual depth can be missed. The pelvic dissection must be pursued until the soft yellow fat within the septum is identified and the entire rectum is freed from the posterior vagina to remove all the disease. In addition, preoperative assessment and postoperative short- and long-term complications are dealt with more efficiently in a multidisciplinary environment.

The purpose of this chapter is to discuss the role of the colorectal surgeon in the laparoscopic management of benign gynaecological conditions and in the associated pre- and postoperative care.

Current status of laparoscopic colorectal surgery in the UK

When surgery is being considered, the laparoscopic route to deliver therapy is becoming increasingly popular and has clearly established benefits such as reduced postoperative pain, faster discharge from hospital and better cosmesis. Currently, in developed countries, a large number of gynaecological procedures are performed on an elective or emergency basis. These include procedures for most benign gynaecological conditions and certain types of gynaecological malignancies as well as innovative procedures designed to treat urogynaecological and adolescent conditions. Although there has been a great emphasis on continuous training and the technology has been constantly improved, laparoscopic procedures are still associated with risks. These mainly comprise visceral, vascular and urogenital injuries. The incidence of complications associated with laparoscopic procedures varies considerably among reports, depending on the experience of the surgeons and the complexity of operations undertaken. Figures range between 1.0/1000 and 12.5/1000 for all complications.[3,4] In the UK, training in gynaecological laparoscopy is overseen by the British Society for Gynaecological Endoscopy in conjunction with the Royal College of Obstetricians and Gynaecologists, and similarly the Royal College of Surgeons and the Association of Coloproctology of Great Britain and Ireland oversees training in laparoscopic colorectal surgery. Similar authorised bodies have been created in most developed countries.

Laparoscopic colorectal surgery still remains investigative to a great extent with a growing but not as yet comprehensive practice by UK colorectal surgeons. Laparoscopic colorectal surgery in the presence of specific gynaecological conditions such as endometriosis is even more technically challenging and remains in the domain of a few specialist centres worldwide. The required skills to adequately perform the myriad operations to treat endometriosis far exceed those necessary for colorectal cancer alone. Few laparoscopic colorectal surgeons would be entirely comfortable with the technical demands to truly perform these operations laparoscopically.

In general, pelvic nonmechanical bowel conditions requiring surgical intervention, such as anorectal cancer and inflammatory bowel disease, invariably involve segmental intestinal resection with or without anastomosis to achieve adequate clearance of the disease. Segmental bowel resection is most frequently performed by open surgery, but advances in stapling devices and minimally invasive instrument technology have encouraged use of the laparoscopic route. Although requiring a different set of skills from open surgery, laparoscopic techniques have become widely accepted following the publication of landmark high-quality trial data from the colorectal cancer setting.[5–10] With benign conditions such as endometriosis (which can affect the rectum in the pelvis), a less radical approach than segmental bowel resection can be offered. From a technical point of view, however, less radical nonsegmental resection (shaving, disc excision or stapling) requires extra technical skills from the operator that are often above and beyond what is experienced by, and familiar to, even dedicated advanced laparoscopic colorectal surgeons during their training period in the UK. The necessity for such extra technical skill along with unfamiliarity with the disease process requires close collaboration between colorectal surgeons and gynaecologists. This has led to a centralisation of practice to a few centres in the UK.

Evolution of laparoscopic colorectal surgery

Early experiences with the laparoscopic technique began in the setting of colonic cancer. The initial results of colectomy were unfavourable: rates of wound tumour implants were higher than expected and there were concerns about oncological outcomes in the short and long term.[4,11] Several international randomised controlled trials were then initiated to address concerns regarding the safety of laparoscopic colorectal surgery. Each trial was designed to primarily test the hypothesis that the control of curable colon cancer achieved with laparoscopic colectomy is equivalent to that achieved with open surgery. Four phase III randomised controlled trials have now been completed and have reported benefits for laparoscopic colectomy: the Barcelona study,[12] the Clinical Outcomes of Surgical Therapy (COST) study,[13] the Colon Cancer Laparoscopic or Open Resection (COLOR) study[14] and the Conventional versus Laparoscopically assisted Surgery in Colorectal Cancer (CLASICC) study.[9,10]

In these studies, laparoscopic surgery significantly prolonged the operating time but reduced the duration of hospital stay compared with open surgery. Laparoscopic surgery significantly reduced the use of narcotics and oral analgesics and sped up the return of bowel function and adoption of a normal diet. Moreover, the laparoscopic approach was associated with a decrease in the number of lymph nodes retrieved, an increase in the risk of anastomotic leakage and a decrease in the risk of operative and perioperative mortality compared with open resection; however, these differences were not statistically significant. Recurrence and survival data have been reported only for the Barcelona and COST trials; these studies show that women treated with laparoscopic colectomy have no survival disadvantage.[9]

Evidence to support laparoscopic rectal resectional surgery is derived almost exclusively from rectal cancer studies.[9,10,14] In people with curable rectal cancer, laparoscopic colectomy is now accepted as an alternative to open colectomy. However, the role of laparoscopic rectal resection in routine practice remains controversial, not just in terms of oncological equivalence but also because of continuing concerns related to technical feasibility.

Colorectal request for benign gynaecological surgery

The assistance of a colorectal surgeon is usually requested before an elective procedure involving pelvic organs and the colorectum or as an emergency related to a visceral complication or unexpected visceral injury. Although colorectal assistance may be requested for a variety of planned surgeries (usually those complicated by adhesions or concomitant pathologies), the most common benign gynaecological condition of the pelvis requiring a joint operative effort is without doubt rectovaginal endometriosis.

Planning for a colorectal intervention

Joint procedures require the desire and ability to work in harmony and adopt different surgical techniques or modifications that best suit the collaborating members of the surgical team. Knowledge of the basic strategy and the most common instruments used by colorectal surgeons allows for a reduction of the operative risk and a better surgical outcome.

Diagnostic tests

Colorectal disorders can broadly be divided into anatomical (luminal obstruction, inflammatory or fistulating disease) and functional disease states. The history often allows the clinician to localise the problem to the right side, the left side or the anorectal region. A small percentage of women, however, present with nebulous symptoms and signs that cannot be localised to a particular site of the bowel. In these situations, a combination of ileocolonoscopy and axial imaging in the form of a computed tomography (CT) or magnetic resonance imaging (MRI) scan can be helpful.

Ileocolonoscopy is the gold standard investigation for luminal bowel disease and has the advantage of being potentially therapeutic and diagnostic. If the history suggests that the clinical problem is likely to be located in the distal (left) colon or rectum, flexible sigmoidoscopy may suffice. Pelvic ultrasound has a limited role in assessing colorectal pathology outside the anus itself, where endoanal ultrasound has been used to assess anal sphincter integrity.

For women presenting with nebulous symptoms, abdominal pain or a mass, a satisfactory ileocolonoscopy is often insufficient to exclude serious pathology and additional axial imaging is essential. The choice of CT versus MRI is a matter of clinical judgement and local availability as both provide similar information with comparable sensitivity and specificity. In younger women of child-bearing age, MRI has advantages in avoiding radiation exposure. CT has the added advantage of being able to provide more detailed information regarding the colon and rectum in the form of a CT pneumocolon (CT colonoscopy with faecal tagging).

Bowel preparation

Oral bowel-cleansing agents have traditionally been prescribed before elective colorectal surgery in an effort to reduce the likelihood of surgical complications arising from anastomotic leakage. This practice is predominantly based on observational data and expert opinion.[15] However, opinion is increasingly divided on the merits of bowel preparation in this context. There is an increasing body of evidence to suggest that bowel preparation is not required for most procedures.[16,17] At present, women who undergo abdominoperineal excision of the rectum, right hemicolectomy, total proctocolectomy or an

TABLE 17.1 **Oral bowel-cleansing agents available in the UK**

Brand name	Manufacturer	Active ingredient(s)
Klen-Prep®	Norgine Pharmaceuticals (Harefield, UK)	Polyethylene glycol
Moviprep®	Norgine Pharmaceuticals (Harefield, UK)	Polyethylene glycol
Fleet Phospho-Soda®	Laboratorios Casen Fleet SLU (Madrid, Spain)	Sodium dihydrogen phosphate dehydrate and disodium phosphate dodecahydrate
Picolax®	Ferring Pharmaceuticals (Langley, UK)	Sodium picosulphate and magnesium citrate
Citrafleet®	Laboratorios Casen Fleet SLU (Madrid, Spain)	Sodium picosulphate and magnesium citrate
Citramag®	Sanochemia (Bristol, UK)	Magnesium carbonate and citric acid

ileoanal pouch operation are generally not prescribed oral bowel-cleansing agents. However, oral bowel-cleansing agents are used more widely in women undergoing anterior resection and left-sided resections. Postoperative rapid recovery programmes are being increasingly employed and usually avoid bowel preparation. In the light of these uncertainties, we recommend that the prescription of oral bowel-cleansing agents is individualised according to the planned surgery. A number of different oral bowel-cleansing agents are currently available in the UK (Table 17.1).

Polyethylene glycols (macrogols) reduce fluid and electrolyte shifts as they are nonabsorbable isosmotic solutions that pass through the bowel without net absorption or secretion. These preparations must be diluted in large volumes of water (up to 4 l), with the initial 2–3 l taken the night before surgery and the remaining 1–2 l the following morning. A proportion of the ingested water is reabsorbed and can in some circumstances lead to water intoxication in predisposed patients. Moviprep® (Norgine Pharmaceuticals, Harefield, UK) allows adequate bowel preparation to be achieved within 12 hours.[18] In addition, pretreatment with domperidone or metoclopramide to facilitate gastric emptying may be considered. Oral sodium phosphate preparations are hyperosmotic and promote colonic evacuation by drawing large volumes of water into the colon (1–1.8 l of water per 45 ml of preparation). These preparations are typically diluted in much smaller volumes of water than the polyethylene glycols (approximately 250 ml). Sodium phosphate preparations have been compared with polyethylene glycols in numerous studies and have generally been found to be safe, equally or more effective, and consistently better tolerated.[19-22] A meta-analysis of eight controlled trials concluded that an 'adequate' preparation was equally likely with sodium phosphate or polyethylene glycol preparations, but that an 'excellent' preparation was more likely with sodium phosphate preparations.[23]

Abdominal entry

Abdominal entry in laparoscopic surgery can be complicated by visceral or vascular injury. At present, four techniques are used to create a pneumoperitoneum: Veress needle insertion, direct trocar insertion, optical trocar insertion and open laparoscopy (Hasson entry). With the first two approaches, entry is blind and the reported complication rate is lower than 1%.[24]

Some studies have revealed a higher rate of visceral injuries with the open-entry technique.[24,25] A 2004 survey identified 106 gynaecologists (57%) who used only the closed-entry technique.[25] There were very few reported complications – 31/31 532 procedures (0.1%) – despite the fact that the pneumoperitoneum was established by the closed-entry technique even in individuals potentially at high risk of entry-related complications (previous laparotomy, obesity). Eighty-one gynaecologists used both entry techniques, but the open-entry technique was used infrequently (in only 2.0% of cases) for suspected adhesions or previous laparotomy (90%) and obesity (7%), or in very thin patients (3%). These 81 gynaecologists reported 20 027 closed-entry procedures and 579 open-entry procedures and complication rates of 0.12% and 1.38%, respectively ($P<0.001$).[25]

Working port positions

Port positioning will be influenced by previous surgery and abdominal wall scarring. If there has been a previous midline incision, there may be small-bowel and omental adhesions that will need to be divided to create space to perform the surgery.

In surgery involving the left side of the colon, commonly employed steps include retraction of the bowel, mobilisation, mesenteric vessel division and, finally, division and anastomosis of the bowel. Retraction of the left side of the colon is achieved by holding the bowel with a 5 mm atraumatic grasper held by the nondominant hand; the grasper is placed through a port in the right upper quadrant. Judicious tilting of the operating table can facilitate retraction of the colon and exposure of the paracolic gutter.

In anterior resection of the sigmoid and the rectum, the splenic flexure often requires mobilisation and the working port placement must reflect that

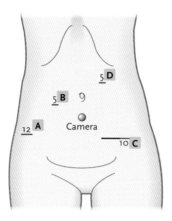

FIGURE 17.1
Laparoscopic port
placement for anterior
resection

(Figure 17.1). A 12 mm trocar is placed in the right lower quadrant (port site A, Figure 17.1). This is used for insertion of a linear stapler. When a low rectal dissection is anticipated, this port should be placed as low as possible on the abdominal wall. Following insertion of the umbilical primary trocar, the right inferior epigastric artery can be identified and avoided. A 5 mm trocar is placed on the right side above the level of the umbilicus (port site B, Figure 17.1). A further 5 mm or 10 mm port is placed at the left lower quadrant for an assistant to provide elevation and traction of the sigmoid colon to facilitate a 'medial to lateral' position of the rectum and sigmoid colon (port site C, Figure 17.1). When splenic flexure mobilisation is anticipated, a further 5 mm port (port site D, Figure 17.1) should be placed more caudally to facilitate the dissection around the splenic flexure. In a standard sigmoid resection, these four ports are sufficient. Port sites A and B will be used by the operator and port sites C and D (Figure 17.1) will be used by the assistant for traction of the mesentery and/or the rectum. Where bowel resection is carried out at the end of a gynaecological procedure, the exact port position may be modified.

Specific instruments

Full videoendoscopy facilities are required. For routine laparoscopic colonic surgery, the following instruments are necessary: two atraumatic bowel graspers (Johann fenestrated grasper or equivalent), a 5 mm cutting device (choice of which depends on the surgeon's preference), a Babcock-type bowel-grasping device and a linear reticulating stapling device that can be used to divide the mesenteric vessels and to divide the bowel with a 45 mm staple line. To facilitate adequate mobility within a narrow pelvis, laparoscopic retractors can be used via a suprapubic port.

A nasogastric tube and urinary catheter are passed when the woman is anaesthetised. All procedures are performed with the woman in the Lloyd–Davies position. A pneumoperitoneum is created using a standard technique and is maintained at 12–15 mmHg by an automatic carbon dioxide insufflator. A 10 mm 0° or 30° laparoscope is inserted through a subumbilical port and an initial diagnostic laparoscopy is performed. Following peritoneoscopy, the other working ports are inserted.

Planned laparotomy

There are no universally accepted criteria regarding when to abandon the laparoscopic approach. A greater body mass index (BMI), operator experience and a higher American Society of Anesthesiology classification have all been implicated as preoperative factors that influence a surgeon's decision to perform a laparotomy from the outset. Adequate management of a large bulky mass on preoperative axial imaging with infiltration or adherence to adjacent structures is very likely to require conversion to laparotomy. Often, once the woman has been anaesthetised and paralysed, subclinical masses become apparent that may influence the surgeon's decision to proceed directly to a laparotomy. Furthermore, manipulation of a large mass with laparoscopic instruments may not be possible and a large abdominal wall incision may be required to extract an en bloc resected specimen. Nevertheless, an initial laparoscopy is often worthwhile.

The majority of studies describe laparoscopic treatment of colorectal endometriosis irrespective of the extent of disease and the surgical procedure. Thus, superficial and disc excision are considered together with colon, or even rectal, resection. The heterogeneity in the mix of procedures makes interpretation of the conversion rates from laparoscopic to open surgery difficult, with rates varying from 0% to 26.3%.[26–35] Data from the rectal cancer setting (the CLASICC trial[10,36]) indicate that conversion rates may be even higher. In this trial, 39% of laparoscopically assisted procedures in women with rectal cancer were converted to open surgery. A high BMI was found to be independently predictive of conversion in a subgroup analysis.[10]

Clearly, a learning curve exists for laparoscopic colorectal resection for endometriosis, with poorer outcomes reported for an early series (fewer than 30 women) versus later cohorts.[37] The rate of laparoconversion, operating time, estimated amount of blood loss and recurrence rate declined as the surgeon's experience increased.[37]

Complications and their management

The complications following colorectal surgery related to gynaecological pathology have now been firmly established. These risks include visceral injury, pelvic autonomic nerve injury, anastomotic leakage, ureteric injury, postoperative infective complications, colovaginal fistulae and stoma formation. The long-term experience with open pelvic segmental resectional surgery allows for reasonably accurate preoperative counselling of women regarding the risks and benefits of any proposed procedure.

The seriousness of vascular injury during abdominal access is high in comparison with visceral injury. Vascular injuries are rare and no evidence-based recommendations for treatment can be given. Injuries to the main vascular structures need an immediate conversion to laparotomy and surgical repair. By contrast, small bowel injuries can be treated laparoscopically. Severe lesions sometimes require segment resections and conversion to open surgery. Injuries of the liver or spleen are manageable with laparoscopic devices. If severe bleeding continues, a laparotomy is recommended.

The choice of incision for laparotomy depends on the area that needs to be exposed, the elective or emergency nature of the operation and the surgeon's preference. A transverse incision is associated with fewer early postoperative complications and a lower incidence of late incisional hernia. However, abdominal or neural dysfunction after transverse access may occur because of nerve, muscle or vessel interruption. A midline incision is still the incision of choice in conditions that require rapid abdominal entry or where the preoperative diagnosis is uncertain, because it is quicker and can easily be extended.

Visceral complications

These can occur during creation of the pneumoperitoneum or during the operative portion of laparoscopy. Both types of injury are more frequent in the face of previous surgery or prior infection that has resulted in the fixation of the bowel to other structures, particularly to the anterior abdominal wall. Approximately 40% of bowel injuries are entry-related and occur with the insufflation needle or with a trocar. The incidence of laparoscopically induced gastrointestinal injury has been reported to be 0.13% by van der Voort and colleagues.[38] In their review, the most common location of injury was the small bowel (55.8%), followed by the large intestine (38.6%) and, less commonly, the stomach (3.9%). Common signs that a bowel injury has occurred include foul-smelling gas, return of bowel contents, high insufflation pressures and asymmetric distension. Early diagnosis of bowel injuries is critical because the associated morbidity and mortality seem to depend on the time at which the injury is identified.[38] If there is concern about anterior wall adhesions, a simple step to preclude a delay in their diagnosis is to view the initial trocar site through an alternative port.

Injury to the gastrointestinal tract may occur during the operative portion of the surgery as well. In the review of 273 bowel injuries by van der Voort and colleagues, three (1.1%) injuries occurred with the grasping forceps and two (0.7%) injuries occurred with the scissors. By contrast, 70 (25.6%) thermal injuries occurred with either a coagulating instrument or the laser.[38] In addition, both electrothermal bipolar vessel sealers and ultrasonic coagulating shears seem to be superior in achieving haemostasis compared with monopolar and bipolar electrocoagulation devices. The former also seem to be safer because lateral thermal injury is more common with monopolar and bipolar instruments. However, lateral thermal injury is possible with any method of coagulation.

Tulikangas and colleagues[39] evaluated characteristics of laparoscopic injuries with several coagulating instruments and documented an average length of injury for various devices. The length of injury for the monopolar cautery was 0.6±0.2 cm for the ureter, 2.1±0.4 cm for the bladder and 1.8±0.3 cm for the rectum. The average length of injury for the bipolar cautery was 0.4±0.2 cm for the ureter, 1.3±0.2 cm for the bladder and 1.3±0.2 cm for the rectum. For the ultrasonic coagulating shears, the average length of injury was 0.5±0.2 cm for the ureter, 0.9±0.2 cm for the bladder and 0.7±0.2 cm for the rectum.

Early perforation develops during or directly after surgery, whereas late perforations may manifest several days to weeks following the surgery. If the diagnosis of a full-thickness perforation is delayed, sepsis, multiorgan failure and even death may occur. Superficial thermal injuries to the bowel can often be repaired by a laparoscopically guided purse-string suture placed beyond the thermally affected tissues. If a perforation has been complete and the site of injury is not directly visible, the surgeon should proceed with laparotomy to adequately explore the perforation site and make sure that a second perforation is not missed.

Pelvic nerve injury

Bladder and sexual dysfunction secondary to pelvic nerve injury are recognised complications of rectal resection. Women have often been excluded from assessment of sexual function after proctectomy in randomised controlled trials. The reasons for the exclusion of women in these trials are not entirely clear. Nevertheless, dyspareunia is clearly recognised as a complication following rectal surgery. Contributing factors such as a tight introitus, a vaginoperineal fistula, uterine prolapse or a displaced uterus have all been documented with an incidence of up to 7% following rectal excision for inflammatory bowel disease.[40]

Anastomotic leak

Anastomotic leak rates following segmental colorectal resection for intestinal endometriosis have been reported to be between 0% and 5.8%.[30,35,41,42]

Anastomotic dehiscence is a recognised complication following both open and laparoscopic intestinal resection. Furthermore, rectal shaving procedures have a recognised delayed perforation rate. Anastomotic dehiscence should be suspected in women who do not make rapid progress following their index surgery and those with a temperature or rising inflammatory markers. The investigation of choice is a CT scan, which is highly sensitive and specific. Anastomotic leakage can result in gas or faecal discharge from the incisional wound, vagina or the drain tract. Faecal peritonitis, an intra-abdominal abscess or a pelvic abscess near the anastomotic site without an obvious faecal fistula need to be considered as well.

Once identified, leaks can be managed conservatively with radiological drainage of pelvic sepsis and antibiotics. Large anastomotic leaks with peritonitis invariably require laparotomy and faecal diversion with a proximal stoma. Many of these women never have intestinal continuity restored.

An anastomotic leak following rectal surgery is associated with a postoperative mortality rate of between 6% and 22%. Furthermore, it has been shown to decrease long-term survival. A recent meta-analysis of randomised controlled trials of anterior resection in the cancer setting has shown that a defunctioning stoma provides a clear benefit because it significantly reduces leakage and reoperation rates. The presence of a defunctioning stoma had no influence on the mortality rate, though.[43] However, a number of points remain to be evaluated critically. First, routine creation of a stoma will reduce quality of life in the subgroup of women who would not have any complications. Second, selective or nonroutine use of faecal diversion is supported by the knowledge that stoma placement itself is a source of morbidity, which is reported to be as high as 30%.[44] These complications may even lead to mortality after elective reversal of the stoma (0–2.3%). Furthermore, the closure of a diverting stoma requires a second hospital stay and additional surgery.

Ureteric injury

After gynaecological procedures, colorectal surgery is the next most common cause of iatrogenic ureteric injuries. Together, low anterior resection (LAR) and abdominal perineal resection (APR) account for 9% of all such incidences.[45] The incidence of ureteral injury during LAR or APR is 0.3–5.7%.[45] The left ureter is involved more often than the right ureter because it may be elevated with the sigmoid mesentery and mistaken for a mesenteric vessel.

Postoperative infective complications

The incidence of postoperative infective complications from colon surgery has been estimated at between 10% and 30% according to selected series.[30,35,46–48] Sepsis of abdominal origin can present as a local or generalised peritonitis or as enterocolitis, septicaemia, an abscess, a phlegmon or another enteric infection. The diagnosis is sometimes difficult, but it is important to differentiate infections that will respond to conservative treatment from those that require surgical intervention.

Rectovaginal fistulae

The reported incidence of rectovaginal fistulae is 3.2–10.3%.[28,31,32,46,49]

Stoma formation

A stoma may be performed electively during surgery or in response to a postoperative complication, such as a fistula (Figure 17.2) Stoma rates quoted in the literature vary between studies. Some series report none, whereas others report overall rates of 2–10%.[50]

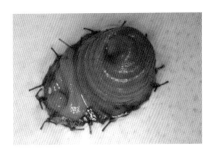

FIGURE 17.2 **Stoma**

Intestinal endometriosis: the colorectal surgeon's view

Intestinal endometriosis is encountered by colorectal surgeons either as an incidental finding in women undergoing emergency surgery for abdominal pain or in the context of a planned resection for established endometriosis that is managed by a multidisciplinary team. The types of procedure that can be performed for intestinal endometriosis include rectal shaving, disc resection and stapled resection.

Rectal shaving

Rectal shaving is performed by excising a serosal disc of endometriosis off the rectal wall laparoscopically.[30,51] This technique requires the operating surgeon to reinforce the excised area with intracorporeal sutures to avoid the risk of fistulation or delayed perforation at the site of treatment.

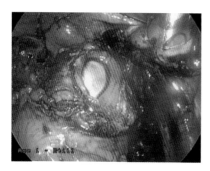

FIGURE 17.3 **Disc resection**

Disc resection

Disc resection is suitable for lesions on the anterior surface of the rectum that involve less than 50% of the circumference of the rectal wall (Figure 17.3). Anterior wall discoid excision using a circular stapler has proved a suitable alternative to shaving procedures. Alternatively, the area can be excised and the defect closed using standard laparoscopic suturing techniques. Disc resection may diminish the risk of serious complications such as bowel fistulae or anastomosis dehiscence.[52]

It is unsuitable for long lesions. For deep endometriosis with rectal muscularis involvement, the debate as to the best approach continues between advocates of the shaving technique versus supporters of bowel resection, despite little evidence for better improvement with bowel resection.

A prospective analysis of 500 cases (under 40 years old) of deep endometriotic nodules excised successfully by laparoscopic nodule resection described very reasonable outcomes for conservative 'shaving' or debulking surgery.[53] In this series, of the 388 women who wished to conceive, 221 (57%) became pregnant naturally and 107 by means of IVF. In total, 328 women (84%) conceived. The overall recurrence rate was 8%, with a significantly lower recurrence rate ($P<0.05$) in women who became pregnant (3.6%) than in those who did not (15%). Severe pelvic pain recurred in 16–20% of women who failed to conceive or who were not interested in conceiving. The incidence of major complications was minimal and included: rectal perforation in seven cases (1.4%); ureteral injury in four cases (0.8%); blood loss of over 300 ml in one case (0.2%); and urinary retention in four cases (0.8%).

These data indicate that in young women, conservative surgery using the shaving technique that preserves organs can yield a high pregnancy rate with low complication and recurrence rates.[53,54] The recurrence rate is, however, significantly lower for segmental versus disc excision.[40,55]

Stapled resection

The decision to resect the diseased rectum (or on occasions the diseased colon) depends on the extent of bowel involvement and, in particular, on whether the lumen of the bowel is in some way compromised. This could be the result of disease itself occluding the lumen but is more often the result of

the fibrosis stricturing the wall of the bowel. Following laparoscopic ablation of endometriosis elsewhere in the pelvis, the
rectum is mobilised around disease present on the anterior
rectal wall. This involves lateral and anterior extraperitoneal
rectal dissection. The latter dissection mobilises the vagina
from the rectum by a sufficient length necessary to allow subsequent anastomosis following resection of the diseased segment. The bowel is then divided distal to the involvement and
the proximal bowel (including disease and colon) delivered
through a small Pfannenstiel incision. The resection takes

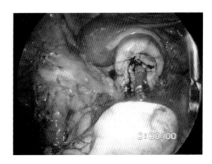

FIGURE 17.4 **Anastomosis**

place extracorporeally and then the bowel is returned to the abdominal cavity
and the pneumoperitoneum re-established prior to the stapled anastomosis
(Figure 17.4).

The first randomised controlled trial of laparoscopically assisted versus
open colorectal resection for endometriosis was published in 2010,[26] focusing on perioperative complications and improvement in symptoms, quality
of life and fertility. In this trial, 52 women with colorectal endometriosis were
randomised to undergo laparoscopically assisted or open colorectal resection
with a primary endpoint of an improvement in dyschesia. The trial identified
significant improvements in digestive symptoms, gynaecological symptoms
and general symptoms such as back pain following both open and laparoscopic surgery. Although no difference in quality of life was noted between
the groups, median blood loss was lower in the laparoscopy group ($P<0.05$)
and the total number of complications was higher in the open surgery group
($P=0.04$); two (7.6%) women in the laparoscopy group required conversion
to open surgery. The pregnancy rate was higher in the laparoscopy group
($P=0.006$), with a cumulative pregnancy rate of 60%. This landmark study
supports the laparoscopic technique as a safe option for women requiring
colorectal resection.

Video 17.1 provides an example of laparoscopic bowel resection.

Conclusion

It is well known that laparoscopic bowel resection carries a risk of major
postoperative complications and that the proper indications for laparoscopic
bowel surgery in women with endometriosis are not yet clear. Laparoscopic
bowel resections should be performed only after careful preoperative evaluation of women's symptoms, a radiological examination of the bowel and
an intraoperative confirmation of the degree of intestinal involvement. In

our opinion, in selected women whose bowel lumen is largely restricted and whose bowel function is greatly reduced, laparoscopic bowel resection can be carried out safely with good long-term results. Although complications are not frequent, when they do occur they can often be serious and long lasting. Therefore, a multidisciplinary approach with a team of gynaecologists and colorectal surgeons currently offers the best solution in assisting women through a mentally and physically demanding journey.

References

1 Pereira R M, Zanatta A, Serafini P C, Redwine D. The feasibility of laparoscopic bowel resection performed by a gynaecologist to treat endometriosis. *Curr Opin Obstet Gynecol* 2010;22:344–53.

2 Pereira R M, Zanatta A, Preti C D, de Paula F J, da Motta E L, Serafini P C. Should the gynecologist perform laparoscopic bowel resection to treat endometriosis? Results over 7 years in 168 patients. *J Minim Invasive Gynecol* 2009;16:472–9.

3 Lam A, Khong S Y, Bignardi T. Principles and strategies for dealing with complications in laparoscopy. *Curr Opin Obstet Gynecol* 2010;22:315–9.

4 Wexner S D, Cohen S M. Port site metastases after laparoscopic colorectal surgery for cure of malignancy. *Br J Surg* 1995;82:295–8.

5 Colon Cancer Laparoscopic or Open Resection Study Group, Buunen M, Veldkamp R, Hop W C, Kuhry E, Jeekel J, Haglind E, et al. Survival after laparoscopic surgery versus open surgery for colon cancer: long-term outcome of a randomised clinical trial. *Lancet Oncol* 2009;10:44–52.

6 Veldkamp R, Kuhry E, Hop W C, Jeekel J, Kazemier G, Bonjer H J, et al.; Colon Cancer Laparoscopic or Open Resection Study Group (COLOR). Laparoscopic surgery versus open surgery for colon cancer: short-term outcomes of a randomised trial. *Lancet Oncol* 2005;6:477–84.

7 Murray A, Lourenco T, de Verteuil R, Hernandez R, Fraser C, McKinley A, et al. Clinical effectiveness and cost-effectiveness of laparoscopic surgery for colorectal cancer: systematic reviews and economic evaluation. *Health Technol Assess* 2006;10:1–141, iii–iv.

8 Lourenco T, Murray A, Grant A, McKinley A, Krukowski Z, Vale L. Laparoscopic surgery for colorectal cancer: safe and effective? – A systematic review. *Surg Endosc* 2008;22: 1146–60.

9 Laparoscopically assisted colectomy is as safe and effective as open colectomy in people with colon cancer Abstracted from: Nelson H, Sargent D, Wieand HS, et al; for the Clinical Outcomes of Surgical Therapy Study Group. A comparison of laparoscopically assisted and open colectomy for colon cancer. N Engl J Med 2004; 350: 2050–2059. *Cancer Treat Rev* 2004;30:707–9.

10 Guillou P J, Quirke P, Thorpe H, Walker J, Jayne D G, Smith A M, et al.; MRC CLASICC trial group. Short-term endpoints of conventional versus laparoscopic-assisted surgery in patients with colorectal cancer (MRC CLASICC trial): multicentre, randomised controlled trial. *Lancet* 2005;365:1718–26.

11 Fleshman J W, Nelson H, Peters W R, Kim H C, Larach S, Boorse R R, et al. Early results of laparoscopic surgery for colorectal cancer. Retrospective analysis of 372 patients treated by Clinical Outcomes of Surgical Therapy (COST) Study Group. *Dis Colon Rectum* 1996;39 10 Suppl:S53–8.

12 Lacy A M, García-Valdecasas J C, Delgado S, Castells A, Taura P, Piqué J M, et al. Laparoscopy-assisted colectomy versus open colectomy for treatment of non-metastatic colon cancer: a randomised trial. *Lancet* 2002;359:2224–9.

13 Clinical Outcomes of Surgical Therapy Study Group. A comparison of laparoscopically assisted and open colectomy for colon cancer. *N Engl J Med* 2004;350:2050–9.

14 COLOR Study Group. COLOR: a randomized clinical trial comparing laparoscopic and open resection for colon cancer. *Dig Surg* 2000;17:617–22.

15 Slim K, Vicaut E, Launay-Savary MV, Contant C, Chipponi J. Updated systematic review and meta-analysis of randomized clinical trials on the role of mechanical bowel preparation before colorectal surgery. *Ann Surg* 2009;249:203–9.

16 Drummond R J, McKenna R M, Wright D M. Current practice in bowel preparation for colorectal surgery: a survey of the members of the Association of Coloproctology of GB & Ireland. *Colorectal Dis* 2011;13:708–10.

17 Fernell J. Review: mechanical bowel preparation before colorectal surgery does not provide any benefit and may be harmful. *Evid Based Nurs* 2009;12:114.

18 Worthington J, Thyssen M, Chapman G, Chapman R, Geraint M. A randomised controlled trial of a new 2 litre polyethylene glycol solution versus sodium picosulphate + magnesium citrate solution for bowel cleansing prior to colonoscopy. *Curr Med Res Opin* 2008;24:481–8.

19 Renaut A J, Raniga S, Frizelle F A, Perry R E, Guilford L. A randomized controlled trial comparing the efficacy and acceptability of phospo-soda buffered saline (Fleet) with sodium picosulphate/magnesium citrate (Picoprep) in the preparation of patients for colonoscopy. *Colorectal Dis* 2008;10:503–5.

20 Ryan F, Anobile T, Scutt D, Hopwood M, Murphy G. Effects of oral sodium picosulphate Picolax on urea and electrolytes. *Nurs Stand* 2005;19:41–5.

21 Yoshioka K, Connolly A B, Ogunbiyi O A, Hasegawa H, Morton D G, Keighley M R. Randomized trial of oral sodium phosphate compared with oral sodium picosulphate (Picolax) for elective colorectal surgery and colonoscopy. *Dig Surg* 2000;17:66–70.

22 Regev A, Fraser G, Delpre G, Leiser A, Neeman A, Maoz E, et al. Comparison of two bowel preparations for colonoscopy: sodium picosulphate with magnesium citrate versus sulphate-free polyethylene glycol lavage solution. *Am J Gastroenterol* 1998;93:1478–82.

23 Hsu C W, Imperiale T F. Meta-analysis and cost comparison of polyethylene glycol lavage versus sodium phosphate for colonoscopy preparation. *Gastrointest Endosc* 1998;48:276–82.

24 Deffieux X, Ballester M, Collinet P, Fauconnier A, Pierre F. Risks associated with laparoscopic entry: guidelines for clinical practice from the French College of Gynaecologists and Obstetricians. *Eur J Obstet Gynecol Reprod Biol* 2011 May 27. [Epub ahead of print].

25 Jansen F W, Kolkman W, Bakkum E A, de Kroon C D, Trimbos-Kemper TC, Trimbos J B. Complications of laparoscopy: an inquiry about closed- versus open-entry technique. *Am J Obstet Gynecol* 2004;190:634–8.

26 Daraï E, Dubernard G, Coutant C, Frey C, Rouzier R, Ballester M. Randomized trial of laparoscopically assisted versus open colorectal resection for endometriosis: morbidity, symptoms, quality of life, and fertility. *Ann Surg* 2010;251:1018–23.

27 Dupree H J, Senagore A J, Delaney C P, Marcello P W, Brady K M, Falcone T. Laparoscopic resection of deep pelvic endometriosis with rectosigmoid involvement. *J Am Coll Surg* 2002;195:754–8.

28 Jerby B L, Kessler H, Falcone T, Milsom J W. Laparoscopic management of colorectal endometriosis. *Surg Endosc* 1999;13:1125–8.

29 Marpeau O, Thomassin I, Barranger E, Detchev R, Bazot M, Daraï E. [Laparoscopic colorectal resection for endometriosis: preliminary results]. *J Gynecol Obstet Biol Reprod (Paris)* 2004;33:600–6. Article in French.

30 Jatan A K, Solomon M J, Young J, Cooper M, Pathma-Nathan N. Laparoscopic management of rectal endometriosis. *Dis Colon Rectum* 2006;49:169–74.

31 Ruffo G, Scopelliti F, Scioscia M, Ceccaroni M, Mainardi P, Minelli L. Laparoscopic colorectal resection for deep infiltrating endometriosis: analysis of 436 cases. *Surg Endosc* 2010;24:63–7.

32 Kossi J, Setälä M, Enholm B, Luostarinen M. The early outcome of laparoscopic sigmoid and rectal resection for endometriosis. *Colorectal Dis* 2010;12:232–5.

33 De Nardi P, Osman N, Ferrari S, Carlucci M, Persico P, Staudacher C. Laparoscopic treatment of deep pelvic endometriosis with rectal involvement. *Dis Colon Rectum* 2009;52:419–24.

34 Daraï E, Bazot M, Rouzier R, Houry S, Dubernard G. Outcome of laparoscopic colorectal resection for endometriosis. *Curr Opin Obstet Gynecol* 2007;19:308–13.

35 Senagore A J, Dupree H J, Delaney C P, Brady K M, Fazio V W. Results of a standardized technique and postoperative care plan for laparoscopic sigmoid colectomy: a 30-month experience. *Dis Colon Rectum* 2003;46:503–9.

36 Jayne D G, Thorpe H C, Copeland J, Quirke P, Brown J M, Guillou P J. Five-year follow-up of the Medical Research Council CLASICC trial of laparoscopically assisted versus open surgery for colorectal cancer. *Br J Surg* 2010;97:1638–45.

37 Carmona F, Martínez-Zamora A, González X, Ginés A, Buñesch L, Balasch J. Does the learning curve of conservative laparoscopic surgery in women with rectovaginal endometriosis impair the recurrence rate? *Fertil Steril* 2009;92:868–75.

38 van der Voort M, Heijnsdijk E A, Gouma D J. Bowel injury as a complication of laparoscopy. *Br J Surg* 2004;91:1253–8.

39 Tulikangas P K, Smith T, Falcone T, Boparai N, Walters MD. Gross and histologic characteristics of laparoscopic injuries with four different energy sources. *Fertil Steril* 2001;75:806–10.

40 Brouwer R, Woods R J. Rectal endometriosis: results of radical excision and review of published work. *ANZ J Surg* 2007;77:562–71.

41 Mereu L, Ruffo G, Landi S, Barbieri F, Zaccoletti R, Fiaccavento A, et al. Laparoscopic treatment of deep endometriosis with segmental colorectal resection: short-term morbidity. *J Minim Invasive Gynecol* 2007;14:463–9.

42 Campagnacci R, Perretta S, Guerrieri M, Paganini A M, De Sanctis A, Ciavattini A, et al. Laparoscopic colorectal resection for endometriosis. *Surg Endosc* 2005;19:662–4.

43 Hüser N, Michalski C W, Erkan M, Schuster T, Rosenberg R, Kleeff J, et al. Systematic review and meta-analysis of the role of defunctioning stoma in low rectal cancer surgery. *Ann Surg* 2008;248:52–60.

44 Nastro P, Knowles C H, McGrath A, Heyman B, Porrett T R, Lunniss P J. Complications of intestinal stomas. *Br J Surg* 2010;97:1885–9.

45 Larach S W, Patankar S K, Ferrara A, Williamson P R, Perozo S E, Lord A S. Complications of laparoscopic colorectal surgery. Analysis and comparison of early vs. latter experience. *Dis Colon Rectum* 1997;40:592–6.

46 Darai E, Thomassin I, Barranger E, Detchev R, Cortez A, Houry S, et al. Feasibility and clinical outcome of laparoscopic colorectal resection for endometriosis. *Am J Obstet Gynecol* 2005;192:394–400.

47 Kaloo P D, Cooper M J, Reid G. A prospective multi-centre study of major complications experienced during excisional laparoscopic surgery for endometriosis. *Eur J Obstet Gynecol Reprod Biol* 2006;124:98–100.

48 Mohr C, Nezhat F R, Nezhat C H, Seidman D S, Nezhat C R. Fertility considerations in laparoscopic treatment of infiltrative bowel endometriosis. *JSLS* 2005;9:16–24.

49 Dubernard G, Piketty M, Rouzier R, Houry S, Bazot M, Darai E. Quality of life after laparoscopic colorectal resection for endometriosis. *Hum Reprod* 2006;21:1243–7.

50 Wills H J, Reid G D, Cooper M J, Tsaltas J, Morgan M, Woods R J. Bowel resection for severe endometriosis: an Australian series of 177 cases. *Aust N Z J Obstet Gynaecol* 2009;49:415–8.

51 Pandis G K, Saridogan E, Windsor A C, Gulumser C, Cohen C R, Cutner A S. Short-term outcome of fertility-sparing laparoscopic excision of deeply infiltrating pelvic endometriosis performed in a tertiary referral center. *Fertil Steril* 2010;93:39–45.

52 Pereira R M, Zanatta A, Reich H, Bianchi P H, Fettback P B, Motta E L, et al. Use of circular stapler for laparoscopic excision of rectosigmoid anterior wall endometriosis. *Surg Technol Int* 2008;17:181–6.

53 Donnez J, Squifflet J. Complications, pregnancy and recurrence in a prospective series of 500 patients operated on by the shaving technique for deep rectovaginal endometriotic nodules. *Hum Reprod* 2010;25:1949–58.

54 Fanfani F, Fagotti A, Gagliardi M L, Ruffo G, Ceccaroni M, Scambia G, et al. Discoid or segmental rectosigmoid resection for deep infiltrating endometriosis: a case–control study. *Fertil Steril* 2010;94:444–9.

55 Remorgida V, Ragni N, Ferrero S, Anserini P, Torelli P, Fulcheri E. How complete is full thickness disc resection of bowel endometriotic lesions? A prospective surgical and histological study. *Hum Reprod* 2005;20:2317–20.

18 Urological aspects of laparoscopic gynaecological surgery

Francis Keeley and Wei Jin Chua

Introduction

Over recent years, laparoscopic techniques in gynaecology have progressed from diagnosis and tubal ligation to major extirpative and reconstructive surgery. These complex procedures are generally associated with lower complication rates than open pelvic surgery, but the nature of the complications can be different. In particular, the use of thermal energy in laparoscopy, whether during electrocautery or during the use of ultrasonic scalpels, can produce ischaemic effects beyond what is apparent laparoscopically. These effects can occasionally cause damage to the urinary tract that can be difficult to recognise.

Urinary tract involvement occurs in 1–2% of women with symptomatic endometriosis. Laparoscopic resection of endometriosis affecting the urinary tract ranges considerably in complexity depending on the extent of invasion. This chapter will address recognition and management of ureteric and bladder involvement from endometriosis as well as prevention of injuries to these structures that can occur during laparoscopic surgery.

Anatomy

The ureter can be divided into either two surgical (proximal and distal) or three radiological (upper, middle and lower) segments. This chapter focuses on surgical issues affecting the distal ureter and hence uses the former classification. The ureter enters the pelvis at the pelvic brim, crossing over the bifurcation of the common iliac artery and vein. It then runs posteriorly, crossing under the uterine artery and matching the level of the cervix. At this point, the ureter lies 1–1.5 cm lateral and anterior to the uterosacral ligament. Although the ureter may often be visualised through the peritoneum in the upper pelvis, it cannot be identified reliably in the area of the uterosacral ligaments. This is particularly true in the presence of diseases such as endometriosis. The presence of uterosacral ligaments that are thickened and nodular can induce a distortion of the normal anatomy of the ureter in this area. Thus, identification of the ureter is most reliably carried out at the pelvic brim, from where it can be traced into the pelvis.

The blood supply of the distal ureter arises from the common iliac, internal iliac, superior vesical and uterine arteries. There are good longitudinal anastomoses between these vessels. The venous drainage follows a pattern similar to that of the arterial supply.

The ureters pass obliquely through the bladder wall at the vesicoureteric junction, the narrowest segment of the ureter. When the bladder distends, the ureters are compressed and flattened, thus preventing reflux of urine and the chance of ascending infections. At cystoscopy, the ureteric orifices are found on the posterior wall near the bladder neck at the lateral aspect of the intertrigonal ridge. The trigone is the only part of the bladder that is fixed. It lies deep within the pelvis in adults, making open surgical exposure difficult.

Principles of ureteric surgery

The ureter is a fine structure that can be injured in a number of ways. Unlike the bladder, the ureter is generally unforgiving when injured. Crucial to its health are the longitudinal anastomoses between the various arteries supplying blood to the ureter. One must recognise that the area with compromised blood supply may be greater than it appears. Furthermore, the ureter tends to retract once it is divided. All of this makes direct anastomosis of the proximal to distal segment of the ureter problematic, frequently leading to a stricture. There are a number of reconstructive techniques designed to overcome these limitations, as discussed later in this chapter.

In the literature, the incidence of ureteric injuries related to gynaecological surgery ranges from 0.12% to 0.25%.[1-3] Ureteric injury is often not caused by complete transection but by thermal energy applied near the ureter, resulting in tissue necrosis with subsequent stenosis and fistula. In addition to causing direct tissue damage, the electrical current may damage the vascular supply to the coagulated tissue. Women tend to present 2–7 days after the operation with symptoms of abdominal pain, peritonitis, leucocytosis and fever.[4] Flank tenderness or haematuria are rarely described. In some women, a raised level of urea and creatinine in the abdominal fluid drainage may aid diagnosis. In some women, the diagnosis is not made until 2 or 3 weeks postoperatively when they present with a ureterovaginal fistula.

Diagnosis

The diagnosis of ureteric obstruction or injury is usually suggested by an abnormal ultrasound, but this requires confirmation by a contrast study: an intravenous urogram (IVU), magnetic resonance imaging (MRI) or a computed tomography (CT) urogram. A contrast study is useful to rule out severe obstruction or, in the case of suspected iatrogenic trauma, extravasation. In women with endometriosis, pelvic MRI is the most useful imaging modality.[5] If ureteric injuries are suspected intraoperatively, intravenous injection of indigo carmine may help to detect the injury. Alternatively, cystoscopic placement of a ureteric catheter can be more definitive and possibly aid in short-term management. Finally, if there are unsuspected abnormalities such as a severely dilated ureter, an on-table IVU may be helpful. In instances of delayed recognition of ureteric injury, placement of a nephrostomy may be necessary to maintain drainage from an obstructed kidney or to divert urine from an area of extravasation.

Management of minor injuries

In women with minor ureteric injury, such as contusion, oedema or mild stenosis, the options for management include observation versus placement of a ureteric catheter or stent. If a ureteric injury is diagnosed intraoperatively, immediate retrograde ureteric stenting is the most expeditious form of management. Often, the diagnosis is made postoperatively and, if the lesion is not too fibrotic, insertion of a ureteric stent can be carried out successfully. Stenting of the ureter allows drainage of urine, resolution of any pelvic urinoma and, in many women, spontaneous healing of the injured site. If technically possible, this method of treatment is preferable in managing most types of ureteric injury.

Ureteric stents have an essential role in the management of ureteric injuries but are associated with severe adverse effects, including hematuria, pain and lower urinary tract symptoms such as urgency, frequency and incontinence.[6] In addition, the stents can be neglected, leading to encrustation, calcification, obstruction and loss of renal function (and litigation). Thus, if a stent is placed, a definitive postoperative plan, including stent removal, must be made. An alternative is to place a temporary external ureteric catheter, which can be attached to a urethral catheter and removed with it. A ureteric catheter, however, cannot be considered a secure method of ensuring adequate drainage in the postoperative period. We commonly place a temporary ureteric catheter in women in whom we expect or find distortion of the ureter, making its identification difficult, especially in instances involving endometriosis. Manipulation of the external portion of the catheter can be used to identify the course of the ureter.

Management of major injuries

Management of a major injury of the ureter or an area of severe involvement with endometriosis depends to a large part on the site of the lesion. Injury below the pelvic brim is generally easiest to manage with a direct anastomosis of the ureter to the bladder. This can be accomplished using a psoas hitch; that is, by fixing the dome of the bladder to the psoas muscle to reduce traction on the anastomosis. For injuries just above the pelvic brim, a Boari flap, using a tubularised strip of bladder to bridge the gap, can be used. In some women who have minimal loss of length and whose ureter has a good blood supply, a direct ureteroureterostomy may be considered, although the risk of long-term stenosis is higher. All of these techniques employ the use of a ureteric stent for a period of 4–6 weeks to protect the anastomosis. Injuries above the pelvic brim involve much more complex options such as ureteroureterostomy, ileal interposition, transureteroureterostomy, autotransplantation and nephrectomy.

Surgical principles

Surgical repair of the ureter typically involves trimming the ureter back to ensure a good blood supply, followed by spatulation of the cut end. A stent is then placed. We place three interrupted sutures at the apex of the spatulation, then running sutures to provide a watertight anastomosis. The repair must be carried out with absorbable sutures, such as polyglycolic acid, and avoid excessive tension on the anastomosis. Follow-up investigations include removal of the stent at 6 weeks and an IVU or CT urogram at 3 months.

Prevention

The best solution remains prevention. Although there are no specific guidelines, the following general points should be considered.

The operator must understand the anatomy of the pelvic ureter and appreciate its proximity to the cervix. A ureteric marker such as a ureteric stent can be placed before starting the operative procedure or ureteral dissection, especially in women with a distorted anatomy. In cases such as complex endometriosis, formal dissection of the ureter may help to avoid complications.

Monopolar diathermy must always be at minimal settings with an understanding of the structures lying under and around the field of application.

Bipolar diathermy or use of an ultrasonic scalpel is preferred to monopolar diathermy because of the reduced distal spread of the current and heat, although no device is completely safe.[7,8] Longer coagulation induces diffusion of thermal energy and the current may damage the vascular supply around the coagulated tissue, leading to delayed tissue necrosis.[9] Bleeding in the area of uterosacral ligaments in particular must be carefully controlled. Surgical clips or sutures may provide a greater margin of safety when controlling bleeding in this area.

Principles of bladder surgery

Iatrogenic injury of the bladder is not thought to be common, but its incidence is not well defined. In a review of the literature (from 1970 to 1996), the incidence of bladder injury during laparoscopic procedures ranged from 0.02% to 8.3%, depending on the type of institution, the case mix and the surgeon's experience.[10] It ranges from 0.01% to 0.06% in more recent large studies.[11] This complication occurs more frequently in women who have a history of caesarean section or previous surgery, or whose bladder is not empty before surgery. The injury can happen during access (insertion of the insufflation needle or trocars) or during the operative procedure, by thermal injury (electrocoagulation, ultrasonic scalpel) and blunt dissection. The urinary bladder, in comparison with the ureter or bowel, is a relatively straightforward organ to repair surgically, provided the bladder neck, ureteric orifices and trigone are avoided.

Diagnosis

Bladder injuries are commonly diagnosed intraoperatively. Urine may be seen in the pelvis, usually secondary to an extraperitoneal perforation or laceration. If bladder injury is suspected but no definitive urine is seen, two tests for diagnosis are possible. First, saline or diluted methylene blue can be administered through a urethral catheter, so the bladder can be checked laparoscopically for leakage. An alternative is to inject 5 ml of methylene blue or indigo carmine intravenously.

Because most of the bladder is hidden within the true pelvis, injuries to the lateral and posterior wall, which are not in direct contact with the peritoneum, may be missed. Therefore, if bladder damage is suspected after the operation, a cystogram should be performed. Approximately 250 ml of contrast is infused into the bladder by gravity and X-ray films are obtained.

Bladder perforations may be seen on the lateral, oblique or drained-out films. Intraperitoneal injuries should be suspected when the contrast medium fills the cul-de-sac, outlines loops of bowel or extends along the paracolic gutter.

Suprapubic pain and fullness, with or without diminished urine output, may suggest bladder injury. If an intraperitoneal bladder injury has been missed, a significant increase in the serum urea level, attributable to urinary contact with the peritoneum, is observed. The definitive diagnosis is made by cystogram.

Thermal injuries to the bladder may not manifest initially. Sudden haematuria, well into the postoperative period, may be a sign of thermal damage. A true perforation may not yet be present and therefore a negative cystogram may be misleading. When suspicion remains high but a cystogram is negative, cystoscopy should be performed to identify any areas of devitalised tissue. The prompt diagnosis of a bladder injury relies on a high degree of suspicion, since the signs and symptoms overlap with other postoperative complications.

Treatment

If there are small tears (less than 2 cm) or extraperitoneal damage, drainage with a urinary catheter for 10–14 days may be sufficient. In other instances, immediate surgical repair is necessary. If damage is recognised intraoperatively, the trocar may be left in place and a purse-string (two-layer) closure may be immediately performed with 2-0 polyglycolic acid sutures. Laparoscopic repair with a two-layer closure should be considered by experienced laparoscopists. If the damage is suspected intraoperatively without any demonstrable leak or intraperitoneal spillage, drainage and observation may be useful. In instances of delayed diagnosis, bladder injuries are handled in the same way as other traumatic ruptures. Intraperitoneal leaks are repaired and drained, whereas extraperitoneal leaks are best managed by a period of catheterisation. Before catheter removal, a cystogram should be performed. The timing of the cystogram depends on the extent of the injury, but it can typically be performed after 7 days. If the leak persists, drainage is prolonged from 14 to 30 days before repeating the cystogram.[12]

Prevention

The first step before inserting the suprapubic trocar is to ensure that the bladder is empty. For short procedures, an in-and-out catheterisation may be sufficient, but it must be carried out in such a way to ensure that the bladder is completely empty. A common mistake is inadequate drainage through a

small-bore catheter. For longer procedures, a Foley catheter should
be inserted. The second step to
prevent trocar damage is to see the
dome of the bladder when inserting the trocar. Women who have
had a previous caesarean section or
who have undergone multiple pelvic surgeries could have a distorted
anatomy. Extra care must be taken
when inserting the ports. In difficult
situations, the insertion site can be
modified and Palmer's point should
be used.

Laparoscopic management of endometriosis of the ureter and bladder

Ureteric involvement

Ureteric involvement occurs in
0.1–0.4% of women with endometriosis. Most commonly it affects
the distal ureter, less commonly the
midureter and rarely the proximal
ureter. The endometriosis can be
extrinsic (deep infiltrating endometriosis compressing the ureter) or
intrinsic (nests of endometrial cells
and stroma in the wall of the ureter). The ratio of extrinsic to intrinsic involvement is reported to be
between 3:1 and 4:1, with the left
ureter more commonly involved
than the right ureter. The woman
may present with symptoms of renal colic, haematuria or silent urinary
obstruction with loss of renal function, resulting in subsequent nephrectomy.
The diagnosis is usually suggested by the presence of hydronephrosis on an
ultrasound and then confirmed by MRI, CT urogram or IVU. MRI is thought

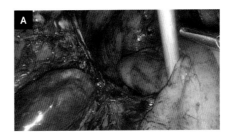
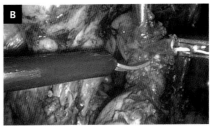
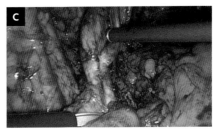
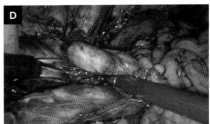
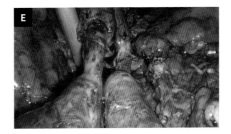

FIGURE 18.1 **Ureteric endometriosis in a duplex collecting system treated by ureterolysis**

(A) Severely dilated ureters seen at the pelvic brim

(B) Endometriotic nodule being sharply dissected off the ureters

(C) Anterior aspect of ureters exposed after excision of endometriosis (note that the serosa of the ureters is intact)

(D) Ureters separated with further sharp dissection to allow for resection of more endometriosis from the posterior aspect of both ureters

(E) Appearance of ureters after ureterolysis

to have the best accuracy but remains relatively insensitive compared with laparoscopy.[13]

Excision of endometriosis adjacent to the ureter not associated with hydronephrosis can be carried out in many women combined with ureterolysis rather than resection of the involved ureter (Figure 18.1). One must keep in mind that the blood supply to the distal ureter comes laterally and that a network of vessels travels along the length of the ureter. Ureterolysis must aim to preserve the adventitia of the ureter. If there is hydronephrosis or the ureter is strictured or ischaemic, segmental resection and reconstruction should be carried out. The decision to resect or perform ureterolysis alone should be based on whether ureteric function seems to be compromised, as evidenced by hydronephrosis or persistent proximal dilatation after ureterolysis.

Bladder involvement

Endometriosis of the bladder and of the ureter seem to be unrelated entities.[14] The bladder is involved roughly twice as often as the ureter and the associated nonurological sites of involvement are different. Within the bladder, the dome and base are nearly equally involved, but endometriosis involving the base is associated with more severe urinary symptoms.[15] Women may present with haematuria, dysuria or irritative voiding symptoms, but nearly 50% are asymptomatic. The diagnosis of bladder endometriosis can be suggested by transvaginal ultrasound or MRI, which are generally accurate but insensitive compared with cystoscopy and laparoscopy (Figure 18.2).[13, 16]

Management of bladder endometriosis begins with an accurate diagnosis. Women with cyclical haematuria, frequency or dysuria associated with symptoms suggestive of endometriosis should undergo cystoscopy in addition to diagnostic laparoscopy. The location and size of the endometriotic nodule within the bladder may require placement of a ureteric catheter or stent if there is involvement of a ureteric orifice or the trigone. Most women are best managed by a laparoscopic partial cystectomy (Figure 18.3), while a minority can be effectively treated by transurethral resection.

The bladder can also be affected following resection of endometriosis because of damage to autonomic nerves in the pelvis.[17] The clinical presentation is of incomplete voiding with a reduced flow, which may lead to urinary

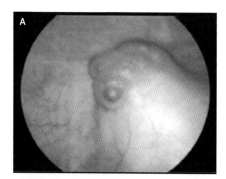

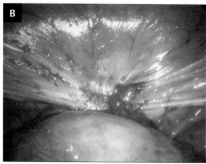

FIGURE 18.2 **Full-thickness bladder endometriosis**

(A) Cystoscopic view of a typical bladder endometriotic nodule

(B) Laparoscopic view in the same woman showing full-thickness endometriosis extending through the bladder and peritoneum

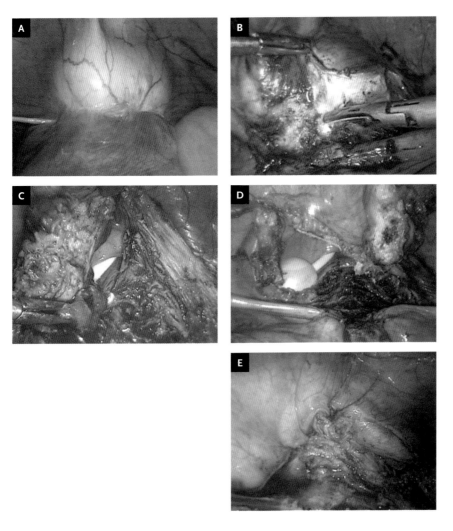

FIGURE

18.3 **Endometriosis of the bladder treated by partial cystectomy**

(A) Another bladder nodule of endometriosis; in this instance, there is no peritoneal endometriosis

(B) The uterovesical peritoneum is opened to mobilise the endometriotic nodule

(C) The nodule has been mobilised and the partial cystectomy started. The catheter is visible inside the bladder

(D) The partial cystectomy has been completed, excising the endometriotic nodule

(E) The bladder defect has been sutured, in this instance in a single layer

frequency, retention and/or urinary tract infections. Bladder dysfunction can result from sympathetic and parasympathetic damage after resection of deeply infiltrating endometriosis involving uterosacral ligaments, rectum and/or the rectovaginal wall. The rate of significant bladder dysfunction after colorectal resection for endometriosis ranges from 15% to 20% and can be as high as 30% after proximal uterosacral ligaments resection. This is explained by the location of the inferior hypogastric plexus at the proximal portion of the uterosacral ligaments. Urodynamic investigations typically demonstrate a hypotonic detrusor and reduced flow rates. Management is directed at avoiding the complications of postvoiding residue, such as infection, and may involve intermittent self-catheterisation. The natural history of hypotonic detrusor is variable and many women recover the ability to void to completion spontaneously.

Video 18.1 provides an example of laparoscopic treatment of an endometrioma of the bladder.

Team working

Women undergoing gynaecological laparoscopy who have suspected involvement of the urinary tract require a team approach to their care. Early involvement of a urologist with reconstructive skills (preferably laparoscopic) is essential. Urological complications resulting from laparoscopic gynaecological surgery in particular demand a team that communicates well. Early recognition of an injury allows for prompt repair in many instances.

Women with endometriosis invading the urinary tract are also best managed by both a gynaecologist and a urologist. A urologist will be interested in the woman's urinary symptoms and the status of the upper urinary tract and bladder. As well as a thorough history, he or she will check for haematuria and, when indicated, perform cystoscopy. In instances where the ureter may be involved, the urologist may recommend placement of ureteric catheters or stents to help identify and protect the ureter. In many instances, an intraoperative consultation may be helpful and reassuring, especially for gynaecologists who do not frequently resect complex endometriosis.

Conclusion

Injuries to the urinary tract are rare but do occur in gynaecological laparoscopy. The incidence has increased during recent years because more complex operations are performed using a laparoscopic technique. Thorough understanding of surgical technique and instruments combined with knowledge of pelvic anatomy can prevent complications. In instances of endometriosis involving the urinary tract, good team working between gynaecologists and urologists can help to plan the most appropriate procedure for the woman undergoing surgery.

References

1 Härkki-Sirén P, Sjörberg J, Kurki T. Major complications of laparoscopy: a follow-up Finnish study. *Obstet Gynecol* 1999;94:94–8.

2 Chapron C, Querleu D, Bruhat M A, Madelenat P, Fernandez H, Pierre F, et al. Surgical complications of diagnostic and operative gynaecological laparoscopy: a series of 29,966 cases. *Hum Reprod* 1998;13:867–72.

3 Jansen F W, Kapiteyn K, Trimbos-Kemper T, Hermans J, Trimbos JB. Complications of laparoscopy: a prospective multicentre observational study. *Br J Obstet Gynaecol* 1997;104:595–600.

4 Grainger D A, Soderstrom R M, Schiff S F, Glickman M G, DeCherney A H, Diamond M P. Ureteral injuries at laparoscopy: insights into diagnosis, management, and prevention. *Obstet Gynecol* 1990;75:839–43.

5 Bosev D, Nicoll L M, Bhagan L, Lemyre M, Payne C K, Gill H, et al. Laparoscopic management of ureteral endometriosis: the Stanford University hospital experience with 96 consecutive cases. *J Urol* 2009;182:2748–52.

6 Joshi H B, Okeke A, Newns N, Keeley F X Jr, Timoney A G. Characterization of urinary symptoms in patients with ureteral stents. *Urology* 2002;59:511–6.

7 Seiler J C, Gidwana G, Ballard L. Laparoscopic cauterization of endometriosis for fertility: a controlled study. *Fertil Steril* 1986;46:1098–100.

8 Baumann H, Jaeger P, Huch A. Ureteral injury after laparoscopic tubal sterilization by bipolar electrocoagulation. *Obstet Gynecol* 1988;71(3 Pt 2):483–5.

9 Jaffe R H, Willis D, Bachem A. The effect of electric currents on the arteries. A histologic study. *Arch Pathol* 1929;7:244–52.

10 Ostrzenski A, Ostrzenska K M. Bladder injury during laparoscopic surgery. *Obstet Gynecol Surv* 1998;53:175–80.

11 Donnez J, Jadoul P, Chantraine F, Nisolle M. Ureteral and bladder injury during laparoscopic surgery. In: Donnez J, Nisolle M, editors. *An Atlas of Laser Operative Laparoscopy and Hysteroscopy*. 2nd edition. New York, NY: The Parthenon Publishing Group, 2001. p. 363–72.

12 Tulikangas P K, Goldberg J M, Gill I S. Laparoscopic repair of ureteral transection. *J Am Assoc Gynecol Laparosc* 2000;7:415–6.

13 Chamié L P, Blasbalg R, Gonçalves M O, Carvalho F M, Abrão M S, de Oliveira I S. Accuracy of magnetic resonance imaging for diagnosis and preoperative assessment of deeply infiltrating endometriosis. *Int J Gynaecol Obstet* 2009;106:198–201.

14 Abrao M S, Dias J A Jr, Bellelis P, Podgaec S, Bautzer C R, Gromatsky C. Endometriosis of the ureter and bladder are not associated diseases. *Fertil Steril* 2009;91:1662–7.

15 Villa G, Mabrouk M, Guerrini M, Mignemi G, Montanari G, Fabbri E, Venturoli S, et al. Relationship between site and size of bladder endometriotic nodules and severity of dysuria. *J Minim Invasive Gynecol* 2007;14:628–32.

16 Savelli L, Manuzzi L, Pollastri P, Mabrouk M, Seracchioli R, Venturoli S. Diagnostic accuracy and potential limitations of transvaginal sonography for bladder endometriosis. *Ultrasound Obstet Gynecol* 2009;34:595–600.

17 Deffieux X, Raibaut P, Hubeaux K, Ismael SS, Amarenco G. [Voiding dysfunction after surgical resection of deeply infiltrating endometriosis: pathophysiology and management]. *Gynecol Obstet Fertil* 2007;35 Suppl 1:S8–13. Article in French.

19 Complications and medico-legal issues

Jonathan Frappell

Introduction

There is a lot of truth in the old surgical aphorism that a surgeon who has no complications is either a liar or has a very timid practice. Complications will inevitably result from our surgery no matter how experienced we are. Not only are serious complications distressing for the affected woman, they can be a cause of great anxiety also for the surgeon, particularly if the woman seeks redress through litigation. This chapter looks at the complications peculiar to laparoscopic surgery, how to minimise their incidence and what to do when they occur. Adherence to the principles of practice contained within this book will benefit women undergoing laparoscopic surgery and hopefully reduce the threat of litigation.

This chapter addresses the subject in the following order:

- the consent process

- the surgery itself

- the medico-legal aspects that may arise when a complication has occurred.

The consent process

Laparoscopic surgery is often perceived as a minor operation and it is this misconception that often leads to litigation. It needs to be appreciated that even a diagnostic laparoscopy can result in serious and life-threatening complications. The most serious example is unrecognised bowel damage at the time of a routine laparoscopy for diagnosis or sterilisation following which the operated woman becomes gravely ill, undergoes a laparotomy, ends up on the intensive care unit and has a prolonged recovery lasting many months. 'You told me this was just a quick look inside my tummy, and look what's happened!' In these circumstances, it is hardly surprising that the aggrieved woman may choose to seek redress through the courts.

In the last 10 years, the attitude to obtaining informed consent has changed out of all recognition. In the past, the somewhat patronising approach was held that a woman with a condition amenable to surgery would only be alarmed by knowing about the risks of the operation. It is now accepted that, for consent to be truly informed, the woman has a right to know all the risks and benefits of the proposed treatment option. Women scheduled for surgery should also be informed of all the alternative choices. This more modern approach is encapsulated in guidance from the General Medical Council.[1]

In 2003, a new consent form was introduced in the National Health Service throughout the UK to aid this process, with specific spaces to document:

- the operation to be performed

- any procedures the woman scheduled for surgery does not want to be carried out

- complications that might arise during or after the operation.

These forms help to focus the consent process and encourage the person taking consent to discuss all aspects of the procedure, including a discussion about the possibility of relatively uncommon but serious complications. What would be done if they were to occur should also be discussed. Giving information at this time is of great benefit to women in determining their choice to have surgery. As surgeons, we naturally find it difficult to accept that complications can and do occur, and the tendency is often to bury our heads in the sand. We all love to celebrate our successes, but it is much harder to confront our failures. This is why it is often so hard to find the true complication rate for many procedures, as poor outcomes are notoriously underreported, particularly in retrospective surveys. A full discussion with the person scheduled for surgery about clearly documented potential complications will remove the burden of unrealistic expectation on the surgeon. However, this does not mean that the surgeon is necessarily relieved of the threat of litigation.

Who can take consent?

Consent does not necessarily have to be taken by the operating surgeon, nor indeed does the person taking consent have to be medically qualified. However, the doctor providing treatment remains responsible for ensuring that the person delegated conforms to the following principles:

- he or she is suitably trained and qualified

- he or she has sufficient knowledge of the proposed investigation or treatment, and understands the risks involved.

As in all situations when consent is required, the woman must have enough time and information to make an informed decision. Ideally, written information leaflets about the procedure and possible complications should be available and given to the woman at the time of the original consultation. This allows her plenty of time to consider the treatment options before signing the consent form.

If the taking of consent is delegated to a more junior member of the team, they should follow a standardised written protocol and be supported by written information leaflets about the procedure.

For more complicated procedures or where the woman is at higher risk, for example following previous abdominal surgery, it is preferable that consent is taken by a surgeon competent at carrying out the procedure, because they will be in a better position to discuss the procedure and any potential complications peculiar to that individual woman.

When should the consent process take place?

Clearly, consent must be given before any treatment has started. However, the 'consent process' is not just the act of the woman signing the consent form but is a process that starts in the consulting room when the woman agrees to undergo an operation. This is a good time to discuss the pros and cons of the procedure and whether any potential benefits might be outweighed by the risks. In the majority of women, the balance of risks will clearly favour having the operation; for example, a young woman with a 7 cm dermoid cyst needs it removing and the risk of serious complications is low. Contrast this with the woman with a past history of a midline laparotomy who presents with pelvic pain and an ultrasound scan showing fluid loculations that might represent an ovarian cyst. If there is no evidence of malignancy, the woman may prefer to put up with the pain rather than accept the chance of serious complications associated with the increased potential for bowel damage.

The initial consultation might be a good time for the woman to sign the consent form if she feels that all her uncertainties have been answered. However, it is often better to sign the consent on a second occasion, to allow time for reflection. Unfortunately, the pressures of the modern National Health Service often limit the number of visits a woman can be afforded. It is helpful to fill out the form in the woman's presence, telling her what is being written down. This is certainly preferable to filling out the form and then sticking it in front of the woman telling her to 'sign here' without giving her the chance to read it first.

What should be discussed?

This is very clearly set out in the Royal College of Obstetricians and Gynaecologists (RCOG) advice document on obtaining consent for diagnostic laparoscopy.[2]

First, briefly run through the mechanics of having a laparoscopy, emphasising the following points:

- The woman will be 'asleep' under a general anaesthetic.

- The 'tummy cavity' needs to be distended with carbon dioxide to obtain a good view of the abdomen and pelvis. This is achieved through a small incision in the umbilicus using either a Veress needle or the open-entry (Hasson) technique.

- Point to where secondary ports are likely to be positioned to enable instruments to be inserted to perform the procedure.

- After the operation, the woman can expect:
  - a sore tummy for a few days
  - the possibility of having shoulder tip pain; explain why it occurs
  - a steady improvement after the first 24 hours
  - a rapid return to normal activities thereafter.

- The surgery might have complications.

In addition to the general complications associated with surgery, such as bleeding and infection, the following issues specific to laparoscopic surgery should be discussed and documented:

- Until insertion of the laparoscope, laparoscopy is a blind procedure. At this time, there is the potential for inadvertent damage from the Veress needle or primary trocar to internal organs, particularly the bowel and blood vessels.

- Open surgery may be required for one or more of the following reasons:

- the intended procedure cannot be carried out laparoscopically for technical reasons
- it is not possible to control intraoperative bleeding using laparoscopic techniques
- it is not possible to repair damage to internal organs using laparoscopic techniques.

When counselling a woman before laparoscopic surgery, the alternative of open surgery should always be discussed, particularly if there is an increased risk of complications. This discussion should be clearly documented in the notes. An additional safeguard to prevent any misunderstanding is to mention this discussion in the letter to the woman's general practitioner, stating that the woman understands these risks, and to send a copy of the letter to the woman for her own information. Most trusts send a copy of all letters to the woman as routine. This helps women to understand their condition and any treatment options recommended.

The language used in any discussion, and indeed on the consent form itself, should ideally avoid technical terms and therefore be readily understood by the woman; for example, it should say 'removal of ovary' instead of 'oophorectomy'. The term 'open surgery' is preferable to 'laparotomy' – I have known aggrieved women maintain they did not understand that consenting to laparotomy as a possible risk of laparoscopy meant that they could end up with a large midline incision when the operation did not go according to plan.

As with any operation, the likely extent of surgery must be discussed and agreed with the woman before the operation. The surgeon should also discuss and document which procedures the woman does not wish to be carried out. In any operation on the ovaries, such as ovarian cystectomy, the circumstances in which it might become necessary to remove the ovary should be discussed and agreed with the woman preoperatively. These may include a strong clinical likelihood of malignancy that had not been anticipated before surgery, or difficulties with securing haemostasis which could only be achieved by removing the entire ovary.

Having mentioned these possible complications, however, it is only right to try and put things in perspective for the woman to avoid unnecessary worry out of all proportion to the real risk. Quoting a risk of three instances in every thousand for inadvertent bowel damage, for example, will usually help to allay unnecessary fears.

Reducing risk at the time of surgery

It is clearly the duty of all doctors not to undertake a procedure for which they are not adequately trained. Equally, it is the responsibility of supervising consultants to ensure that procedures are delegated only to those with the appropriate level of skill and experience, unless the person undertaking the procedure is being directly supervised as part of their training programme.

The risks peculiar to the laparoscopic approach will be minimised by a sound and thorough knowledge of the principles of surgery outlined in this book. The following considerations are particularly pertinent and should be kept in mind at all times.

Understanding the technology

In contrast to open surgery, minimal access surgery (MAS) uses a lot of relatively complicated and sophisticated equipment. A competent MAS surgeon must have a sound understanding of how it all works and be able to supervise the theatre team in its set-up and operation. It is not acceptable for a surgeon to use any item of equipment, particularly energy devices or tissue morcellators, without understanding the underlying physical principles and having undergone some training in its use. Manufacturers and suppliers are becoming increasingly sensitive to the likelihood that they could be found vicariously liable if a woman suffers a complication from the misuse of their equipment, and are developing training courses and accreditation programmes with certification. Surgeons would be wise to avail themselves of these opportunities rather than rely on the outmoded 'see one, do one, teach one' approach. In the event of a complication arising from the use of specialised equipment, failure to show evidence of training in the use of that equipment would make it difficult to defend the case in the event of litigation.

Entry technique

The choice of entry technique should be in accordance with advice in the RCOG Green-top Guideline No. 49 on safe entry techniques.[3]

Although adherence to these guidelines and the use of techniques such as Palmer's test to confirm the correct placement of the Veress needle in the peritoneal cavity will help to minimise risk, inadvertent damage to the bowel can still occur at an estimated rate of approximately 3/1000.[4] It is good practice to make a brief note of the primary entry technique, documenting the intra-abdominal pressure used (for example 25 mmHg) and noting that a

360° view of the abdominal cavity was undertaken immediately after insertion of the laparoscope to exclude the possibility of inadvertent damage from the Veress needle or primary trocar.

Clear documentation of these details may help to protect against subsequent litigation in the event of an unidentified bowel injury. Using a proforma to record these operative details with each and every woman can be very helpful.[5]

Alternative sites and methods of primary entry

It is vital that all laparoscopic surgeons are familiar with the Hasson or open technique as an alternative to the so-called closed technique using the Veress needle. The indications for using the Hasson technique are:

- The woman is very thin so there is a significantly increased risk of damage to the major blood vessels on the posterior abdominal wall when using the closed technique.

- Attempts to enter the peritoneal cavity with the Veress needle through the umbilicus have been unsuccessful. Recourse to the Hasson technique is recommended after two failed attempts with the Veress needle.

- The woman has midline abdominal laparotomy scars.

When there are midline abdominal scars, the risk of small or large intestine being tethered to the underside of the scar is high. The Hasson open-entry technique will not necessarily protect from inadvertent entry to the intestine, but if it does happen the surgeon is more likely to recognise the problem. The damage can be repaired and subsequent problems with peritonitis are less likely. It should be noted that the Hasson entry technique can be employed at any site on the abdominal wall and it does not have to be in the midline. It is common practice among general surgeons to site the Hasson entry well away from the midline, usually just lateral to the lateral edge of the rectus muscle. In this way, it is usually possible to avoid going anywhere near bowel that might be adherent to the underside of a midline laparotomy scar.

The alternative option in this situation is to use the Veress needle through Palmer's point, which is situated 1–2 cm below the left costal margin in the midclavicular line. This has been shown to be the site where adhesions are least likely to occur,[6] of course with the exception of women who have had surgery in the left upper quadrant. Once the pneumoperitoneum of 25 mmHg is established with the Veress needle, a 5 mm port can be inserted through Palmer's point and a 5 mm laparoscope used to view the peritoneal cavity. To minimise the risk of damage to underlying organs in this position, it is prudent to deflate the stomach with a nasogastric tube. If the woman is at risk of splenic enlargement, an ultrasound scan of the spleen should be obtained before surgery.

Whatever entry technique is employed, the woman should be flat on the table until a good view is obtained through the primary trocar. Once this is achieved, the woman can be put in the head-down Trendelenburg position.

Secondary port insertion

Theoretically, no damage should occur from secondary ports because they should only be inserted under direct vision. In fact, damage to inferior epigastric arteries in the anterior abdominal wall is one of the most common causes of litigation relating to laparoscopy. It is vital, therefore, to understand the anatomical relationships that allow identification of the position of the inferior epigastric artery, and to place the secondary ports either well lateral or in the midline to avoid damaging these blood vessels.

From the medico-legal point of view, it is very difficult to defend injuries caused by the insertion of secondary ports, particularly to anatomically normal organs. Injury to the fundus of the bladder can be minimised by catheterisation and emptying the bladder before the insertion of the suprapubic port. It is also important to insert secondary trocars at 90° to the skin so that they traverse the shortest distance possible between the skin and the underlying peritoneum. If the port is inserted at an oblique angle, the tip of the port can penetrate the peritoneum a significant distance away from the skin incision. This is how many injuries to the inferior epigastric arteries and the fundus of the bladder are caused.

A quick method to tamponade bleeding is to pass a Foley catheter down the trocar. Inflate the balloon and then pull it up tightly against the anterior abdominal wall, holding it in place with artery forceps on the outside of the abdominal wall. This gives time to assess the situation and obtain haemostasis with bipolar diathermy or a suture.

Identification of bladder and bowel injury

Bladder

Identification of the bladder itself can sometimes be difficult and may be made easier by filling the bladder with 100 ml of dilute methylene blue. If there is any concern about bladder injury, the integrity of the bladder wall must be tested by instilling dilute methylene blue through a catheter and looking for any leaks. Bladder injuries can be repaired laparoscopically with absorbable sutures (for example 2-0 polydioxanone) and an indwelling catheter left in place for 7–14 days while the bladder heals. Depending on the size of the defect, it may be advisable to check for integrity via a cystogram before catheter removal.

Bowel

Where dissection of bowel is required, for example during adhesiolysis, the bowel wall must be closely inspected for signs of damage. Following extensive dissection of the rectosigmoid where integrity may have been compromised, the bowel wall should be tested using the so-called jacuzzi test. Fill the pelvis with water using the suction/irrigation wand and then insufflate the rectum with air, using either a sigmoidoscope or, more simply, a 50 ml bladder syringe, having first obstructed the sigmoid lumen with a soft Johann forceps or by compressing it against the pelvic brim. If any bubbles are seen, a perforation has occurred.

Remember that even though the mucosa may be intact, damage to the seromuscular layer can cause an area of weakness and may result in a mucosal perforation during the postoperative period.

If there is any doubt as to whether repair is required, the opinion of a bowel surgeon should be sought.

Port closure

Closure of the deep layer, which is usually the rectus sheath, must be performed in all ports of 10 mm or more, particularly those away from the midline. This is frequently done with the aid of a J-shaped needle, but it is difficult to be certain that complete closure has been obtained with this method, particularly in obese women.

Using a J needle is almost always sufficient to close the primary port site in the umbilicus where required, but for 10 mm port sites elsewhere the use of a port closure device aids closure. This is in effect a suture carrier that is inserted under direct laparoscopic vision so that closure of all layers, including the peritoneum, can be undertaken quickly and effectively. These are available as inexpensive single-use items.

Postoperative recovery

Following laparoscopy, steady recovery of the woman is the norm. If the woman's condition fails to improve, or indeed deteriorates, after the first 24 hours, one should suspect the possibility of visceral damage and take steps to establish or refute the diagnosis of peritonitis. As the woman may well have been discharged home very soon after surgery, it is important that she has written instructions setting out the expected pattern of recovery and the level of pain and discomfort she might be expected to feel. If the woman begins to feel unwell, she must have ready access to coming back to the hospital for review with relevant contact details to enable her to do this.

There is frequently delay in the diagnosis of peritonitis from inadvertent damage to bowel or bladder. The average length of time is 1.3 days from the surgery with a range of 0–4 days.[7] This is partly because the clinical signs can be vague and nebulous, and partly because of a reluctance to resort to exploratory laparoscopy or laparotomy until the diagnosis becomes obvious. This of course means that by the time the woman comes to laparotomy, she can be seriously compromised.

Failure of any woman to recover as expected after the first 24 hours should set alarm bells ringing. Increasing abdominal pain, nausea, abdominal distension, vomiting and reduced bowel sounds are all highly suspicious signs and symptoms pointing to a possible diagnosis of peritonitis. Frequently, in the early stages, the woman will have a normal temperature and white blood cell count, which can be falsely reassuring.

If there is any suspicion of peritonitis, the following plan should be enacted:

- 4-hourly measurements of temperature, pulse and respiration

- daily full blood count and C-reactive protein levels

- regular review (every 4–6 hours) by senior medical staff to assess trends in the woman's signs and symptoms

- intravenous administration of fluids and 'nil by mouth' except for plain water

- early general surgical opinion following computed tomography scan of the abdomen.

It can be difficult to balance the desire to avoid a negative laparotomy, which in retrospect turns out to have been unnecessary, with delay, which results in the woman becoming profoundly unwell.

It is acceptable to carry out a diagnostic laparoscopy to assess the situation, particularly when one's general surgical colleague is a skilled laparoscopic surgeon. However, it may well be impossible to identify the site of any bowel damage laparoscopically and an exploratory laparotomy may therefore be necessary to identify and repair the problem.

Arrangements for help when things go wrong

Major vascular injury

There should be a written protocol in the operating theatre for the action to be taken in the event of a major vascular injury occurring during surgery, usually at the time of the primary trocar insertion. This is a rare event, but when it does happen, prompt action can save the woman's life. The situation is very similar to that encountered in massive obstetric haemorrhage and a similar chain of events needs to occur:

- immediate midline laparotomy and pressure on site of bleeding

- summon help using a 'crash call' through the hospital switchboard; ask for immediate presence of the following personnel:
  - on-call gynaecology consultant
  - consultant vascular surgeon
  - consultant anaesthetist (even if a consultant is giving the anaesthetic, they will need help to stabilise and resuscitate the woman)
  - staff and instruments from the vascular theatre

- liaise with a consultant haematologist
  - urgent cross-match of 8 units of blood
  - type o negative blood.

Whatever the adverse effect, a multidisciplinary approach with help from surgeons, urologists, the imaging team and intensive care specialists may be needed to correct the problem.

In addition to leading the multidisciplinary team, the supervising consultant is responsible for providing an open and honest account of what happened to the woman. This should be combined with a plan of management so that the woman and her family know what to expect in the coming days and weeks.

An expression of regret and apology where appropriate is to be encouraged. This is not an admission of negligence or liability and in fact may well save the surgeon from litigation in the future.

If there were problems during the operation, a detailed operation note should be made by the supervising surgeon. This is not something that should be delegated to a more junior member of the team.

Moreover, it is sensible to produce a contemporaneous report of events to inform the risk management process within the surgeon's own department and hospital, and as an aide memoire in case of future litigation.

It is also wise, particularly in independent practice, for the surgeon to contact their medical defence society, who will offer advice and support.

Skills training

Endoscopic surgery lends itself to learning and updating technical skills by practising on simulators. These can range from a simple skills box, available in many hospitals, to the sophistication of virtual-reality computerised simulation and to operating on fresh cadaveric specimens or in animal laboratories.

Practising even simple hand–eye coordination exercises in a skills box will accelerate the learning curve dramatically, making surgery on the woman both quicker and safer.

When moving onto more advanced techniques, the wise surgeon will avail themselves of opportunities to learn by attending training courses with hands-on practice in simulated conditions, by visiting colleagues who are performing the technique and by having an experienced colleague with them in theatre when undertaking their first few procedures. All trust governance departments should have clear guidelines on how to introduce new procedures into the trust.

Suturing is one of the more difficult techniques to perform laparoscopically but should be incorporated into a surgeon's skills training from the very start. This not only enables the surgeon to take on more advanced techniques, but also enhances confidence levels enormously and improves the ability to deal laparoscopically with complications such as bladder injury.

Because suturing may be performed only infrequently in some surgeons' practice, it is a good idea to spend time each week practising this skill on a simple laparoscopic skills training box.

Chapter 6 covers training in more detail.

Medico-legal aspects

It is important for surgeons to understand that, just because the woman has signed a consent form that documents the risks of the procedure, this does not necessarily protect them from litigation if an adverse effect does occur. Proper consent, however, will defend the surgeon against the charge that the woman did not understand the implications of the procedure and that they would not have had it done if they had understood what it involved.

Just as with open surgery, if damage occurs to a normally situated organ during a straightforward procedure, this may be difficult to defend. Damage to bowel from a Veress needle or primary trocar during primary entry may be defensible as long as adherence to sound surgical principles, as previously outlined, has been clearly documented in the notes. Conversely, inadvertent damage arising from secondary trocar insertion can be difficult to defend because secondary trocars should be inserted under direct vision and therefore damage should not occur.

A survey by the Medical Defence Union[8] of clinical negligence claims against gynaecologists in the independent sector over a 10-year period (1998–2008) shows that such claims are not as common as one might think – approximately one claim per surgeon is made every 8 years, the same rate as that for orthopaedic surgeons. One-quarter of all claims involved a laparoscopic procedure, which reflects the common use of laparoscopic surgery in gynaecology. The most common procedures involved were hysterectomy and sterilisation and the most common reason for litigation was tissue damage; that is, damage to organs such as bowel, bladder, ureters and blood vessels. This review by the Medical Defence Union showed that the year-on-year increase in claims seen during the first half of this 10-year period levelled off during the second half, although the cost of claims increased by 10% per year, far above the annual rate of inflation.

Laparoscopic surgeons have often felt that they are unfairly singled out by litigants when there are complications that might not have led to litigation had the procedure been performed by open surgery. This may have been true in the past, when some medical experts were sceptical of the benefits of laparoscopic surgery and indeed when the skill levels of laparoscopic surgeons generally were probably lower than is the norm currently. This would suggest that laparoscopic surgery is now accepted as mainstream practice, rather than being considered as an experimental technique performed only by mavericks. As the benefits of laparoscopic surgery become ever more apparent, there will be increased demand for MAS techniques from women and, possibly, from commissioners. Surgeons will naturally want to respond to these demands. By ensuring that they are properly trained, keep their skills updated and follow sound surgical principles, surgeons will be well placed to protect the women they operate on from unintended harm and themselves from unwanted litigation.

References

1 General Medical Council. *Consent: Patients and Doctors Making Decisions Together.* London: GMC; 2008 [www.gmc-uk.org/guidance/ethical_guidance/consent_guidance_index.asp].

2 Royal College of Obstetricians and Gynaecologists. *Diagnostic Laparoscopy.* Consent Advice No. 2. London: RCOG; 2008 [www.rcog.org.uk/diagnostic-laparoscopy].

3 Royal College of Obstetricians and Gynaecologists. *Preventing Entry-related Gynaecological Laparoscopic Injuries.* Green-top Guideline No. 49. London: RCOG; 2008 [www.rcog.org.uk/womens-health/clinical-guidance/preventing-entry-related-gynaecological-laparoscopic-injuries-green-].

4 Richardson R E, Sutton C J E. Complications of first entry: a prospective laparoscopy audit. *Gynaecol Endosc* 1999;8: 327–34.

5 Raheem M, Afifi Y. Standards of documentation at laparoscopic entry. *Gynecol Surg* 2008;5:299–302.

6 Audebert A J M. The role of microlaparoscopy for safer wall entry: incidence of umbilical adhesions according to past surgical history. *Gynaecol Endosc* 1999;8:363–7.

7 Härkki-Sirén P, Kurki T. A nationwide analysis of laparoscopic complications. *Obstet Gynaecol* 1997;89:108–12.

8 Roberts K. Avoiding negligence claims in gynaecology. *MDU Journal* 2009;25:18–21.

Index

Note: page numbers in *italics* refer to figures, those in **bold** refer to tables.